# MUSCULOSKELETAL EMERGENCIES

# MUSCULOSKELETAL EMERGENCIES

## Bruce D. Browner, MD, MS, FACS

Gray-Gossling Chair, Professor and Chairman Emeritus
Department of Orthopaedic Surgery
New England Musculoskeletal Institute
University of Connecticut Health Center
Farmington, Connecticut;
Director of Orthopaedics
Hartford Hospital
Hartford, Connecticut

## Robert P. Fuller, MD, FACEP

Associate Professor
Department of Emergency Medicine
University of Connecticut School of Medicine;
Emergency Medicine Clinical Chief of Service
John Dempsey Hospital
Farmington, Connecticut

With 591 illustrations

**ELSEVIER**
SAUNDERS

1600 John F. Kennedy Blvd.
Ste 1800
Philadelphia, PA 19103-2899

Musculoskeletal Emergencies ISBN: 978-1-4377-2229-1

**Library of Congress Cataloging-in-Publication Data**
Musculoskeletal emergencies / [edited by] Bruce D. Browner, Robert Fuller.
    p. ; cm.
Includes bibliographical references and index.
ISBN 978-1-4377-2229-1 (hardcover : alk. paper)
I. Browner, Bruce D.  II. Fuller, Robert, 1964-
[DNLM: 1. Musculoskeletal System—injuries—Handbooks. 2. Emergencies—Handbooks. 3. Orthopedic Procedures—methods—Handbooks. 4. Wounds and Injuries—diagnosis—Handbooks. WE 39]
617.4'7044—dc23

2012018273

*Executive Content Strategist:* Dolores Meloni
*Content Development Specialist:* Julie Mirra
*Publishing Services Manager:* Catherine Jackson
*Senior Project Manager:* Rachel E. McMullen
*Design Direction:* Steve Stave

Printed in China

Last digit is the print number:   9  8  7  6  5  4  3  2  1

*To my wife, Barbara Thea Browner; to my children, Jeremy Todd Browner, Esq, Nina Mikhelashvili Browner, MD, Nicole Browner Samuel, and Marc Aaron Samuel, Esq; and to my grandsons, Benjamin Noah Browner, Zachary Myer Samuel, and Dylan Jethro Samuel.*

*In memory of my mother, Mona Alexander Browner.*

*In appreciation of support and encouragement from my father, Irwin Eric Browner, and his wife, Adele Doris Browner, and my mother-in-law, Betty Appleman Jacowsky.*

Bruce D. Browner

*To my wife, Natalie Colemen-Fuller, PhD; to my children, Sarah Noel Fuller, Julia Coleman Fuller, and Ellen Roselyn Fuller; and to my parents, Bob and Patricia Fuller.*

Robert P. Fuller

# Contributors

**Paul A. Anderson, MD**
Professor
Department of Orthopedic Surgery and Rehabilitation
University of Wisconsin
Madison, Wisconsin

**Michael Aronow, MD**
Associate Professor
Department of Orthopaedic Surgery
University of Connecticut School of Medicine
Farmington, Connecticut

**Sarah Axler, MD**
Resident
Department of Orthopaedic Surgery
University of Connecticut Health Center
Farmington, Connecticut

**Nicholas A. Bontempo, MD**
Resident
Department of Orthopaedic Surgery
University of Connecticut Health Center
Farmington, Connecticut

**John C. Brancato, MD**
Assistant Professor
Departments of Pediatrics and Emergency Medicine
University of Connecticut School of Medicine and
    Connecticut Children's Medical Center
Hartford, Connecticut

**Robert T. Brautigam, MD, FACS**
Interim Director, Neuroscience, Neurosurgery/Trauma
    Intensive Care Unit
Department of Surgery
Hartford Hospital
Hartford, Connecticut

**Bruce D. Browner, MD, MS, FACS**
Gray-Gossling Chair, Professor and Chairman Emeritus
Department of Orthopaedic Surgery
New England Musculoskeletal Institute
University of Connecticut Health Center
Farmington, Connecticut;
Director of Orthopaedics
Hartford Hospital
Hartford, Connecticut

**Fernando Checo, MD**
Fellow, Spine Surgery
New England Baptist Hospital
Boston, Massachusetts

**Anat Cohen, MD**
Resident
Pediatric Medicine
Case Western Reserve University
Cleveland, Ohio

**Megan Cummings, MD**
Emergency Medicine Residency Program
University of Connecticut
Hartford, Connecticut

**Thomas M. DeBerardino, MD**
Associate Professor
Department of Orthopaedic Surgery
University of Connecticut Health Center
Farmington, Connecticut
Team Physician, Orthopaedic Consultant
University of Connecticut Athletic Department
Storrs, Connecticut

**Andrew S. Erwteman, MD, DPT**
Resident
Department of Orthopaedic Surgery
University of Connecticut Health Center
Farmington, Connecticut

**Benjamin H. Evenchik, MD**
Physician
Department of Emergency Medicine
University of Connecticut
Hartford, Connecticut

**Deborah Feldman, MD**
Assistant Professor
Department of Obstetrics and Gynecology
University of Connecticut
Attending Perinatologist
Department of Obstetrics and Gynecology
Hartford Hospital
Hartford, Connecticut

**Joel V. Ferreira, MD, MA**
Resident
Department of Orthopaedic Surgery
University of Connecticut Health Center
Farmington, Connecticut

**Michael J. Finn, MD**
Assistant Professor
Department of Neurosurgery
University of Colorado School of Medicine
Aurora, Colorado

# Acknowledgments

The editors would like to thank the following people from Elsevier for their contributions to the conception, construction, and marketing of this work.

- Dolores Meloni, Executive Content Strategist. Dolores conceptualized the book with the editors and did all of the market research and budget development. She obtained approval for the project and worked with us to get it started.
- Julie Mirra, Content Development Specialist. Julie helped develop the direction of the content and design and corresponded with all contributors to get the material in the door on time and looking fabulous.
- Rachel McMullen, Senior Project Manager. Rachel oversaw the copyediting and typesetting of the chapters. She also handled review until all pages were perfect.

- Steven Stave, Design Manager. Steve designed the interior and the cover on this project.
- Carla L. Holloway, Marketing Manager. No one would know about this book without Carla and her team.
- David Dipazo, Video Specialist. David worked to perfect the edited video sent from the editors. He then posted the videos on our Expert Consult website for all to see.

We would also like to thank our executive assistants for their support in organizing meetings and communicating with authors and the publisher. Dr. Browner and Dr. Fuller had help from their assistants Sue Ellen Pelletier and Lynda Burns at the University of Connecticut Health Center and Dr. Browner's assistant, Kaye Straw, at Hartford Hospital.

# A Thumbnail Assessment of Emergency Medicine in the United States

## THE START

Access to emergency room (ER) care across the United States in the 1950s and 1960s did not keep up with the needs of the growing postwar population. The numbers of practicing physicians had not kept pace with the growth. Many began to use the ER as their primary source of medical care. Understaffed, underfunded, and underequipped, the ERs were serious problems for most hospitals. Practicing physicians who staffed community hospitals were pressured by demands for their time. They were on-call to the ER during their nonclinic hours. Hospitals and their affected physician staff became open to ideas that might ease the situation.

In 1961 an overburdened practicing physician, James D. Mills in Alexandria, VA, decided to limit his practice to ER coverage. He pulled together a few of his colleagues and they covered the ER around the clock. James Mills (1920-1989), respected General Practitioner and proper gentleman, is credited as being the "father of emergency medicine." The success of the "Alexandria Plan" caused several similar groups to form across the country. Chief among them was a group led by John G. Wiegenstein (1930-2004), in Lansing, Michigan. Wiegenstein and seven others boldly formed a society called the American College of Emergency Physicians (ACEP) in 1968. ACEP is now widely accepted as the most effective sounding board for the practice of emergency medicine while strongly encouraging scientific progress. The vision of these few men and women lives on. They looked forward to residency training for emergency physicians and the attainment of primary board status for emergency medicine.

## ACADEMIA STUMBLES FORWARD

Meanwhile, academic institutions responsible for the big-city teaching hospitals assigned responsibility for their ERs to the departments of Surgery and Medicine. Although their residency training programs provided some medical manpower, the need for clinical experience in their specialties did not justify staffing the ER solely with their residents. The ER was as serious a problem in the "city hospitals" as it was in community hospitals. The obvious solution was to create a residency program for emergency medicine. This was not an option because it would have encroached on the privileges and scarce resources provided to the existing specialties. A crisis was needed to make a change.

The race riots in Cincinnati, Ohio, in the late 1960s provided a crisis. The University of Cincinnati's Cincinnati General Hospital ER was crowded with patients who perceived their care as poor and were dissatisfied with long waits. Hospital leaders assigned two residents, one in internal medicine and one in neurosurgery, to come up with a plan. They recommended starting a residency in Emergency Medicine (EM). Of course, they were turned down, but they had developed a curriculum and had even selected a resident, Bruce Janiak, in 1970. The two originators went on to practice their specialties. The "residency" struggled on for a few years and almost disappeared but managed to produce leaders in emergency medicine. Richard Levy, a recent graduate, became its head in 1977 and developed a strong education and research oriented department while putting community dissatisfaction to rest. It remains one of the strongest EM residency programs in the United States.

The news that a Residency in Emergency Medicine had begun at the University of Cincinnati was reported in 1970 in a national news magazine. Five new residencies in Emergency Medicine began, more or less simultaneously in 1971-1972 in these teaching hospitals: Los Angeles County General Hospital; Hennepin County General Hospital in Minneapolis; Medical College of Pennsylvania in Philadelphia; Louisville General Hospital; and the University of Chicago. The ERs were now called Emergency Departments (EDs). Just 3 years later, 32 EM residency programs were in operation.

## WELL-EARNED RESPECT

Emergency physicians were considered itinerant know-nothings by the elite of some specialties in the 1960s. Board status was needed for emergency medicine. ACEP appointed members to a committee on board establishment in 1974. This group worked with the American Board of Medical Specialties (ABMS) to gain acceptance as a primary board. Committee member, Peter Rosen, EM Director at the University of Chicago and a staunch enemy of indecisiveness, famously answered endless wavering from the specialties with blunt invective. Nevertheless, progress was painfully slow. The first step was to develop and administer an oral and written examination designed to certify that an emergency physician was capable of making good decisions in any emergency situation. This test was to be the American Board of Emergency Medicine (ABEM) examination. It was successfully administered in

1980 and those who passed it became board certified by an EM "Conjoint Board."

Preparing for such an examination was a daunting challenge for both test takers and those trying to condense the large quantities of useful information into the essentials the emergency physician needed to safely rescue and manage all emergency cases. In 1979 ACEP published *Emergency Medicine, a Comprehensive Study Guide*, the brainchild of Judith E. Tintinalli, EM Residency Director at Wayne State/Detroit Receiving. Ronald Krome, Director of EM at Wayne State/Detroit Receiving, and myself were co-editors. The three of us enlisted the expert opinions of many specialists to assure that the most current and most useful information was being provided. We had no difficulty obtaining their input. Many excellent chapters were submitted. We received much unsolicited positive feedback from test takers. What seemed to be a crushing weight was now liftable. They found themselves confident in their fund of knowledge across a wide scope and their ability to make use of it.

With the Fellow of the College of Emergency Physicians (FACEP) letters after his or her name, the emergency physician felt pride in having met the test of competence administered by his and her peers.

## NOW WHAT

Emergency medicine, and all of medicine, is going through of period of needed change. There may be less compartmentalization of practice. Acute and chronic care may be less distinct as advances in technology improve communications and an emphasis on long-term health comes to the forefront. These processes are well underway in many areas. Many primary care clinics consider themselves "medical homes" where primary care physicians work with a skilled ancillary staff to coordinate care of patients with multiple health issues. Ideally, many community resources can be made available to care coordinators to help patients weather bad times and thus avoid hospitalization and excessive use of the Emergency Department and in-patient services.

Emergency Physician Robert Fuller and Orthopaedic Surgeon Bruce Browner have the opportunity to address some of these complex issues in their text *Musculoskeletal Emergencies*. Emergency physicians and orthopedists share many frustrations (patient obesity, alcoholism, homelessness, and so on). Once again, EM physicians and their colleagues in all of the specialties should formulate and address the essentials of what they need to know to lead patients into a healthier life. Asking their primary care colleagues and clinics for information about how to assist in this effort is the obvious starting point.

In Minnesota, a rural Emergency Medical Services (EMS) provider is attempting to serve as a medical clinic and Emergency Department extender, providing some basic contact and care to patients unable to travel. Primary care providers are the traditional leaders in this field, but every specialty can contribute, and must contribute if the overall health of our population is to improve. I look forward to reading the text. I want to learn more about the possibilities resulting from the collaborative approach between the specialties.

**Ernie Ruiz, MD**

# Contents

# *Video Contents*

**These brief videos will review the common presentations, exam findings, radiographic findings, techniques for reduction, post-reduction x-ray, exam, and care.**

Shoulder Dislocation
*See Chapter 9: Shoulder*

Elbow Dislocation
*See Chapter 10: Elbow and Distal Humerus*

Wrist Fracture
*See Chapter 11: Wrist and Forearm*

Hip Dislocation
*See Chapter 13: Hip and Thigh*

Foot Dislocation
*See Chapter 16: Foot*

# PART I
# General Principles

# Chapter 1

# *General Principles of Initial Care*

Michael A. Miranda and Randy L. Olson

Orthopedic injuries are common presentations to the emergency department. Most injuries are traumatic in nature, resulting in pain and deformity. Emergency medicine physicians need to be able to recognize the gravity of the injury and resources needed to take care of the patient. The assessment begins with a thorough history and proceeds with a tailored examination to create a differential diagnosis and generate a treatment plan.

## HISTORY

As with any medical encounter, the patient's history is key. Obtaining details such as mechanism, timing, and initial symptoms can be helpful. Some patients may be unable to speak because of their injuries, necessitating the reliance on family, friends, witnesses, and emergency personnel such as paramedics or police officers who accompany the patient to the trauma bay to relay vital information. When obtaining an orthopedic history, the clinician should determine the chief complaint, the events as best recollected, the mechanism of the injury, the energy or speed of injury, timing, function after the injury, neurologic status changes, reductions or manipulations already performed, pain generators, concomitant injuries, and new limitations. The history should also include a complete medical (including allergies and current medications), surgical, and social history. Occupation and prior activity level are important to establish. Aspects of this broader history may alter the treatment plan.

### *Traumatic Presentation*

The history may be very limited in situations where the patient is already intubated and few witnesses are available. Emergency personnel may be the only source of injury information. These personnel should be used to assist in understanding the nature and severity of the injury. Information about the scene and energy of the injury entailed can be approximated by asking questions such as the following: Was it a motor vehicle crash at highway speed or a fender-bender at a local intersection?

Was it a fall from a ladder or multiple stories of a building? Did an airbag deploy, and were hydraulic extraction tools needed? Was it a prolonged extrication? What was the penetrating object? What type of gun was used? Is there an open wound and what has been done to it? All of these questions can help the clinician assess the severity of the traumatic situation to establish the diagnostic and treatment pathways to pursue.

### *Limb-Specific Presentation*

Most patients with musculoskeletal injury present to the emergency department in a less emergent fashion with injuries from simple falls, sports-related injuries, or injuries from other low-energy incidents. Common injuries include hip fractures in elderly adults, wrist fractures from a fall on an outstretched hand, and ankle fractures. The complaint is often localized to one limb or joint. A more focused history may be pursued after quickly determining that there are no other injuries. Similar questions may be tailored to the individual's injury. Determining the mechanism and what currently hurts is the first step. The patient can be asked demonstrate the mechanism with the contralateral extremity if he or she is able to do so. The clinician can ask the following questions: When did the pain begin? Was there associated swelling or numbness? Does either of the adjacent joints hurt? Did you feel a "pop" or a joint dislocate? Has there already been a manipulation or reduction to a dislocated joint? Elderly patients often present from a skilled nursing facility, and dementia may limit the history the clinician is able to obtain from the patient. A quick phone call to a caretaker at the facility may yield information important to the injury.

### *Spine Presentation*

Injuries to the spine are often part of a traumatic presentation. Neck or back pain may be the chief complaint of some patients. Establishing whether there was an acute injury to cause the pain or the pain is a chronic condition is a key beginning point. It is crucial to discover new neurologic deficits. Also, new-onset bowel and bladder dysfunction, which may reflect an emerging cauda equina syndrome, is a crucial diagnostic finding.

## PHYSICAL EXAMINATION

The orthopedic physical examination of a patient includes assessment of the axial and appendicular skeleton and the pelvis. The extent of the examination depends in part on the awareness of the patient and his or her ability to interact with the clinician. Early examination of a patient involved in trauma is critical to assess the body before soft tissues become distorted from swelling. Evaluation should proceed in a systematic way to minimize chances of missed injuries and maximize efficiency and reproducible results. The trauma bay is a very active place with many different personnel partaking in the care of the patient. This activity may make the physician's job more difficult, but doing things systematically ensures completeness.

In the trauma setting, all clothing should be removed to perform a complete examination. Obvious open fractures and deformity should prompt immediate orthopedic surgery consultation. Initial examination should adhere to tenets of advanced trauma life support with attention to the ABCs—*A*irway, *B*reathing, and *C*irculation. The musculoskeletal examination can then proceed in a stepwise fashion, as follows:

- *Visual Inspection*
  Note deformity, wounds, burns, ecchymosis, sources of bleeding, entry and exit wounds from penetrating trauma, and use or disuse of an extremity by the patient
- Palpation
  It is critical to palpate all long bones, joints, and areas of wounds to assess for crepitation, false motion, and soft tissue defects such as a quadriceps tendon rupture. This palpation is especially important in an unresponsive patient because abnormal motion is the only way to find an injury and image and treat it appropriately. Pain is produced by this examination, but this is the time to be as complete as possible.
- Head
  Palpate the face, mandible, and cranium.
- Cervical Spine
  While maintaining spinal precautions, palpate the cervical midline, noting any pain or stepoffs.
- Upper Extremity
  Palpate the shoulders, humeri, elbows, forearms, wrists, hands, and each individual finger.
- Pelvis
  Examine the pelvis with gentle compression of the iliac wings in the anteroposterior plane, mediolateral plane, and on the pubis.
- Lower Extremity
  Palpate the hips, groin, femora, knees, tibiae, ankles, feet, and each toe.
- Spine
  Using a coordinated team effort to ensure spinal precautions, logroll the patient and palpate the thoracic, lumbar, and sacral spine feeling for vertebral stepoffs and paraspinal areas of tenderness. While the patient

is in this position, you may also palpate the scapulae and any other area of visible trauma.
- Range of Motion
  Take each limb and its joints through a full range of motion to assess for blockage to movement.
- Muscle Examination
  The muscular examination may be limited because of pain, but documentation of function is important to guide treatment. Minimal movement or response to a noxious stimulus is enough to assess the presence of volitional muscular function. Obvious trauma to an area warrants a more thorough and specific examination. Grossly, the upper extremity should be tested for the following:
  - Deltoid—axillary nerve
  - Biceps—musculocutaneous nerve
  - Triceps—radial nerve
  - Extensor pollicis longus—radial nerve
  - Flexor pollicis longus—anterior interosseous branch of the median nerve
  - Intrinsics—median and ulnar nerves
  The lower extremity should be tested for the following:
  - Quadriceps—femoral nerve
  - Tibialis anterior—deep peroneal nerve
  - Gastrocnemius and soleus complex—tibial nerve
  - Extensor hallucis longus—deep peroneal nerve
  - Flexor hallucis longus—tibial nerve
  Each muscle can be graded on a numerical scale. This documentation helps in treatment decision making and in rehabilitation. Table 1-1 shows the grading system.
- Neurologic Examination
  Further neurologic assessment beyond motor function involves sensory testing of major nerves and dermatomes, including the C5-T1 dermatomes and distal sensation in the median, radial, and ulnar distributions in the hand. In the lower extremity, the L2-S2 dermatomes and femoral, sural, saphenous, tibial, and deep and superficial peroneal distributions are assessed. Perianal sensation is assessed during the rectal examination. Reflexes to test include the biceps, triceps, brachioradialis, patellar tendon, and Achilles tendon. Other reflexes directed more at the spinal examination include the Babinski reflex, perianal "wink," and bulbocavernosus reflex. Classification systems to assess head injury in trauma patients are available. The best-known classification is the Glasgow Coma Scale (GCS); the GCS

**TABLE 1-1** Muscle Grading System

| 5 | Normal | Complete range of motion against gravity with full resistance |
|---|--------|---------------------------------------------------------------|
| 4 | Good | Complete range of motion against gravity with some resistance |
| 3 | Fair | Complete range of motion against gravity |
| 2 | Poor | Complete range of motion with gravity eliminated |
| 1 | Trace | Evidence of contractility; no joint motion |
| 0 | Zero | No evidence of contractility |

score ranges from 3 to 15 and is made up of three individual scores for eye opening, verbal response, and motor response (Table 1-2). A score of 8 or less requires intubation to secure the airway.

■ Special Consideration

In female patients, when pelvic trauma is suspected or visualized on pelvic radiographs, a vaginal examination is warranted to rule out occult open fracture into the vagina.

Patients with more routine limb or spine injuries and a nontraumatic presentation still should have a complete examination from the cervical spine to the toes because the main injury may distract from another, less painful area of injury. All examinations of upper extremity injury should begin with the cervical spine to rule that out as a possible cause of injury.

## RESUSCITATION

Resuscitation of a trauma patient is carried out under the guiding principles of the American College of Surgeons Committee on Trauma, including the primary, secondary, and tertiary survey. The primary survey can be easily remembered as *ABCDE*:

*A*irway and cervical spine precautions

*B*reathing and ventilation

*C*irculation with hemorrhage control

*D*isability/dysfunction

*E*xposure/environmental control (prevent hypothermia)

■ Airway

The cervical spine should be stabilized manually or with a cervical collar while the airway is evaluated and secured. Clear any obstructions to the airway, and use a chin lift or jaw thrust to help establish an airway; do not manipulate the cervical spine. An oropharyngeal or nasopharyngeal airway may be placed or definitive endotracheal or nasotracheal intubation may be established for patients with a GCS score less than 8, combative patients with an altered mental status, or patients who are hemodynamically unstable. If an airway cannot be established, a surgical airway may need to be created by performing a cricothyroidotomy and placing a tracheostomy tube. After an airway is established, supplemental oxygen can be started to help normalize physiologic status.

■ Breathing

Adequate ventilation not only provides oxygen to the tissues but also expels carbon dioxide waste products. If a patient is not breathing on his or her own, bag-valve ventilators or ventilation machines can be used to deliver oxygen. A trauma surgeon, if available, should evaluate the patient's chest. Monitor chest wall rise, respiratory rate and depth, use of accessory muscles, and presence of cyanosis to assess breathing. Special attention should be paid to:

• Tension pneumothorax—immediate needle thoracostomy and chest tube placement needed
• Open pneumothorax—three-sided occlusive dressing and chest tube needed
• Flail chest and pulmonary contusion—loss of chest wall integrity from multiple rib fractures
• Massive hemothorax

■ Circulation

Hypotension after trauma is primarily hypovolemic in nature owing to blood loss and fluid shifts. Monitor the patient closely because mental status, coloration, and pulses are good indicators of hemodynamic status. Open fractures, especially of long bones, are often sources of significant blood loss. Apply direct pressure to bleeding sources, and elevate the extremity if possible. A tourniquet may be needed until more definitive management can address the problem. Pelvic fractures or pelvic and abdominal trauma creating internal hemorrhage can hide a significant amount of blood causing hemodynamic instability. Either of these situations can result in hemorrhagic shock. Table 1-3 provides a classification of hemorrhagic shock. Shock needs to be dealt with expeditiously. Two large-bore intravenous catheters are placed in both antecubital fossae. A

**TABLE 1-2** Glasgow Coma Scale

| Eye Opening | | Incomprehensible sounds | 2 |
|---|---|---|---|
| Spontaneous | 4 | None | 1 |
| To voice | 3 | **Motor Response** | |
| To pain | 2 | Obeys command | 6 |
| None | 1 | Localized pain | 5 |
| **Verbal Response** | | Withdraws to pain | 4 |
| Oriented | 5 | Flexion to pain | 3 |
| Confused | 4 | Extension to pain | 2 |
| Inappropriate words | 3 | None | 1 |

**TABLE 1-3** Hemorrhagic Shock

| Class | Blood Loss | BP | HR | pH | Respiration | UOP | CNS |
|---|---|---|---|---|---|---|---|
| I | <15% (<750 mL) | Normal | Normal | Normal | Normal | >30 mL | Anxious |
| II | 15%-25% (750-1500 mL) | Normal | ↑ | Normal | ↑ | 20-30 mL | Irritable, confused, combative |
| III | 25%-40% (1500-2000 mL) | ↓ | ↑ | ↓ | ↑ | 5-15 mL | Irritable, lethargic |
| IV | >40% (>2000 mL) | ↓ | ↑ | ↓ | ↑ | <5 mL | Lethargic, coma |

*BP,* Blood pressure; *CNS,* central nervous system; *HR,* heart rate; *UOP,* urine output.
From Malinzak R, Albritton M: Orthopaedic trauma. In First aid for the orthopaedic boards, New York, 2006, McGraw-Hill, p 31.

central line may be needed for rapid volume infusion. Resuscitation is undertaken beginning with 2 L of lactated Ringer solution or normal saline. If the patient is still unstable, blood should be infused, and ongoing monitoring should be continued to re-evaluate the hemodynamic status. Loss of hemodynamic stability requires continued searching for a bleeding source. Ideally, crossmatched blood is given, but often the trauma situation is more emergent and life-threatening mandating use of universal donor O– blood.

- Disability/Dysfunction

  Assess the patient's level of consciousness. Neurologic status can be assessed quickly using the mnemonic *AVPU* (Alert, responds to *Voice*, responds to *Pain*, Unresponsive). Decline in neurologic status requires re-evaluation and possible therapeutic intervention. The cervical spine is maintained in a collar, whereas a backboard is used to maintain stabilization of the thoracic and lumbar spine. You can ask alert patients to follow quick simple commands to assess gross motor function.

- Exposure/Environment

  All clothing is removed to allow a head-to-toe examination. After the examination, the patient is covered to prevent hypothermia. Patients from hypothermic or hyperthermic situations require special protocols to return their core body temperature to normothermic levels. Foreign material on the patient's body may need to be removed and copiously irrigated or neutralized.

After the primary survey, the secondary survey is immediately begun. Most of the musculoskeletal examination as previously described is done at this time. Additional ultrasound examination (focused abdominal sonography for trauma [FAST]) of the chest and abdomen can quickly identify free fluid around the heart and in the abdomen and pelvis. A pelvic radiograph may show an unstable pelvic fracture that requires stabilization. Orthopedic surgical intervention to place an external fixator on the pelvis may be needed to decrease the pelvic volume and stabilize the patient. Additional radiographs in orthogonal planes are obtained for every area of gross or suspected musculoskeletal injury. Early reduction of limb deformity contributes to hemodynamic stabilization and analgesia. Steady inline traction or injury-specific maneuvers help reduce a fracture or dislocation. Wound management and splinting are performed during the secondary survey.

Fractures, especially in the lower leg and in the forearm, can lead to compartment syndrome. A high index of suspicion is warranted. The five "P's"—pain out of proportion, pain with passive stretch, pulselessness, paresthesias, and pallor—are monitored regularly for impending compartment syndrome. Emergent surgical intervention may be needed to decompress the affected compartments.

## WOUND MANAGEMENT

Traumatic musculoskeletal wounds in patients presenting to the emergency department are often the result of an open fracture. Other wounds include simple and deep lacerations. In 2005, more than 11 million wounds were treated in emergency departments throughout the United States in 2005.[1] Open fractures result from high-energy trauma such as motor vehicle crashes, falls from a height, and crush injuries. Lower energy injuries may result in open fractures especially in anatomic regions of limited soft tissue coverage, such as around the ankle. The primary goal in all wound management is prevention of infection. Patzakis and Wilkins[2] found 64% of 1104 open fractures had culture-positive bacterial contamination. All open fractures should be considered contaminated because the skin is traumatically violated and subcutaneous tissues are exposed to the environment. Prevention of infection includes early wound management and antibiotic administration.

Gustilo and Anderson[3] proposed a classification system for open fractures in 1976; this was modified in 1984 and is widely used today (Table 1-4).[4] Type I fractures result from low-energy trauma and are less than 1 cm in length with minimal contamination or muscle damage. Type II fractures are 1 to 10 cm in length with moderate soft tissue injury. Bone coverage is adequate, and fracture comminution is minimal. Type III open fractures are divided into subtypes A, B, and C. Type IIIA injuries have extensive soft tissue damage regardless of wound size, and the bone coverage is adequate. Heavily contaminated wounds with severe comminution and segmental fractures are also considered type IIIA. Type IIIB fractures have extensive soft tissue damage and significant contamination with periosteal stripping and bone exposure requiring soft tissue flaps. Type IIIC fractures have associated arterial injury requiring repair. Classification of an open fracture can be done only after the initial débridement when the full extent of the injury is known.

Irrigation of wounds is a leading principle in wound management. The "solution to pollution is dilution" dictum highlights the need for copious irrigation of traumatic wounds to remove as much foreign debris and contamination as possible to prevent infection. There is no definitive protocol on the volume needed, delivery method, or irrigation solution to use.[5] Anglen proposed a protocol of 3 L of irrigation for type I fractures, 6 L for

**TABLE 1-4** Gustilo and Anderson Classification of Open Fractures

| Type | Description |
| --- | --- |
| I | <1 cm, clean wound |
| II | 1-10 cm, mild to moderate soft tissue damage with adequate bone coverage, mild comminution |
| IIIA | Extensive soft tissue damage, flaps or avulsions despite wound size with adequate bone coverage, heavily contaminated |
| IIIB | Extensive soft tissue damage with periosteal stripping requiring soft tissue coverage, massive contamination |
| IIIC | Arterial injury requiring repair |

type II fractures, and 9 L for type III fractures based on the availability of 3-L irrigation bags. In the emergency department, this protocol may be dictated by the resources available. Simple bulb syringe or pouring from a saline bottle is the most straightforward approach and the most readily available. Gravity flow saline or sterile water is another option. Pulsatile lavage is often used, but this has not been shown to result in more efficacious removal of contamination. Whether low-pressure or high-pressure lavage should be used is debated. High-pressure irrigation is more effective at removing bacteria and debris, but it comes at the price of more damage to bone and local host healing potential.[6] An open fracture is an orthopedic emergency, and the patient needs to be taken to the operating room in expedited fashion based on his or her overall condition. Practical management considerations for the trauma bay include the following:

- Quickly assess the open fracture to determine the nature of the injury better
- Remove gross contamination by hand or using instruments
- Copiously irrigate the wound to remove as much contamination as possible
- Reduce any reducible fractures
- Cover the wound with moist gauze
- Splint or immobilize the fracture

Multiple examiners should be avoided because repetitive uncovering of the wound increases the chance of introducing bacteria and causing an infection. One thorough temporization of the wound should be performed before proceeding to the operating room.

Additives to saline irrigation have been used without great supporting evidence of their efficacy. Antiseptics such as hydrogen peroxide and povidone-iodine (Beta-dine) are not recommended because multiple animal studies have shown greater deleterious toxic effects to the host tissues than benefits. Antibiotics such as bacitracin, polymyxin, and Neosporin have been used but have not proven to be beneficial in preventing infection. These agents incur greater cost, have the potential for allergic reaction, and may lead to greater bacterial resistance.

Lacerations constitute an even greater proportion of wounds managed in the emergency department. The area around the wound can be anesthetized with a local anesthetic such as lidocaine or bupivacaine and the wound can be gently explored with a cotton-tipped sterile probe. If tendon laceration is involved, the on-call orthopedic surgeon should be consulted regarding the details of the injury and loss of function to determine if orthopedic intervention in the emergency department is needed. The wound should be irrigated with saline. A clean laceration may be loosely closed with interrupted nylon sutures to allow the wound to drain. If the skin edges are damaged, simple excision of 1 to 2 mm of tissue followed by loose closure is warranted. Coverage of the wound consists of a nonadherent dressing such as a petrolatum gauze and dry sterile gauze. If there is loss of skin coverage, a small wound may be irrigated and left to heal by secondary intention. These wounds are covered with a damp-to-dry dressing.

## ANTIBIOTIC AND TETANUS PROPHYLAXIS

### Antibiotics

The term *prophylaxis* is more correctly used in the surgical setting before skin incision. In the emergency setting of the trauma bay, open fractures, as previously discussed, should be considered already contaminated, and antibiotics are used as treatment. Antibiotics should be given as soon as possible in patients with open fractures. They serve as an adjunct to débridement and irrigation. Patzakis and Wilkins[2] found a 4.7% infection rate in open fractures when antibiotics were initiated within 3 hours of injury. This rate increased to 7.4% in cases where antibiotics were delayed at least 3 hours after injury. Brown et al.[7] showed similar support for early antibiotic administration using a 2-hour initial time point. A Cochrane database review by Gosselin et al.[8] found the use of antibiotics had a protective effect against early infection compared with no antibiotics or placebo with a risk ratio of 0.43. A comprehensive meta-analysis by the Eastern Association for the Surgery of Trauma (EAST)[9] published in 2000 provided practical guidelines for antibiotic administration for open fractures. Adapted recommendations include the following:

- *Type I and II fractures:* Administer a first-generation or second-generation cephalosporin to cover gram-positive organisms. A quinolone such as ciprofloxacin may be used in cases of known allergy to cephalosporins.
- *Type III fractures:* Add gram-negative coverage with an aminoglycoside. If there is concern for fecal or dirt contamination, such as in a farm injury, raising suspicion for possible clostridial contamination, high-dose penicillin should be added.

An often used regimen for adults in the trauma bay includes 1 g of cefazolin and, if warranted, tobramycin or gentamicin, 3 to 5 mg/kg. Gentamicin can be administered as a daily dose or in divided doses every 8 hours.[10]

### Tetanus Prophylaxis

Tetanus prophylaxis is administered to prevent life-threatening clostridial infection. Tetanus is caused by neurotoxins from *Clostridium tetani*. Prophylaxis against tetanus was started in soldiers in World War I, and immunization programs began in 1924. Tetanus immunoglobulin (TIG) provides temporary immunity by antibodies directly binding toxins. Tetanus toxoid (Tt) given in the emergency department does not ensure protection from tetanus, and it does more for tetanus immunity in subsequent injuries than the current one.[11] Wounds prone to tetanus include open fractures, crush injuries, tissues with oxygen deficiency, devitalized tissues, and wounds contaminated with dirt or rust. Recommendations from the Immunization Practices Advisory Committee for tetanus administration are provided in Table 1-5.[12]

**TABLE 1-5** Immunization Practices Advisory Committee Recommendations for Tetanus Prophylaxis in Wound Management

| History of Adsorbed Tetanus Toxoid (Doses) | Non–Tetanus-Prone Wounds | | Tetanus-Prone Wounds | |
|---|---|---|---|---|
| | Td* | TIG | Td | TIG |
| Unknown or <3 doses | Yes | No | Yes | Yes |
| ≥3 doses† | No‡ | No | No§ | No |

*Note:* Tetanus toxoid and TIG should be administered with different syringes at different sites.

*For children <7 years old, diphtheria tetanus pertussis (DTP, DT if pertussis vaccination is contraindicated) vaccination is preferred to tetanus toxoid alone. For persons 7 years or older, Td is preferred to tetanus toxoid alone.

†If only three does of fluid toxoid have been given, a fourth dose of toxoid, preferably an absorbed toxoid, should be given.

‡Yes, if >10 years since last dose.

§Yes, if >5 years since last dose.

*Td,* Tetanus and diphtheria toxoids adsorbed; *TIG,* tetanus immunoglobulin.

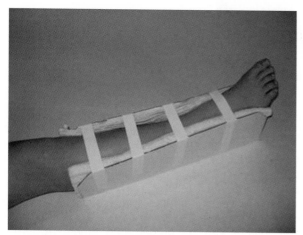

**FIGURE 1-1.** Temporary emergency cardboard splint.

## SPLINTING AND IMMOBILIZATION

Patients often present to the emergency department in some sort of immobilization, either homemade or commercial. Emergency personnel may place an extremity in a temporary field splint made out of cardboard (Fig. 1-1) or another material or use commercial splints such as a hare traction splint for stabilization of lower extremity fractures (Fig. 1-2). Stabilization of fractures helps alleviate pain and improves hemodynamics. These temporary splints are intended for transport to the emergency department until examination and more definitive or robust splinting can be applied by emergency or orthopedic clinicians. The emergency department physician should obtain an orthopedic consultation as soon as he or she knows a patient has a fracture so that an early examination can be performed and the fracture can be stabilized.

Whenever splinting a fracture, the adjacent joints should be immobilized as well to minimize motion at the fracture site; this helps to maintain alignment and provide pain control. Splints can be made out of off-the-shelf premade splinting material, such as fiberglass with padding that is dipped in water and molded on the body. A better, more well-fitting splint often can be made from plaster or

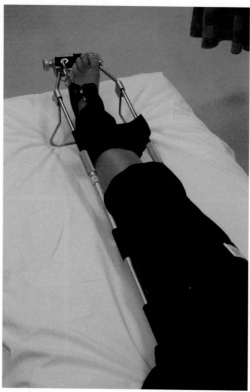

**FIGURE 1-2.** Hare traction splint. *(From Marx JA, editor: Rosen's emergency medicine: concepts and clinical practice, ed 7, Philadelphia, 2009, Mosby.)*

fiberglass, cast padding, and an elastic bandage. When making a splint, certain cautions should be kept in mind, as follows:

- All bony prominences should be well padded to prevent pressure ulcers.
- All skin should be covered with adequate cast padding to prevent thermal burns from the exothermic reaction of the plaster or fiberglass. It is helpful to let the patient know that the area being splinted will start to feel warm as the splint sets.
- Circumferential plaster or tape should be avoided in the acute setting to allow expansion with subsequent swelling.

For painful joints without facture and soft tissue injuries such as a quadriceps tendon or patella ligament rupture, simple immobilization of the affected joint maintains flexibility and function in the adjacent joints. Symptomatic relief is also provided to the affected joint such as the knee.

In cases where splints would provide inadequate fracture stabilization, skeletal traction may be used. This traction is often used for femoral fractures and unstable acetabular fractures. Traction pins can be placed in the trauma bay. Traction pins are placed from areas of more anatomic concern to areas of less concern. Femoral traction pins are placed in the distal femur from medial to lateral to avoid neurovascular structures, whereas tibial traction pins are placed in the proximal tibia from lateral to medial. Calcaneal pins are placed lateral to medial.

The workhorse methods of immobilization are shown in Figure 1-3 and include knee immobilizer, wrist cock-up

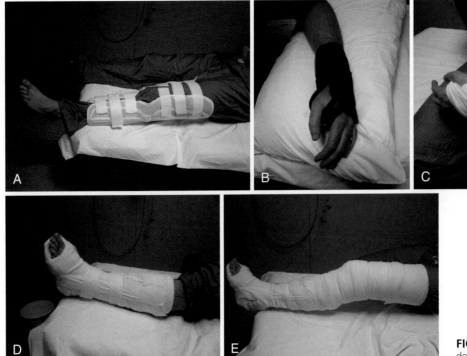

**FIGURE 1-3. A-E,** Workhorses of emergency department stabilization.

splint, sugar-tong forearm splint, and short and long leg splints.

## PRIORITIES

When considering each individual patient, both emergency physicians and orthopedic surgeons need to prioritize the injuries and address them in a systematic fashion. Life-threatening injuries always come before limb-threatening ones. As discussed earlier, advanced trauma life support guidelines take initial precedence to stabilize a patient. Orthopedic intervention may be required to help manage life-threatening injuries such as exsanguination from fracture lacerations of major vessels or severe pelvic trauma or major crush injuries that could lead to significant coagulopathy.

After life-threatening injuries have been stabilized, less threatening musculoskeletal injuries can be addressed. These injuries can be divided into emergent, urgent, semielective, and elective as outlined in Box 1-1.[13] An ischemic limb is the next priority after addressing

---

### Box 1-1 Musculoskeletal Injury Prioritization

**Emergent**

*Life-Threatening*
   Exsanguinating injuries
     Traumatic amputations
     Near amputations
     Pelvic crush fractures
   Massive crush causing coagulopathy
**Limb-Threatening**
   Vessel injuries
     Vessel compromise from fractures or dislocations
     Compartment syndrome
   Joint dislocations
   Progressive neurologic lesions
**Urgent**
   Open fractures
   Traumatic arthrotomies
   Fractures contributing to ARDS, fat embolism, hemorrhage
     Long bones
     Major pelvic disruptions

   Fractures associated with massive swelling
   Fractures at risk for avascular necrosis
**Semielective**
   Fractures preventing patient mobilization
     Lower extremity
     Acetabulum
     Minor pelvis
     Major upper extremity
   Open soft tissue injuries
     Lacerations
     Tendon and ligament lacerations
**Elective**
   Minor upper extremity fractures
   Minor foot and ankle fractures
   "Nonoperative" fractures operatively stabilized to ease nursing care
   Closed soft tissue injuries
     Ligament and tendon tears

From Kennedy JP, Blaisdell FW: Initial assessment and general management. In Blaisdell FW, Trunkey DD, editors: Trauma Management Volume VI: Extremity Trauma, ed 1, New York, 1992, Thieme, p 12.
*ARDS,* Acute respiratory distress syndrome.

life-threatening situations. Vascular injury or compromise and compartment syndromes lead to an ischemic limb. Fracture reduction may be sufficient to restore blood flow to a compromised area. Joint reductions should be accomplished as soon as possible. Reductions are often less traumatic and easier to perform in the early time frame of management. Fracture reduction is likely to help pain management and may contribute to the stability of the patient.

Urgent injuries include open fractures, traumatic arthrotomies, and fractures potentially causing harm to surrounding tissues and other organ systems. Semielective injuries include mobility-altering fractures, such as hip fracture commonly seen in elderly patients. These injuries typically require hospital admission. Many of the musculoskeletal complaints seen in the emergency department are classified under the elective group. These include minor fracture and soft tissue injuries that can be stabilized in the emergency department and followed up in the orthopedic clinic. Surgery may or may not be warranted; this can be determined and arranged by the orthopedic surgeon. These injuries include hand, wrist, foot, and ankle injuries.

The musculoskeletal system constitutes just one aspect of the human biologic system. It accounts for many patient presentations to emergency departments worldwide. Whether simple injuries or massive trauma, emergency physicians and personnel and orthopedic surgeons alike need to have a firm foundation on how to prioritize and treat these injuries.

## References

1. Abubaker AO: Use of prophylactic antibiotics in preventing infection of traumatic injuries. Oral Maxillofac Surg Clin North Am 21:259–264, 2009.
2. Patzakis MJ, Wilkins J: Factors influencing infection rate in open fracture wounds. Clin Orthop Relat Res 243:36–40, 1989.
3. Gustilo RB, Anderson JT: Prevention of infection in the treatment of one thousand and twenty-five open fractures of long bones: retrospective and prospective analyses. J Bone Joint Surg Am 58:453–458, 1976.
4. Gustilo RB, Mendoza RM, Williams DN: Problems in the management of type III (severe) open fractures: a new classification of type III open fractures. J Trauma 24:742–746, 1984.
5. Anglen JO: Wound irrigation in musculoskeletal injury. J Am Acad Orthop Surg 9:219–226, 2001.
6. Bhandari M, Schemitsch EH, Adili A, et al: High and low pressure pulsatile lavage of contaminated tibial fractures: an in vitro study of bacterial adherence and bone damage. J Orthop Trauma 13:526–533, 1999.
7. Brown KV, Walker JA, Cortez DS, et al: Earlier debridement and antibiotic administration decrease infection. J Surg Orthop Adv 19:18–22, 2010.
8. Gosselin RA, Roberts I, Gillespie WJ: Antibiotics for preventing infection in open limb fractures. Cochrane Database Syst Rev 4:1–21, 2009.
9. EAST Practice Management Guidelines Work Group: Practice management guidelines for prophylactic antibiotic use in open fractures. Available at: http://www.east.org/tpg/openfrac.pdf. Accessed September 21, 2010.
10. Sorger JL, Kirk PG, Ruhnke CJ, et al: Once daily, high dose versus divided, low dose gentamicin for open fractures. Clin Orthop Relat Res 366:197–204, 1999.
11. Rhee P, Nunley MK, Demetriades D, et al: Tetanus and trauma: a review and recommendations. J Trauma 58:1082–1088, 2005.
12. Diphtheria, tetanus, and pertussis: recommendations for vaccine use and other preventive measures of the Immunization Practices Advisory Committee (ACIP). Available at: http://www.cdc.gov/mmwr/preview/mmwrhtml/00041645.htm. Accessed September 23, 2010.
13. Kennedy JP, Blaisdell FW: Initial assessment and general management. In Blaisdell FW, Trunkey DD, editors: Trauma Management Volume VI: Extremity Trauma, ed 1, New York, 1992, Thieme, pp 1–15.
14. Court-Brown C, McQueen M, Tornetta P: The multiply injured patient. In Tornetta P, Einhorn TA, editors: Orthopaedic Surgery Essentials: Trauma, ed 1, Philadelphia, 2006, Lippincott Williams & Wilkins, pp 12–18.
15. Brautigam RT, Ciraulo DL, Jacobs LJ: Evaluation and treatment of the multiple-trauma patient. In Browner BD, Jupiter JB, Levine AM, et al, editors: Skeletal Trauma, ed 3, Philadelphia, 2003, Saunders, pp 120–132.
16. Bosse MJ, Kellam JF: Orthopaedic management decisions in the multiple-trauma patient. In Browner BD, Jupiter JB, Levine AM, et al, editors: Skeletal Trauma, ed 3, Philadelphia, 2003, Saunders, pp 133–146.
17. Smith WR, Agudelo JF, Parekh, et al: Musculoskeletal trauma surgery. In Skinner HB, editor: Current Diagnosis and Treatment in Orthopaedics, ed 3, New York, 2006, Lange Medical Books/McGraw-Hill, pp 81–162.

Chapter 2     # *Radiographic Imaging*

Alisa Kanfi, Douglas Montgomery, Susan O'Brien, Mary Norton, and Marinella M. Russell

## ORDERING BASICS

Imaging is an important step in evaluating musculoskeletal complaints. Physical examination, history of the present illness, and the mechanism of injury guide the anatomic area of interest. Two projections are the minimum for localizing a fracture and assessing its orientation. In a trauma setting, two orthogonal views are recommended (i.e., anteroposterior [AP] and cross-table lateral). Imaging the joint above and below the area of injury can identify an occult fracture. For example, imaging the knee in a comminuted ankle fracture may reveal a fibular head fracture (Maisonneuve fracture) (Figs. 2-1 and 2-2).

In the trauma setting, the patient's clinical condition, the mechanism and location of trauma, and the clinical suspicion of injury often determine the best modality for initial imaging. After an initial assessment of a relatively unstable patient following a motor vehicle collision, a computed tomography (CT) scan of the head, cervical spine, chest, abdomen, and pelvis may be indicated. With current technology, image postprocessing of the raw data from a trauma CT scan can be manipulated to reformat areas of interest with high detail. Multiplanar and three-dimensional reformatting may show an abnormality not otherwise appreciated on radiographs or axial acquisitions. For example, a particular costochondral fracture was difficult to visualize on the axial images; however, three-dimensional reformatted images clearly showed the alignment and extent of the fracture (Figs. 2-3 through 2-5). In the case of a trauma patient with a complex scapula fracture, the images from the initial CT scan can be reformatted in multiple planes using the highly detailed bone algorithm and provide the surgeons with a three-dimensional image of the scapula, without having the patient undergo a second scan (Figs. 2-6 and 2-7).

It often may be difficult to decide which is the best initial test to order to evaluate a complaint. Radiographs can be an excellent preliminary evaluation with high resolution of a painful extremity; however, injuries can be radiographically occult or obscured based on the superimposition of structures. Difficulties in patient positioning, particularly in patients with large body habitus, can pose challenges for adequate radiographic images.

If there is high clinical suspicion for pathology that is not visualized on the radiographs, a CT scan or magnetic resonance imaging (MRI) may aid in these situations. CT scan has excellent spatial resolution and shows osseous detail with precision. It can also aid in imaging difficult patients. In an older patient with extensive degenerative changes or in a patient in whom adequate visualization of the lower cervical spine cannot be achieved, a CT scan may be the best initial test for evaluation of the cervical spine.

The value of MRI is its superior contrast resolution, which detects soft tissue injury and sometimes radiographically occult fractures (Figs. 2-8 through 2-10). It is the modality of choice for evaluating for spinal cord injury. MRI also has the benefit of emitting no ionizing radiation and can be used in patients in whom radiation exposure is a concern, such as pregnant patients and children. However, hairline fractures may not be as evident with the inferior spatial resolution of MRI compared with CT.

The American College of Radiology (ACR) has established the ACR Appropriateness Criteria, which are evidence-based guidelines to assist referring physicians and other providers in making the most appropriate imaging or treatment decision for a specific clinical condition. By employing these guidelines, providers enhance quality of care and contribute to the most efficacious use of radiology. The guidelines were developed by expert panels in diagnostic imaging, interventional radiology, and radiation oncology. Each panel includes leaders in radiology and other specialties. The ACR Appropriateness Criteria have been incorporated in the following sections to

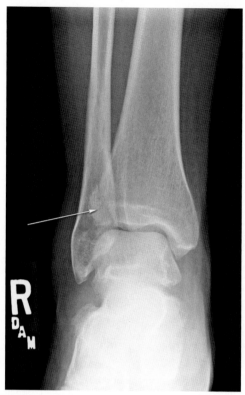

**FIGURE 2-1.** Anteriorposterior (AP) radiograph of the right ankle demonstrates a nondisplaced intraarticular fracture at the lateral aspect of the distal tibia (*arrow*). There is minimal widening of the ankle mortise. Given the findings and the mechanism of injury, further examination of the entire length of the fibula may be warranted.

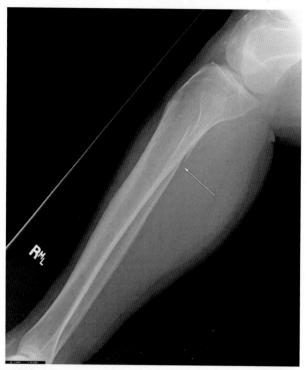

**FIGURE 2-2.** Lateral radiograph of the tibia and fibula on the same patient now reveals an obliquely oriented fracture of the fibula, consistent with a Maisonneuve fracture (*arrow*).

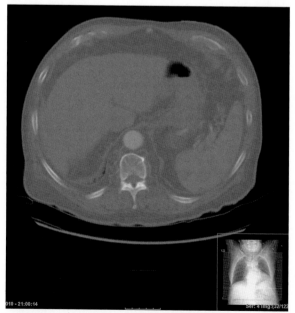

**FIGURE 2-3.** Axial contrast-enhanced CT scan of the chest on the bone window setting is unremarkable and does not show a displaced fracture.

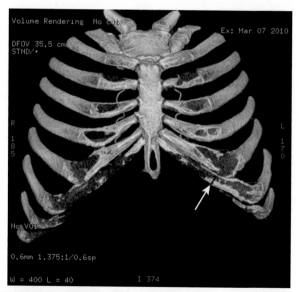

**FIGURE 2-4.** Volume-rendered reformatted image of the same patient as shown in Figure 2-3 reveals a subtle, nondisplaced fracture of the costochondral cartilage *(arrow)*, which is easily overlooked on the source images.

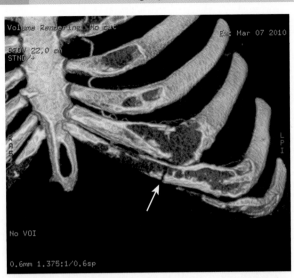

**FIGURE 2-5.** A nondisplaced fracture of costochondral cartilage *(arrow)* is further highlighted on the obliquely oriented, coned-in view on the reformatted image.

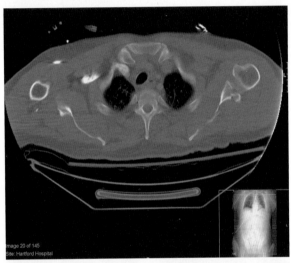

**FIGURE 2-6.** Noncontrast CT scan of the chest using the bone algorithm of a trauma patient shows a comminuted fracture of the left scapula with extension to the glenoid articular surface.

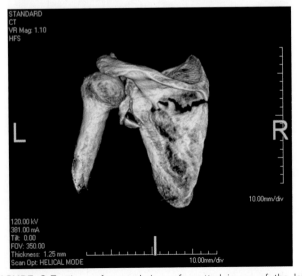

**FIGURE 2-7.** The surface-rendering reformatted image of the left scapula of the same patient as shown in Figure 2-6 using the source data from the initial trauma CT scan better delineates the extent of the fracture, which can improve preoperative surgical planning.

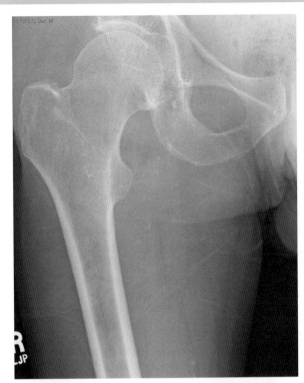

**FIGURE 2-8.** Initial AP radiograph of the right hip acquired after a fall does not show a fracture. Clinical suspicion for an occult hip fracture remained high, and MRI was subsequently performed.

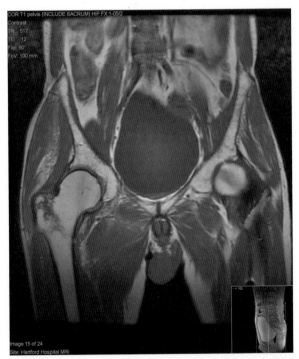

**FIGURE 2-9.** Coronal T1-weighted image of the pelvis shows a linear area of decreased signal in the right femur, consistent with a nondisplaced, radiographically occult, proximal femoral fracture.

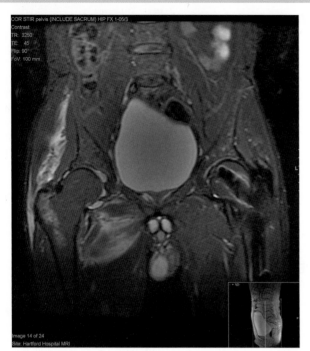

**FIGURE 2-10.** Coronal, fluid-sensitive, STIR MRI of the right femur shows associated high signal bone marrow edema. MRI also reveals injury to the adjacent musculature. Artifact from prior left hip pinning is visible.

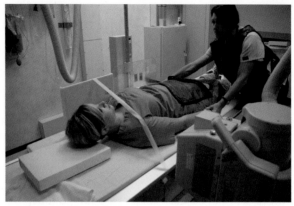

**FIGURE 2-11.** Appropriate patient positioning for a lateral radiograph of the cervical spine, with traction provided by the radiology technologist.

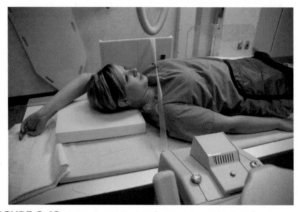

**FIGURE 2-12.** Patient positioning for a swimmer's view for improved visualization of the lower cervical spine.

aid in identifying the most appropriate imaging tool for evaluation of musculoskeletal injuries.

- ACR Appropriateness Criteria Rating Scale
  - 1, 2, 3—usually not appropriate
  - 4, 5, 6—may be appropriate
  - 7, 8, 9—usually appropriate

## SPINE

### Cervical Spine

- ACR Appropriateness Criteria
  In cases of suspected acute cervical spine trauma, imaging is indicated by clinical criteria (National Emergency X-radiography Utilization Study [NEXUS] or Canadian Cervical Spine Rule [CCR]).
  - CT scan of the cervical spine without contrast agent

    With sagittal and coronal reformats (ACR rating 9)

    High-resolution, thin-section slices (1-mm minimum thickness)

  - X-ray of the cervical spine: Lateral view only (ACR rating 6) (Figs. 2-11 and 2-12)

    If plain films are inadequate, CT scan is often indicated.

    Patient is clinically unevaluable more than 48 hours after injury.

  - MRI of the cervical spine without contrast agent (ACR rating 9)

    To look for ligamentous injury, cord pathology, and edema

    Sequences: T1 to assess for blood products or fracture lines, T2 and short tau inversion recovery (STIR) sequence to evaluate for cord edema and bone and soft tissue edema, T2* gradient-recalled echo (GRE) sequence to evaluate for hemorrhagic cord contusion

    If there is a suspicion of ligamentous injury, MRI is indicated.

  - CT scan of the cervical spine without contrast agent (ACR rating 9)

    Often both CT and MRI are needed (ACR rating 8) to evaluate soft tissue and ligamentous damage

    X-ray of the cervical spine is sometimes useful for surgical planning.

    If clinical or imaging findings suggest arterial injury, CT and angiography are indicated.

- CT scan of the cervical spine without contrast agent, with sagittal and coronal reformatting (ACR rating 9)
- CT angiography or magnetic resonance angiography (MRA) of the head and neck (ACR rating 9)

    CT angiography or MRA can be performed based on institutional preference.

    Imaging may be performed without gadolinium-based contrast agents if they are contraindicated because of prior severe allergic reaction or severe renal dysfunction with glomerular filtration rate less than 30 (mL/min/1.73m$^2$).

- MRI of the cervical spine without contrast agent is performed if neurologic deficit is present (ACR rating 8).
- ACR Scenario
  Follow-up imaging is indicated for a patient with no unstable injury shown on initial imaging but who is kept in a cervical collar for neck pain.
  - X-ray, with additional views (ACR rating 7)

    AP, lateral, open-mouth obliques, and extension and flexion views; individualized based on clinical findings

  - CT not indicated unless follow-up radiographs or clinical examination suggests an abnormality.
  - CT and MRI may be appropriate if radiographs suggest a further problem.


### Pediatric Spine

- Atlanto-occipital dislocation or dissociation
  This injury is 10 times more common in children 1 to 10 years old.
    The false-negative rate for a single cross-table lateral radiograph ranges from 21% to 26%. Complete evaluation with either conventional radiography or CT is necessary.
  - When performing trauma head CT, include C2.
  - When performing neck CT, include clivus through T1.

    Sagittal and coronal reformats

  - MRI should include STIR sequence and MRA.

    T1 useful for identifying blood products

    T2 best sequence for cord edema and ligament integrity

    STIR delineates soft tissue and bone edema

    Consider CT angiography or MRA for evaluation of associated vascular injury if a cervical fracture is present.

- Known Cervical Fracture
  If there is a known cervical fracture, ACR Appropriateness Criteria recommends CT of the thoracic and lumbar spine without contrast agent (ACR rating 9).
    For injury of the thoracic and lumbar spine, x-ray is the preferred modality (ACR rating 8).


### Thoracic Spine and Lumbar Spine

- CT Scan of Thoracic or Lumbar Spine Without Contrast Agent (ACR Rating 9)
  - Dedicated images with sagittal and coronal reformat or derived from trauma thorax-abdomen-pelvis scan
- MRI of Thoracic or Lumbar Spine Without Contrast Agent
  - Depends on clinical findings and results of CT scan
  - To assess for cord abnormalities or soft tissue injury
- X-ray for Localizing Signs (ACR Rating 3)
- Neurologic Abnormalities
  - CT scan without contrast agent and MRI without contrast agent (ACR rating 9)
  - Myelography and postmyelography CT (ACR rating 7)


## PELVIS

- X-ray
  A radiograph of the pelvis is a good place to start when assessing for a pelvic fracture. A variety of views can be obtained.
  - AP View
  - Inlet View, Caudad

    Best shows ring configuration of pelvis, and narrowing or widening of diameter of ring is immediately apparent

    Evaluates for posterior displacement of pelvic ring or opening of pubic symphysis

    Patient is positioned as in AP view of pelvis with beam tilted 40 degrees caudally; central ray passes through the midpelvis

    Best radiographic view to show posterior displacement

  - Outlet View, Cephalad

    Shows anterior ring superimposed on posterior ring

    Evaluates for vertical shift of pelvis (migration of hemipelvis)

    Proximal or distal displacements of anterior or posterior portion of ring are best appreciated on this view

    Patient is positioned as in AP view of pelvis with the beam tilted 40 degrees cephalad; x-ray beam is centered to the symphysis pubis, with inclusion of entire pelvis

  - Judet Views

    Also known as internal and external oblique views

    Shows iliopectineal and ilioischial lines, anterior and posterior column, and anterior and posterior wall

    Patient is supine with involved side of the pelvis rotated anteriorly 45 degrees; x-ray beam is directed vertically toward affected hip (Fig. 2-13)

- CT Scan
  CT scan almost always should be considered when there is an acetabular fracture to assess for small

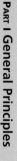

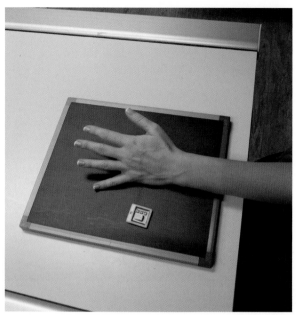

**FIGURE 2-24.** Proper positioning for oblique view of the left hand.

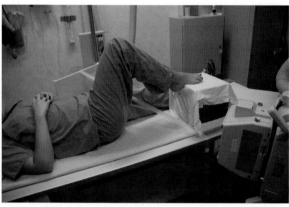

**FIGURE 2-25.** Proper patient positioning for a cross-table lateral view of the left hip. This view is favored in the trauma setting. The patient's unaffected right leg is elevated out of the plane of the x-ray beam.

- Hip fractures can often be subtle, or occult, particularly in elderly patients with superimposed degenerative changes and osteopenia.
- ◼ MRI and CT Scan
  - If there is high clinical suspicion for a fracture and initial radiographs are negative, MRI is the most sensitive test and is considered the next best test.
  - If MRI is contraindicated or unavailable, CT scan without contrast agent can add additional information.

## *Femur*

- ◼ X-ray
  - Standard x-ray views: AP and lateral
  - Hip and knee joints are included on field of view

## *Knee*

- ◼ ACR Appropriateness Criteria
  - In a patient of any age (excluding infants) with a fall or twisting injury with focal tenderness, effusion, or inability to bear weight, or a combination of these, first study is x-ray of the knee (ACR rating 9)

    Standard views: AP, lateral, and bilateral oblique

    MRI of the knee without contrast agent as an initial test may be appropriate (ACR rating 5).

  - In a scenario of injury 2 days prior of unknown mechanism, with focal patellar tenderness, effusion and ability to walk, best initial test is x-ray of the knee (ACR rating 9)
  - In a patient with significant trauma to the knee from a motor vehicle accident, and posterior knee dislocation (dashboard injury) is suspected

    X-ray of the knee is initial examination to assess overall injury (ACR rating 9)

    MRI of the knee without contrast agent is necessary to evaluate extent of damage to the ligaments and other supporting structures of knee (ACR rating 9).

    Arteriography of the knee performed interventionally as MRA or as CT angiography may be appropriate (ACR rating 7).

  - Evidence of a fat-fluid level joint effusion indicates fracture because fatty marrow has leaked into the joint fluid; if fracture is not visualized, further evaluation with CT scan or MRI may be necessary.
  - Certain fractures of the knee have a high association with internal derangement.

    Small avulsion of the lateral tibial plateau (Segond fracture) has a high association with anterior cruciate ligament tears.

    Avulsion of the fibular head (arcuate sign) is evidence of posterolateral corner injury.

    These soft tissue injuries are further assessed with MRI.

  - Patellar fractures can be difficult to detect on radiographs, particularly if inadequate views are obtained (Figs. 2-26 and 2-27).

    If patellar fracture is suspected, sunrise view of the knee would be suggested.

    Patellar fractures also would be easily detected on CT.

## *Tibia and Fibula*

- ◼ X-ray
  - Standard views: AP and lateral
  - Images include knee and ankle articulations
- ◼ Other Imaging
  - Stress fractures of the tibia may be subtle, in which case, MRI could provide additional information.
  - Nuclear medicine bone scan is also sensitive for stress fracture

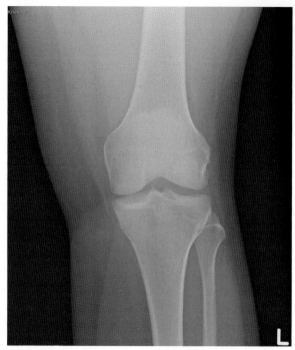

**FIGURE 2-26.** Initial AP view of the left knee does not reveal the underlying patellar fracture.

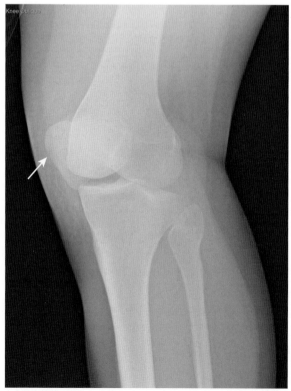

**FIGURE 2-27.** Oblique projection of the left knee in the same patient as shown in Figure 2-26 shows a cortical irregularity at the medial aspect of the patella, consistent with a fracture. There is associated edema and injury in the soft tissues.

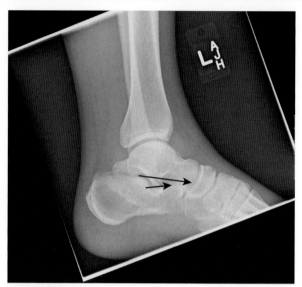

**FIGURE 2-28.** Complex fracture involving the body of the calcaneus. A decreased Bohler angle is evident.

## Ankle

- ACR Appropriateness Criteria Use Ottawa Ankle Rules
  - Ottawa ankle rules

    Inability to bear weight immediately after the injury *or*

    Point tenderness over the medial malleolus or the posterior edge or inferior tip of the lateral malleolus or talus or calcaneus *or*

    Inability to ambulate for four steps in the emergency department

  - X-ray of the ankle is indicated (ACR rating 9)
  - Standard views: AP, lateral, and mortise
  - Three-view ankle radiographic examination is good at identifying fractures that need immobilization or surgical or other intervention
  - If radiograph is negative, clinical follow-up is warranted for ruling out an ankle injury that may eventually need treatment

## Calcaneus

- X-ray
  - Dedicated views of the calcaneus are recommended if there is clinical suspicion for fracture based on clinical symptoms and mechanism of injury (jumping) (Figs. 2-28 and 2-29)

## Foot

- X-ray
  - Routine views: AP, lateral, and oblique
  - Classically, the foot is imaged with flexion; if patient is unable to flex the foot because of injuries or pain, x-ray beam and image receptor can be angled (Fig. 2-30)

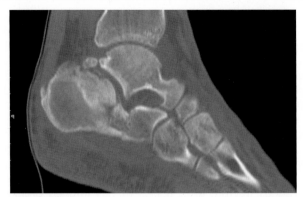

**FIGURE 2-29.** Extent of the comminuted, complex calcaneus fracture of the same patient as shown in Figure 2-28 is better visualized on a noncontrast CT scan. A depressed Bohler angle is again noted.

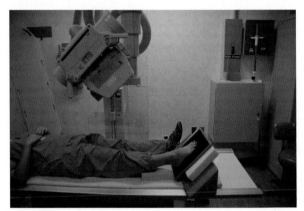

**FIGURE 2-30.** In the setting of trauma, the patient may be unable to flex the foot adequately for AP radiographic imaging. This problem can be circumvented by angling the x-ray beam and image receptor.

- Appropriate positioning is essential to ensure the absence of a fracture or subluxation—Lisfranc deformity can be subtle and is often overlooked (Figs. 2-31 and 2-32).
- CT scan or MRI to delineate occult fractures

## INTERPRETING IMAGES

It is crucial to evaluate all aspects of the radiograph and all views provided. Be careful to analyze the entire image and avoid the so-called satisfaction of search by identifying the initial abnormality. For example, ankle injuries are often associated with a fracture of the base of the fifth metatarsal. The lateral image of the ankle series may be the only view in which the bases of the metatarsals are visualized. It is important that the base of the fifth metatarsal is included with appropriate positioning because this may be the only view in which the fracture can be visualized. Evaluating each image in a patterned approach can limit this error.

## TIPS

- Use soft tissue swelling and mechanism of injury as a guide.

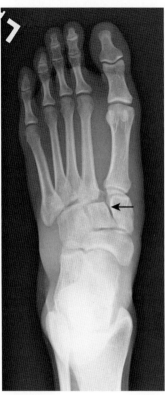

**FIGURE 2-31.** AP and oblique views of the left foot reveal a Lisfranc deformity with additional fractures involving the base of the second, third, and fourth metatarsals.

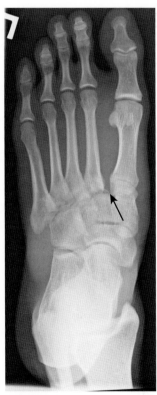

**FIGURE 2-32.** AP and oblique views of the left foot reveal a Lisfranc deformity with additional fractures involving the base of the second, third, and fourth metatarsals.

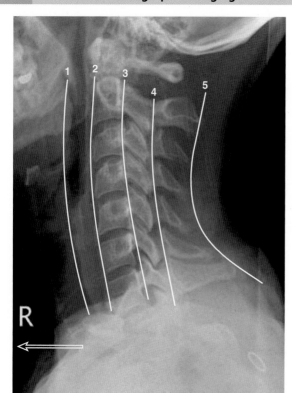

**FIGURE 2-33.** Lateral radiograph of the cervical spine outlines the essential lines to assess on all examinations: prevertebral soft tissue line (*1*); anterior vertebral line (*2*); posterior vertebral line (*3*); spinolaminar line (*4*); interspinous line (*5*). Any disruption of the lines should raise the suspicion for fracture or ligamentous injury.

■ Be aware of common secondary signs that have a high association with radiographically occult fractures.
  • Sail sign of the anterior fat pad in the elbow
  • Posterior fat pad sign in the elbow
  • Fat-fluid level in the knee joint
  • Prevertebral soft tissue swelling (Fig. 2-33)
  • Paraspinal hematoma
■ As discussed previously, certain fractures have a high association of soft tissue or ligamentous injury.

## COMMUNICATING FINDINGS

It is important to describe the orientation of the fracture line and aspect of the bone it involves. Important findings include whether is it comminuted, distracted, or angulated. A compound fracture should be clinically apparent. A pertinent positive finding is whether the fracture involves or extends to the articular surface; if so, the percent of involvement of the articular surface or the degree of depression may be valuable to the orthopedic surgeon.

It is also important to recognize potential complicating factors of the fracture. If there is posterior translocation of the tibia in a "dashboard injury," there may be a role for CT angiography or angiography of the lower extremity to assess the integrity of the popliteal artery. If there is a calcaneus fracture after a patient has jumped or fallen from a height, it may be useful to recommend imaging the lower thoracic or lumbar spine for possible vertebral body fractures.

Finally, communication and frequent interaction between the ordering practitioner, the radiologist, and the radiology technologist is essential. The radiology technologist can assist with appropriate positioning of the patient and determine which views may not be attainable or adequate, obviating the need for cross-sectional imaging. This communication also enables the radiologist to answer the clinical question fully and potentially to highlight a more suitable examination. Open communication between all members of the health care team is crucial to ensure the best care for the patient.

## Bibliography

American College of Radiology: ACR Appropriateness Criteria. Available at: http://acr.org/ac.Accessed Feb 14, 2012.

Baker C: Evaluation of pediatric cervical spine injuries. Am J Emerg Med 17:230–234, 1999.

Bontrager KL, Lampignano JP: Textbook of Radiographic Positioning and Related Anatomy, St Louis, 2005, Elsevier Mosby.

Brant WE, Helms CA: Fundamentals of Diagnostic Radiology, Philadelphia, 2007, Lippincott Williams & Wilkins.

Donnelly LF: Fundamentals of Pediatric Radiology, Philadelphia, 2001, Saunders.

Greenspan A: Orthopedic Imaging: A Practical Approach, Philadelphia, 2011, Lippincott Williams & Wilkins.

Lustrin ES, Karakas SP, Ortiz AO, et al: Pediatric cervical spine: normal anatomy, variants, and trauma. Radiographics 23:539–560, 2003.

Oka M, Monu JU: Prevalence and patterns of occult hip fractures and mimics revealed by MRI. AJR Am J Roentgenol 182:283–288, 2004.

Sonin A: Diagnostic Imaging. Musculoskeletal: Trauma, Salt Lake City, 2010, Amirsys.

Wheeless' Textbook of Orthopaedics. Available at: http://www.wheelessonline.com/.Accessed Feb 14, 2012.

# Chapter 3 · *Infections Involving the Musculoskeletal System*

Ankita S. Kadakia, Cristina Fe G. Mondragon,
and Edward L. Pesanti

## NONTRAUMATIC SKIN AND SOFT TISSUE INFECTIONS

This section reviews infections of the skin and musculo-skeletal system that have developed without major antecedent trauma. Such infections are among the most common infections that are encountered in the emergency department and warrant prompt recognition. They have a wide spectrum of disease severity ranging from localized lesions involving skin and soft tissues, joints, bones, or implanted prostheses to rapidly spreading processes that involve the fascial planes. We discuss here infections that affect the limbs and trunk.

### Common Infections Limited to Skin and Subcutaneous Tissues

#### Folliculitis, Furuncles, and Carbuncles
Folliculitis appears as pruritic, small, white-headed lesions around one or more hair follicles (Fig. 3-1). *Furuncles* (Fig. 3-2) form as a result of suppuration and extension into the subcutaneous tissue. These lesions can coalesce to form larger masses called *carbuncles* (Fig. 3-3).

■ Folliculitis is commonly caused by *Staphylococcus aureus*.
■ Folliculitis caused by *Pseudomonas aeruginosa* can be seen in certain settings (i.e., hot tub folliculitis); this generally does not require antibiotic treatment.
■ Folliculitis can be treated with topical antimicrobials and does not typically require systemic antibiotics: 1% clindamycin, 2% erythromycin, or 2% mupirocin
■ Furuncles and carbuncles require drainage and systemic antibiotics directed at *S. aureus* and other skin bacteria.

#### Cellulitis
Cellulitis refers to a diffuse, rapidly spreading skin infection that extends to involve the subcutaneous tissues with areas of edema, redness, and heat. Cellulitis is sometimes accompanied by lymphangitis and inflammation of regional lymph nodes (Fig. 3-4). Vesicles, bullae, and cutaneous hemorrhage in the form of petechiae or ecchymoses may develop. Systemic manifestations can accompany cellulitis. Fever and leukocytosis can be present, and serious reactions such as hypotension and mental status changes may be seen.

Treatment options are as follows:

• Outpatient treatment, methicillin-resistant *S. aureus* (MRSA) suspected: clindamycin, doxycycline
• Trimethoprim/sulfamethoxazole (TMP/SMX)
• Outpatient treatment, MRSA not suspected: cephalexin, dicloxacillin, amoxicillin/clavulanate
• Inpatient treatment: vancomycin, clindamycin

Most infections are caused by *Streptococcus pyogenes*, typically group A but also other groups such as B, C, or G. *S. aureus* may cause cellulitis, usually in association with furuncles, carbuncles, or abscesses.

After minor injuries occurring in seawater, an aggressive form of cellulitis caused by *Vibrio* species that may progress to necrotizing fasciitis may occur. Treatment is with vancomycin. Systemic antibiotic treatment is occasionally warranted. Intravenous antibiotics may be required if the severity of the infection necessitates hospitalization.

In patients with neutropenia, *P. aeruginosa* can cause painful ulcerations called *ecthyma gangrenosum*, which warrant directed treatment with antipseudomonal antimicrobials.

#### Herpetic Whitlow
A primary infection with herpes simplex may manifest as inflammation limited to a finger, known as herpetic whitlow (Fig. 3-5). Although these lesions typically are erythematous with irregular vesicles, the vesicles are not evident in many patients. Typically, the digit is swollen, erythematous, and uncomfortable but not painful. Health

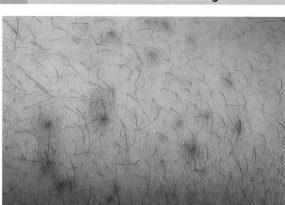

FIGURE 3-1. Folliculitis. *(From Zitelli BJ, Davis HW: Atlas of pediatric physical diagnosis, ed 5, St Louis, 2007, Mosby.)*

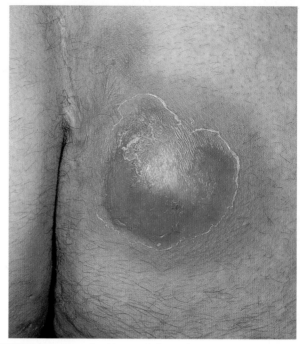

FIGURE 3-2. Furuncle. *(From Habif TB: Clinical dermatology, ed 5, St Louis, 2009, Mosby.)*

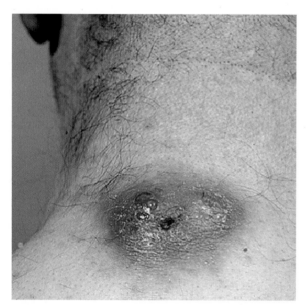

FIGURE 3-3. Carbuncle. *(From Buttaravoli P: Minor emergencies, ed 2, St Louis, 2006, Mosby; borrowed from White G, Cox N: Diseases of the skin, ed 2, St Louis, 2006, Mosby.)*

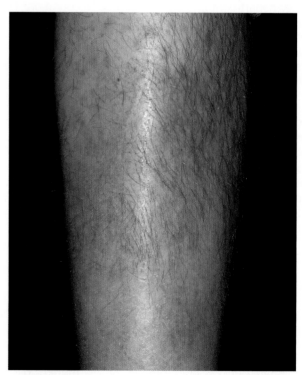

FIGURE 3-4. Cellulitis. *(From Habif TB: Clinical dermatology, ed 5, St Louis, 2009, Mosby.)*

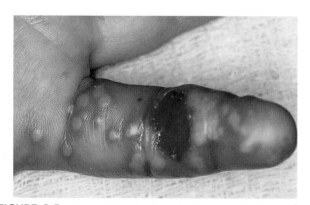

FIGURE 3-5. Herpetic whitlow. *(From Zitelli BJ, Davis HW: Atlas of pediatric physical diagnosis, ed 5, St Louis, 2007, Mosby.)*

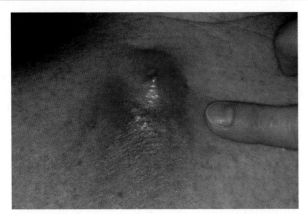

**FIGURE 3-6.** Abscess. *(From Pfenninger JL: Pfenninger and Fowler's procedures for primary care, ed 3, St Louis, 2010, Saunders.)*

care workers, particularly dentists and dental hygienists, are more commonly affected with herpetic whitlow than other people. Treatment with acyclovir is followed by rapid resolution.

## Indolent Infections Primarily Affecting the Fingers

Infection of the digit manifests as an uncomfortable—not described as painful—swelling of a finger with dusky erythema and can persist for days to weeks before the patient seeks medical care. These infections are caused by accidental inoculation of organisms pathogenic for other animal species. *Mycobacterium marinum* should be suspected if there is exposure to fish, amphibians, or reptiles. *Erysipelothrix rhusipathiae* should be suspected if there is a history of exposure to fish, cattle, deer, or elk. If these conditions are suspected, consultation with an infectious disease specialist should be obtained.

## *Infections of the Skin That Extend Below the Subcutaneous Tissues*

### Abscess

Abscesses are painful and tender collections of pus within the dermis and deeper skin tissues that usually manifest as red nodules, often surmounted by a pustule with a rim of erythematous swelling (Fig. 3-6).

- The cause is typically polymicrobial and reflects the normal regional skin flora.
- *S. aureus* as a single pathogen is seen in about 25% of cutaneous abscesses, and it is usually a major component in abscesses from which mixed flora are isolated.
- Drainage of abscesses is usually adequate treatment, unless there is significant inflammation of surrounding soft tissue or systemic manifestations of infection, especially fever.
- When warranted, antibiotic therapy should be directed at *S. aureus*.

## Necrotizing Fasciitis

Necrotizing fasciitis refers to deep and devastating infections that involve the fascial or muscle compartments or both with major destruction of tissue. Extension from a skin lesion is seen in 80% of cases, but there is no visible skin lesion in 20%. Examination of the involved area usually reveals a "wooden-hard" feel of subcutaneous tissues; pain is often quite severe and disproportionate to the examination findings. Necrotizing fasciitis is usually accompanied by high fever and other systemic manifestations, such as tachycardia, hypotension, change in mental status, or impaired tissue perfusion. Necrotizing fasciitis is typically polymicrobial (*S. pyogenes* plus anaerobic bacteria plus aerobic gram-negative organisms).

- Urgent surgical evaluation for possible operative débridement is mandatory.
- Broad-spectrum intravenous antibiotics should be initiated as soon as possible with careful consideration of common pathogens:
  - Vancomycin and penicillin and clindamycin *or*
  - Vancomycin and imipenem or meropenem or piperacillin or ticarcillin

## *Clinical Approach to Soft Tissue Infections*

After a specific diagnosis is made, a proper clinical assessment of disease severity is crucial to facilitate appropriate management. Clinical assessment should address the following elements:

- Severity and anatomic extent of infection
- The environment in which the infection developed (e.g., marine exposure, farm animals)
- Host factors such as diabetes and conditions that compromise the immune system
- Need for urgent surgical evaluation for operative débridement

Physical examination findings that suggest a more severe infection include the following:

- Pain disproportionate to physical findings
- Abnormal vital signs
- Violaceous bullae
- Cutaneous hemorrhage
- Skin sloughing
- Skin anesthesia
- Rapid progression
- Gas in tissues

Imaging studies including plain films, computed tomography (CT), and magnetic resonance imaging (MRI) are used to supplement a careful physical examination and are helpful in revealing deeper foci of infection, such as abscesses in large muscles or myonecrosis. However, the absence of radiographic findings may be misleading in the early stages of infection and should not preclude aggressive treatment in appropriate situations. Ultrasound is evolving as a useful adjunct in diagnosing deep tissue infections.

Common comorbidities must be considered in the assessment of these infections. Patients may require

PART I General Principles

**TABLE 3-1** Soft Tissue Infections

| | Usual Microbes | Systemic Antibiotics* | Surgical Consult/ Intervention |
|---|---|---|---|
| Cellulitis | *Streptococcus pyogenes* *Vibrio* species† | Amoxicillin, macrolide Ciprofloxacin | Not necessary |
| Folliculitis | Skin flora; *Pseudomonas aeruginosa* | Not indicated | |
| Abscess | *Staphylococcus aureus* | TMP/SMX or doxycycline | Incision and drainage |
| Furuncle | *S. aureus* | | |
| Carbuncle | *S. aureus* | | |
| Necrotizing fasciitis | *S. pyogenes,* anaerobic bacteria, other aerobes | Intravenous broad-spectrum antibiotics, including coverage for anaerobes | Immediate consultation mandatory |

*Oral antibiotics are appropriate if outpatient therapy is planned.
†Consider *Vibrio* species if there was marine exposure before onset.
*TMP/SMX,* Trimethoprim/sulfamethoxazole.

directed treatment of clinical entities such as diabetic keto-acidosis, hyperosmolar nonketotic state, neutropenia, human immunodeficiency virus (HIV), and other conditions that result in an immunocompromised state (e.g., long-term steroid treatment, use of tumor necrosis factor-α inhibitors) and would warrant a more aggressive initial approach (Table 3-1).

## *Septic Arthritis*

Native joint septic arthritis usually occurs through hematogenous spread of infection into a joint usually from bacteremia, which is generally transient and asymptomatic. Trauma involving a joint, including cuts, scrapes, and open wounds, and contiguous spread of infection from surrounding soft tissue can lead to septic arthritis. Patients with rheumatologic diseases are prone to developing septic arthritis. These patients also tend to be taking immunosuppressive and biologic agents, which can lead to more frequent infections or infections that are more difficult to treat. Bacterial infection in a joint can lead to destruction of the joint and should be treated urgently to avoid loss of joint function.[1]

Septic arthritis tends to be monarticular; however, more than one joint can be involved in cases of preceding bacteremia. Septic joints are typically painful and swollen and are often red and hot. Patients are typically febrile. However, any inflammatory arthritis may manifest in an identical fashion.

Most native joint infections are caused by *S. aureus* including MRSA. Patients with inflammatory arthritis (e.g., rheumatoid arthritis) who develop septic arthritis usually have *S. aureus* as the causative agent of bacterial arthritis. Infections with *Streptococcus* species are the second most

common infections followed by infections with gram-negative bacilli, infections with anaerobic species, and polymicrobial infections.

Intravenous drug abusers tend to present with staphylococcal or streptococcal septic arthritis. Diabetic patients are also prone to staphylococcal or streptococcal infections and gram-negative bacilli such as *P. aeruginosa.* Regardless of the type of patient or injury to the joint, MRSA antimicrobial coverage should be given because of the high prevalence rate in the community setting. Empiric intravenous antibiotic selection should include activity against gram-positive organisms including MRSA and gram-negative organisms; antibiotic choice can be tailored when results of Gram staining or culture of synovial fluid become available.

Another important cause of septic arthritis is gonococcal arthritis. Gonococcal arthritis should be in the differential diagnosis of organisms causing septic arthritis especially in young, sexually active patients. Two clinical forms exist: primarily monarticular joint swelling or tenosynovitis later in the disease process and polyarthralgia with little joint effusion earlier in the disease process.[36]

Synovial fluid culture should be tested for *Neisseria gonorrhoeae* but is not always positive, particularly in multiarticular disease. As with other causes of septic arthritis, the synovial leukocyte counts for gonococcal arthritis are usually greater than 50,000 cells/mm³. Nucleic acid testing for *N. gonorrhoeae* can be performed on urine samples. Patients with suspected gonococcal arthritis should be initially treated with ceftriaxone, 1 g intravenously.

The possibility of inflammatory arthritis secondary to autoimmune conditions (e.g., rheumatoid arthritis and its variants, systemic lupus erythematosus, psoriatic arthritis), metabolic abnormalities (e.g., gout, pseudogout), and Lyme disease must be considered. A careful history, examination of the patient for other joint abnormalities and skin changes, and evaluation of the joint fluid assist in excluding these conditions.

### Diagnosis

Prompt evaluation of the joint fluid obtained by arthrocentesis is mandatory. Normal joint fluid is viscous and clear, whereas infected fluid is typically watery and cloudy. The fluid must be analyzed for cell count (typically >25,000 white blood cells/mm³) and differential (typically >90% neutrophils). Joint fluid in septic arthritis typically has high protein and lactate dehydrogenase and low glucose, but these values are of lesser value than the cell count and differential in establishing the diagnosis. Samples must be submitted for microbial culture and sensitivity testing. A radiograph of the affected joint should be considered. Synovial fluid leukocyte counts greater than 25,000 cells/ mm³ are suggestive of septic arthritis; however, lower synovial leukocyte counts do not exclude infection, especially in patients who are receiving biologic agents, such as anti–tumor necrosis factor agents.

### Therapy

Treatment of septic arthritis is usually straightforward and requires attention to three issues:

**TABLE 3-2** Septic Arthritis

| Organism | Consider In | | Joint Fluid Gram Stain | Empiric Antibiotic | |
|---|---|---|---|---|---|
| | | | | In ED | At Home If Not Hospitalized |
| *Neisseria gonorrhoeae* | Sexually active patient | Monarticular Polyarticular | Usually + Usually − | Ceftriaxone Ceftriaxone | Doxycycline Doxycycline |
| *Staphylococcus aureus* | Any patient, especially IVDU, DM, and prior inflammatory arthritis | | Usually + | Vancomycin* | Doxycycline, TMP/SMX or linezolid |
| *Streptococcus pyogenes, Streptococcus pneumoniae* | Any patient | | Usually + | Penicillin G, ampicillin, or cephalosporin* | Amoxicillin, cephalexin, or azithromycin |
| Gram-negative rods (e.g., *Pseudomonas aeruginosa*) | Any patient, especially IVDU, prior inflammatory arthritis, immunosuppressant therapy | | Usually + | Ceftazidime, quinolone* | Ciprofloxacin, other quinolone |
| Other bacteria (e.g., *Haemophilus* species) | | | Usually + | | TMP/SMX, doxycycline, or ciprofloxacin |
| Fungi (e.g., *Candida albicans*) | | | Usually − | Await identification of organism; empiric choice problematic; may start with fluconazole | |
| *Borrelia burgdorferi* | Patient living in area endemic for Lyme disease | | Always − | Doxycycline or amoxicillin | Doxycycline or amoxicillin |

*If hospital admission is under consideration; otherwise may initiate planned outpatient regimen.
*DM,* Diabetes mellitus; *ED,* emergency department; *IVDU,* intravenous drug use; *TMP/SMX,* trimethoprim/sulfamethoxazole.

1. An appropriate antibiotic must be administered (Table 3-2).
2. Because joint destruction is mediated by acidic joint fluid under pressure, the fluid must be removed. Fluid removal can be done by arthrocentesis, which may have to be repeated multiple times, or surgically. Septic arthritis of the hip requires orthopedic surgical intervention because needle aspiration, which may need to be repeated several times, is very difficult. Patients presenting to the emergency department with septic arthritis should be seen by a qualified internist or orthopedic surgeon at the time of presentation or the next day. The involved joint or joints must be depressurized at the initial encounter and as often as necessary during follow-up.
3. Discomfort is due to the inflammatory reaction and pressure. Pain relief is usually evident after arthrocentesis, but some patients may require supplemental non-steroidal anti-inflammatory drug (e.g., ibuprofen or naproxen) or acetaminophen therapy.

## Prosthetic Joint Infections

Prosthetic joint infections usually occur as a result of local introduction of bacteria to the joint at the time of surgery or by hematogenous spread at any time. The latter is the most common etiology. Although instrumental implementation, such as dental, genitourinary, or gastrointestinal procedures, can introduce bacteria into the bloodstream, theoretically leading to hematogenous spread of bacteria to a prosthetic joint space, the origin of the bacterial contaminants is usually not evident.

Coagulase-negative staphylococci and *S. aureus* including MRSA are the most commonly implicated organisms, together accounting for 40% to 80% of infections. Streptococci, enterococci, gram-negative rods, and diphtheroids (*Corynebacterium* and *Propionibacterium*) together account for the remainder.

Prosthetic joint infections require a complex evaluation and treatment plan. Treatment or suppression of these infections largely depends on the type and extent of the infection and qualities of the patient's prosthesis, such as ease of removing the prosthesis, and how long the patient has had symptoms of infection.

For an acutely ill patient thought to have involvement of a prosthetic joint, emergency diagnosis and treatment should be focused on ailments that may accompany or lead to infection of the prosthesis. Common infections such as urinary tract infections, pneumonia, and cellulitis should be considered with appropriate evaluation and treatment. Any patient with a painful prosthetic joint and signs of an accompanying infection should be referred to an orthopedic surgeon skilled in management of the implant. If immediate treatment of the patient's illness is believed to be necessary, hospital admission is warranted. For less severe cases, consultation with an orthopedic surgeon and infectious disease specialist and careful follow-up may be appropriate.

## INFECTIONS RELATED TO TRAUMATIC INJURIES

Injuries have many possible etiologies that can range from trauma related to home and recreational activities (e.g.,

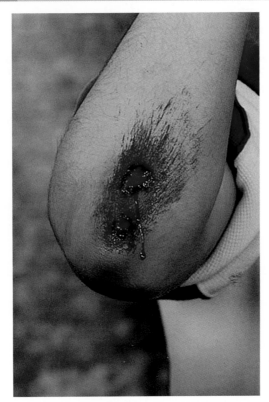

**FIGURE 3-7.** Abrasions.

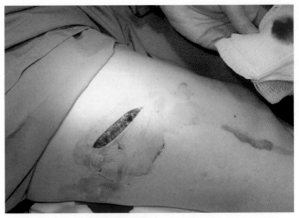

**FIGURE 3-8.** Lacerations.

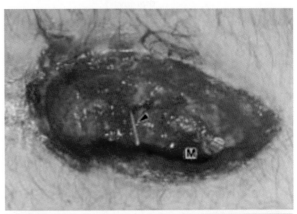

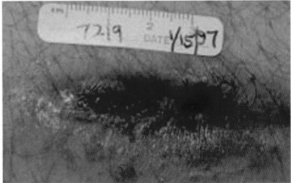

**FIGURE 3-9.** Crush wounds.

falls in the home and animal bites from domestic pets) to motor vehicular accidents, to injuries sustained from assault and violence (e.g., gunshot wounds, knife wounds, or human bite wounds).[2] Wounds resulting from traumatic injuries may lead to infectious complications. Rates of infection vary, however, depending on the circumstances of the injury. Consequently, the approach to management and evaluation of different traumatic injuries should be individualized. Infection risk in traumatic injuries is not uniform, and these injuries manifest different disease states.

## Mechanism of Injury

Mechanical forces that result in soft tissue injury include shear, tension, and compression. Types of wounds are determined by the magnitude and direction of the injuring force and the volume of tissue that is involved. Resulting wounds are typically categorized into the following types:[3]

1. Abrasions are wounds that result from forces applied in opposite directions resulting in loss of epidermis and possibly dermis (Fig. 3-7).
2. Lacerations either are caused by shear forces with little tissue damage at the wound edge resulting in sharp margins or result from tensile and compressive forces that produce jagged and contused margins (Fig. 3-8).
3. Crush wounds are caused by the impact of an object against tissue with resulting compression; tissue may be contused or partially devitalized (Fig. 3-9).
4. Puncture wounds are caused by a combination of forces and usually manifest with a small opening such

that depth and extent of injury cannot be entirely visualized (Fig. 3-10).
5. Avulsions are wounds that have separation of a portion of tissue through shear and tensile forces (Fig. 3-11).
6. Combination wounds have configurations usually resulting from a combination of shear, tensile, and compressive forces.

## Bacterial Contamination

Regardless of wound type, virtually all traumatic wounds are considered to be contaminated with bacteria. Bacterial contamination of wounds can result from external or endogenous bacterial pathogens.[3,4] Exogenous pathogens

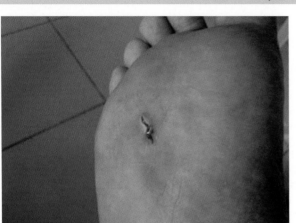

**FIGURE 3-10.** Puncture wounds.

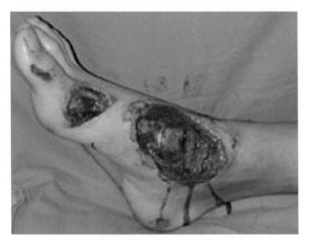

**FIGURE 3-11.** Avulsions.

in wounds generally originate from the environment where the injury occurred. Examples are *Clostridium* species associated with soil contamination, *Vibrio vulnificus* or *Aeromonas* species from water-related injuries, and *S. aureus* infections from fomites. Exogenous pathogens can also originate from normal flora of the skin or colonization at a site adjacent to the injury, such as with *S. aureus* or *S. pyogenes.*[4]

Endogenous bacteria are derived from the skin and the polymicrobial flora of the oropharynx, gastrointestinal tract, and vagina where anaerobic bacteria predominate over facultative organisms. *S. aureus* and *S. pyogenes* must be considered likely pathogens in any soft tissue infection. Anaerobic bacteria are also likely pathogens in infections resulting from injuries potentially contaminated with mouth, gut, or vaginal flora.[4]

The quantity of bacteria present at the time of wound closure has been associated with development of infection. In a series by Krizek and Robson,[5] traumatic wounds containing less than $10^5$ bacteria/g of tissue in patients presenting less than 3 hours after injury were shown to heal without infection. In the same series, wounds in which infections developed after closure showed more than $10^5$ bacteria/g of tissue. Experimental models showed that fewer bacteria are required to infect wounds that are caused by a compressive force ($\geq 10^4$ bacteria/g tissue)

compared with wounds that are caused by a shear force ($\geq 10^6$ bacteria/g tissue). In addition, animal models have provided valuable knowledge showing that crush wounds, burst stellate lacerations, and wounds contaminated with soil are associated with increased infection rates.[3-5]

Quantity of bacteria present in a wound is often determined by the nature and amount of foreign debris contaminating a traumatic wound. Visible contamination of a wound increases risk of infection, and undetected foreign bodies in sutured wounds are likely to result in infection. Bacterial proliferation may also result from the presence of devitalized and necrotic tissue.[3]

Lastly, bacterial contamination can result from medically installed devices such as catheters, tubes, surgical drains, and vascular devices used for treatment of traumatic injuries. These devices allow pathogens to circumvent the skin and mucosal barriers and persist on their surfaces.[6]

## Risk Factors for Wound Infections

Risk factors for infection of wounds relate to the nature of the host and the characteristics of the wound. Host risk factors for infection include the following:

1. Age
2. Diabetes mellitus
3. Chronic renal failure
4. Malnutrition
5. Obesity
6. Immune-compromising conditions
7. Corticosteroid use
8. Chemotherapeutic agents

Wound risk factors for infection include the following:

1. High bacterial counts
2. Oil contamination
3. Crush injury
4. Wound depth, configuration, and size
5. Involvement of joints, bones, and tendons
6. Intraoral involvement
7. Puncture wounds
8. Most bite wounds (high risk of infection)
9. Presence of foreign material

The above-listed risk factors suggest that prevention of infection in traumatic injuries should be considered multifaceted; reliance on antibiotics should *not* be the primary focus. A multifaceted approach to prevention of infection includes the following steps:

1. The wound must be thoroughly cleaned and irrigated with potable water.
2. Careful débridement of any devitalized tissue must be performed.
3. Any foreign debris must be meticulously removed.
4. Only after the aforementioned steps, judicious use of antibiotics targeted to the likely infecting organisms may be considered.

## Antimicrobial Prophylaxis

Routine use of antimicrobial prophylaxis in the setting of injuries, although a common practice, is controversial, and a brief review of current evidence is warranted. Various studies have been undertaken to investigate the value of prophylactic antimicrobials in the setting of different types of injuries. These studies looked at antibiotic prophylaxis in injuries ranging from simple, nonbite wounds, to closed fractures, to penetrating abdominal trauma. Not unexpectedly, the individual studies were heterogeneous and often small in size; however, more recently, large meta-analyses have provided valuable insight into this topic.

Overall, there is little evidence to support the administration of prophylactic antibiotics in the setting of simple, nonbite wounds and nonhuman mammalian bite wounds. However, limited evidence exists to support the use of antibiotic prophylaxis in the setting of human bite wounds and in mammalian bite wounds of the hand.[7,8]

In the setting of complex injuries, various studies showed antibiotic prophylaxis to be useful in reducing infection rates. In both open fractures and closed fracture surgeries, antibiotic prophylaxis reduced the incidence of superficial and deep surgical site infections.[9] There is also evidence to support antibiotic prophylaxis in patients with severe burns; in such patients, there was a significant reduction in all-cause mortality when antibiotic prophylaxis was administered for 4 to 14 days.[10]

It is important that prophylactic antibiotics be chosen on the basis of sensitivities of organisms likely to be causative of infection should infection develop. At the present time, approximately one half of infections caused by *S. aureus* are due to oxacillin-resistant *S. aureus* (MRSA). Use of empiric antibiotics that rely on cephalexin or ampicillin/sulbactam for coverage of *S. aureus* provides no coverage of MRSA. It is also important to consider the patient's ability to purchase the antibiotics. Antibiotic regimens that provide good coverage against MRSA may cost $10 for a 1-month supply (TMP/SMX, doxycycline) or approximately $5000 for the same duration (linezolid) if purchased at one of the major drug store chains (Table 3-3). To be effective, antibiotics must attain therapeutic blood levels and inhibit the growth of likely bacterial pathogens. These objectives can be achieved after either oral or intravenous administration of currently available antibiotics. Because oral antibiotics are prescribed to complete a course of therapy for most patients seen after the injuries discussed in this chapter, there is no reason to mandate that the first dose be given intravenously.

## Bite Wounds

### Animal Bites
#### Cat Bite
Cat bite wounds usually are more common on upper extremities but can occur on lower extremities and the face. Cat bites tend to result in infection more frequently than dog bites owing to cats' long, narrow, front teeth, which tend to cause deeper puncture wounds and soft tissue abscesses.[11] These wounds can be particularly troublesome if near or overlying a joint because there is an

**TABLE 3-3** Approximate Retail Costs of Oral Antibiotics

| Antibiotics Available for <$10/mo | Useful for Infections Caused by: | Alternatives | Approximate Cost for 1 Month |
|---|---|---|---|
| Amoxicillin | *Streptococcus, Enterococcus, Haemophilus* species | Ampicillin/sulbactam | $450 |
| Cephalexin | *Streptococcus,* oxacillin-sensitive *Staphylococcus* species | Cefuroxime axetil | $300 |
| Ciprofloxacin | *Pseudomonas* species, other gram-negative rods | Levofloxacin | $1500 |
| Erythromycin | *Streptococcus* species | Azithromycin | $400 |
| Doxycycline | *Staphylococcus* species including MRSA, many GNR, *Pasteurella, Haemophilus* species | Linezolid* | $5100 |
| Metronidazole | Anaerobes | Clindamycin | $240 |
| Penicillin V | *Streptococcus* species, some anaerobes | | |
| SMX/TMP | *Staphylococcus* species including MRSA, many GNR, *Pasteurella, Haemophilus* species | Linezolid* | $5100 |
| Tetracycline | *Staphylococcus* species including MRSA, many GNR, *Pasteurella, Haemophilus* species | Linezolid* | $5100 |

Note: Pharmacies in national chains (e.g., Walmart, Walgreen's, CVS) make many generic medications, including antibiotics, available at a modest cost. For the agents listed, a 10-day course, often adequate for treatment of wounds, can cost only $4, and a supply sufficient for a 1-month course can be obtained for $10. Current listings are posted on the websites of individual pharmacies. For uninsured patients, the cost of antibiotics may be a major consideration.
*Not used for *Pasteurella* species, *Haemophilus* species, or other GNRs.
*GNR,* Gram-negative rods; *MRSA,* methicillin-resistant *Staphylococcus aureus; TMP/SMX,* trimethoprim/sulfamethoxazole.

*Vibrio* species can cause rapidly progressive cellulitis leading to necrotizing fasciitis. Bullae and erythema are often present. Early surgical intervention with débridement may be necessary.[20] Doxycycline, fluoroquinolones, and third-generation cephalosporins are active against *Vibrio* species.

*M. marinum* infections generally occur as a result of injury on the hands or extremities that have been in contact with aquariums, injury from a fish or shellfish, or injury in saltwater or brackish water. Usually cutaneous lesions are seen, which can be long-standing owing to the long incubation period of *M. marinum*.[21] If *M. marinum* infection is suspected, consultation with an infectious disease specialist should be sought.

*Aeromonas* species, especially *A. hydrophila,* infections tend to occur after penetrating trauma in freshwater or trauma associated with fish or marine animals. *Aeromonas* infection can manifest similarly to gangrene caused by clostridia with rapid onset and progression of cellulitis leading to myonecrosis. Bullae, edema, and erythema are often present. Treatment is similar to treatment of infection with *Vibrio* species; early surgical intervention with débridement is often necessary. TMP/SMX and ciprofloxacin are generally active against *Aeromonas* species. Third-generation cephalosporins, carbapenems, and aztreonam have been used, although some β-lactamase-producing strains hydrolize carbapenems and cephalosporin classes (Fig. 3-12 and Table 3-6).[15]

## USE OF ANTIBIOTICS

Table 3-7 outlines usual dosages and some practical tips concerning the use of various commonly prescribed antibiotics.

## References

1. Mandell GL, Bennet JE, Dolin R, editors: Principles and Practice of Infectious Diseases, ed 7, Philadelphia, 2010, Churchill Livingstone.
2. Centers for Disease Control and Prevention: Injury, violence, and safety. Available at: http://cdc.gov/InjuryViolenceSafety.
3. Roberts J, Hedges J: Clinical Procedures in Emergency Medicine, ed 5, St Louis, 2010, Elsevier.
4. Brook I, Frazier EH: Aerobic and anaerobic microbiology of infection after trauma. Am J Emerg Med 16:585–591, 1998.
5. Krizek T, Robson M: Evolution of quantitative bacteriology in wound management. Am J Surg 30:579–584, 1975.
6. Abubaker AO: Use of prophylactic antibiotics in preventing infection of traumatic injuries. Dent Clin North Am 53:707–715, 2009.
7. Cummings P, Del Beccaro MA: Antibiotics to prevent infection of simple wounds: a meta-analysis of randomized studies. Am J Emerg Med 13:396–400, 1995.
8. Medeiros I, Saconato H: Antibiotic prophylaxis for mammalian bites. Cochrane Database Syst Rev (2):CD001738, 2001.
9. Gillespie WJ, Wallencamp GH: Antibiotic prophylaxis for surgery for proximal femoral and other closed long bone fractures. Cochrane Database Syst Rev (3):CD000244, 2010.
10. Avni T, Levcovich A, Ad-El DD, et al: Prophylactic antibiotics for burns patients: systematic review and meta-analysis. BMJ 340:c241, 2010.
11. Oehler RL, Velez AP, Mizrachi M, et al: Bite-related and septic syndromes caused by cats and dogs. Lancet Infect Dis 9:536, 2009.
12. Compendium of Animal Rabies Prevention and Control, 2011: National Association of State Public Health Veterinarians, Inc. MMWR Recomm Rep 60(RR06):1–14, 2011.
13. Tregle RW, Jr, Loe CL, Earhart RH, et al: Cercopithecine herpesvirus 1 risk in a child bitten by a bonnet macaque monkey. J Emerg Med 41:e89–e90, 2010.
14. Garg A, Sujatha S, Garg J, et al: Wound infections secondary to snake bite. J Infect Dev Ctries 3:221–223, 2009.
15. Stevens DL, Bisno AL, Chambers HF, et al: Practice guidelines for the management of skin and soft-tissue infections. Clin Infect Dis 41:1373–1406, 2005.
16. Volgas DA, Stannard JP, Alonso JE: Current orthopaedic treatment of ballistic injuries. injury. Int J Care Injured 36:380–386, 2005.
17. Simpson BA, Wilson RH, Grant RE: Antibiotic therapy in gunshot wound injuries. Clin Orthop Relat Res 408:82–85, 2003.
18. Luchette FA, Borzotta AP, Croce MA, et al: Practice management guidelines for prophylactic antibiotic use in penetrating abdominal trauma. J Trauma 48(3):508–518, 2000.
19. Pennycook A, Makower R, O'Donnell AM: Puncture wounds of the foot: can infectious complications be avoided? J R Soc Med 87:581–583, 1994.
20. Patterson TF, Bell SR, Bia FJ: Vibrio alginolyticus cellulitis following coral injury. Yale J Biol Med 61:507–512, 1988.
21. Jernigan JA, Farr BM: Incubation period and sources of exposure for cutaneous Mycobacterium marinum infection: case report and review of literature. Clin Infect Dis 31:439–443, 2000.
22. Boenning DA, Fleisher GR, Campos JM: Dog bites in children: epidemiology, microbiology, and penicillin prophylactic therapy. Am J Emerg Med 1:17–21, 1983.
23. Keiser H, Ruben F, Wolinsky E, et al: Clinical forms of gonococcal arthritis. N Engl J Med 279:234–240, 1968.

## Bibliography

Brakenbury PH, Muwanga C: A comparative double blind study of amoxycillin/clavulanate vs placebo in the prevention of infection after animal bites. Arch Emerg Med 6:251–256, 1989.
Brand M, Goosen J, Grieve A: Prophylactic antibiotics for penetrating abdominal trauma. Cochrane Database Syst Rev (4):CD007370, 2009.
Bratzler DW, Houck PM; Surgical Infection Prevention Guideline Writers Workgroup: Antimicrobial prophylaxis for surgery: an advisory statement from the National Surgical Infection Prevention Project. Am J Surg 189:395–404, 2005.
Brown KV, Walker JA, Cortez DS, et al: Earlier debridement and antibiotic administration decrease infection. J Surg Orthop Adv 19:18–22, 2010.
Cheung JP, Fung B, Wong SS, et al: Mycobacterium marinum infection of the hand and wrist. J Orthop Surg (Hong Kong) 18:98–103, 2010.
David MZ, Daum RS: Community-associated methicillin-resistant Staphylococcus aureus: epidemiology and clinical consequences of an emerging epidemic. Clin Microbiol Rev 23:616–687, 2010.
Finkelstein R, Oren I: Soft tissue infections caused by marine bacterial pathogens: epidemiology, diagnosis, and management. Curr Infect Dis Rep 13:470–477, 2011.
García-De La Torre I, Arnulfo Nava-Zavala A: Gonococcal and nongonococcal arthritis. Rheum Dis Clin North Am 35:63–73, 2009.
Gerhardt RT, Matthews JM, Sullivan SG: The effect of systemic antibiotic prophylaxis and wound irrigation on penetrating combat wounds in a return-to-duty population. Prehosp Emerg Care 13:500–504, 2009.
Ho J, Taylor DM, Cabalag MS, Ugoni A, et al: Factors that impact on emergency department patient compliance with antibiotic regimens. Emerg Med J 27:815–820, 2010.
Kennedy J, Tuleu I, Mackay K: Unfilled prescriptions of Medicare beneficiaries: prevalence, reasons, and types of medicines prescribed. J Manag Care Pharm 14:553–560, 2008.
Kirking DM, Lee JA, Ellis JJ, et al: Patient-reported underuse of prescription medications: a comparison of nine surveys. Med Care Res Rev 63:427–446, 2006.
Masini BD, Murray CK, Wenke JC, et al: Prevention and treatment of infected foot and ankle wounds sustained in the combat environment. Foot Ankle Clin 15:91–112, 2010.
Melvin JS, Dombroski DG, Torbert JT, et al: Open tibial shaft fractures: I. evaluation and initial wound management. J Am Acad Orthop Surg 18:10–19, 2010.
Margaretten ME, Kohlwes J, Moore D, et al: Does this adult patient have septic arthritis? JAMA 297:1478–1488, 2007.
Morgan MS: Diagnosis and management of necrotising fasciitis: a multiparametric approach. J Hosp Infect 75:249–257, 2010.
Schmitz GR, Bruner D, Pitotti R, et al: Randomized controlled trial of trimethoprim-sulfamethoxazole for uncomplicated skin abscesses in patients at risk for community-associated methicillin-resistant

Staphylococcus aureus infection. Ann Emerg Med 56:283–287, 2010.

Shirtliff ME, Mader JT: Acute septic arthritis. Clin Microbiol Rev 15:527–544, 2002.

Singer AJ, Dagum AB: Current management of acute cutaneous wounds. N Engl J Med 359:1037–1046, 2008.

Smack DP, Harrington AC, Dunn C, et al: Infection and allergy incidence in ambulatory surgery patients using white petrolatum vs bacitracin ointment: a randomized controlled trial. JAMA 276:972–977, 1996.

Steere AC: Lyme disease. N Engl J Med 345:115–125, 2001.

Yun HC, Blackbourne LH, Jones JA, et al: Infectious complications of noncombat trauma patients provided care at a military trauma center. Milit Med 175:317–323, 2010.

# Chapter 4

# *Analgesia, Conscious Sedation, Regional Blocks, and Anesthesia*

### Robert P. Fuller, Richard Sheppard, and Richard Gannon

Musculoskeletal injuries and diseases can be extremely painful, and a compassionate and thoughtful approach is required to provide adequate pain and anxiety relief. Depending on the patient's underlying illness and clinical needs, the proper selection of type of analgesia and anxiolysis can have a significant impact on the outcome.

## GENERAL CONCEPTS FOR PAIN MANAGEMENT

1. Pain reduction should be an early goal.
2. Pain reduction should be planned anticipating further management so as to improve, not impede, that management.
3. Modalities that work fast with the least systemic effects should be chosen.
4. Emergency department pain reduction should be transitioned to the outpatient or the inpatient pain management plan.

## ANALGESIA

### Mild Pain

Patients with acute traumatic or nontraumatic musculoskeletal complaints can be offered oral analgesia with acetaminophen (Tylenol) or a nonsteroidal anti-inflammatory drug (NSAID) early in presentation or in triage. These medications reduce pain with very few side effects, and there is no evidence that a single oral dose would impact further pain management, sedation, or anesthesia decisions.

### Moderate Pain

Patients with more severe pain from acute traumatic or nontraumatic musculoskeletal complaints should be offered parenteral narcotic pain medications if there is no other method for better pain control. Pain medication generally should be administered before imaging studies and other diagnostic interventions. Better pain control methods may include splinting, ice, reduction of dislocation, hematoma block, arthro-block, or regional block.

### Severe Pain

Trauma to an extremity with obviously deformed fractures or fracture-dislocations of the wrist, elbow, or ankle is best managed with early arthro-block or hematoma block and splinting for stability. Arthro-block or hematoma block offers excellent pain relief very quickly with no systemic side effects. Often there is no need for parenteral pain medication after adequate block. Patients with obvious or likely long bone fractures (i.e., hip, shoulder) or axial injuries (i.e., back, pelvis) are likely to require parenteral narcotic pain medications before studies. A patient with a clinically obvious simple dislocation often can undergo reduction before any studies are done. Reductions dramatically improve patients' pain, reduce the risk of time-related complications of displacement, and reduce or eliminate the need for parenteral pain medications.

For nontraumatic injuries, when arthrocentesis is part of the diagnostic work-up, planning to place local anesthetic (lidocaine or bupivacaine without epinephrine with or without steroid) at the time of the therapeutic or diagnostic aspiration can greatly improve short-term pain relief and make examination for ligament stability and range of motion possible.

## MEDICATIONS FOR PAIN

### Opioids

For severe pain, patients may require initial dosing with intravenous opioids every 15 to 30 minutes to control pain. If the only routes available are intramuscular or subcutaneous routes, doses could be repeated every 30 to 60 minutes. The most common side effects with opioids include nausea, vomiting, sedation, delirium, hypotension, constipation, pruritus, urine retention, and respiratory depression.

Patients frequently claim to be opiate allergic, but careful discussion often reveals a side effect rather than a true allergic reaction. In this instance, switching to any other opioid may decrease the risk of side effects. Patients can develop diffuse pruritus and hives especially at an intravenous injection site. This side effect is most likely due to histamine release and can be controlled by an antihistamine.

## Morphine

Morphine is the most commonly used parenteral opioid analgesic. The starting dose is 0.05 to 0.1 mg/kg (intravenous, intramuscular, or subcutaneous route). The analgesic equivalent oral dose is two to three times the parenteral dose. Morphine is available as immediate-release tablets, sustained-release tablets and capsules, liquid, liquid concentrate, and suppository. The liquid concentrate (20 mg/mL) can be given sublingually to provide analgesia. More recently, an abuse-resistant tablet Embeda (morphine with naltrexone) became available. Elderly patients and patients with impaired renal function require careful consideration for repeated doses of morphine because of decreased elimination. These metabolites provide analgesia but also cause nausea, vomiting, myoclonus, sedation, delirium, and respiratory depression.

## Hydromorphone

The usual initial dose of hydromorphone is 0.0075 to 0.015 mg/kg (0.5 to 1 mg) administered intravenously, subcutaneously, or intramuscularly. The equivalent oral dose is approximately four times the parenteral dose. Parenteral hydromorphone is approximately five times more potent than parenteral morphine. Hydromorphone has only one weakly active metabolite, and it is a good choice in elderly patients and patients with impaired renal or liver function. It is available as an injection, immediate-release tablet, oral solution, suppository, and sustained-release tablet.

## Fentanyl

The usual initial dose of fentanyl is 0.5 to 1 µg/kg administered intravenously, subcutaneously, or intramuscularly. It is a lipophilic drug, and it has a rapid onset and a short duration of action (<1 hour); this makes it easy to titrate and an excellent choice for patients who are likely to have significant improvement in their discomfort during the emergency department visit (i.e., pain is greatly reduced after joint reduction). Fentanyl is also well absorbed via the nasal route and the inhalation route, which has great utility in pediatric patients. Fentanyl has only minimally active metabolites, which coupled with its short duration of action makes it suitable for elderly patients and patients with liver disease or renal insufficiency.

## Oxycodone

The usual dose of oxycodone is 5 to 10 mg in an immediate-release tablet. It is available as a sustained-release, tamper-resistant tablet (OxyContin); liquid; and liquid concentrate. The liquid concentrate (20 mg/mL) is useful for sublingual administration. Various commercial preparations of oxycodone with acetaminophen (different strengths) and ibuprofen are available.

## Methadone

Methadone can be used for analgesia and to prevent opioid abuse. When used for analgesia, methadone needs to be given in divided doses (every 8 hours or every 6 hours). When used to prevent opioid abuse, it needs to be given only once per day. Methadone is generally not prescribed by emergency physicians.

## Buprenorphine and Buprenorphine-Naloxone (Suboxone)

Buprenorphine is an opioid partial agonist. Buprenorphine and the combination of buprenorphine and naloxone are used to treat opioid addiction and are generally not prescribed by emergency physicians.

## *Non-Narcotic Pain Medications*

## Acetaminophen

Acetaminophen is widely available and useful as a non-prescription analgesic for mild to moderate pain and as an antipyretic. The usual adult dose is 650 mg orally or rectally every 4 hours as needed or 1 g every 6 hours as needed. The suggested maximum daily dose of acetaminophen at the present time is 4 g/day with a lower maximum dose (<2 g/day) for patients taking warfarin. Doses higher than 4 g/day can lead to hepatotoxicity. The combination of an NSAID with acetaminophen provides better analgesia for somatic and visceral pain than either agent alone.

## Nonsteroidal Anti-inflammatory Drugs

Multiple NSAIDs are available to treat somatic and visceral pain. These agents do not work well for neuropathic pain. NSAIDs exert their pharmacologic effect by reversibly inhibiting prostaglandin formation through nonselective inhibition of cyclooxygenase enzymes I and II (COX-I and COX-II). Aspirin is the only NSAID that irreversibly binds to COX-I. COX-I is responsible for maintenance of normal physiologic functions (i.e., gastric mucosal barrier, platelet aggregation); COX-II is an inducible enzyme that is found at sites of tissue injury. If NSAIDs are prescribed, it is probably best to give them around-the-clock initially because NSAIDs inhibit a process from occurring: prostaglandin generation → cytokine release → edema, inflammation, and pain.

NSAIDs should not be given to patients after the 30th week of pregnancy, patients with congestive heart failure, or patients with renal dysfunction. Giving an NSAID to a patient who is already receiving a high-dose corticosteroid

## Chapter 6  *Perioperative Assessment*

Nicole Silverstein and Richard Sheppard

A preoperative evaluation is a comprehensive review of a patient. It is done to determine a patient's stability for surgery and how to optimize existing medical conditions for the proposed surgery. Actions taken to optimize medical conditions may include, but are not limited to, making changes in medications, suggesting preoperative tests or procedures, and proposing higher levels of postoperative care. The ultimate decision to plan for surgery is in the hands of the surgeon, the anesthesiologist, and the patient. A medical evaluation helps gather information to limit the risks and supply knowledge to the surgeon, anesthesiologist, and patient to enable informed consent. Anesthesia is an important aspect of medicine, and knowledge is required of risks, surgical procedures and complications, and perioperative care of the patient.

## PREOPERATIVE CARDIAC RISK ASSESSMENT

One of the first areas often addressed in a preoperative evaluation is the patient's cardiac status. This evaluation includes both the patient's diagnoses and risk factors and the risk of the proposed surgery. The American College of Cardiology and the American Heart Association (ACC/AHA) published an algorithm with Guidelines on Perioperative Cardiovascular Evaluation and Care for Noncardiac Surgery in 2007 that help assess this risk (Fig. 6-1).[1]

The first step requires determination of the urgency of the surgery. Emergent surgeries do not warrant preoperative evaluation. Patients should be taken directly to the operating room with no further cardiac assessment. They should be assessed and monitored after surgery for any optimization of their medical conditions.

When it is determined that the proposed surgery is not emergent; the patient's current cardiac condition is assessed to detect any active cardiac conditions, such as the following:

1. Active decompensated heart failure
2. Unstable angina

3. Recent myocardial infarction, defined as either non–ST segment elevation or ST segment elevation myocardial infarction within the past month
4. Severe valvular disease, most notably severe aortic stenosis
5. Significant arrhythmia, such as supraventricular tachycardia, rapid atrial fibrillation, or ventricular tachycardia; rate-controlled atrial fibrillation is not considered a significant arrhythmia

If any of the above-listed conditions are present, they should be evaluated and treated before the operation. After these cardiac conditions have been adequately treated, the patient should be reassessed for surgery.

If there are no active cardiac conditions present, the type of surgery is determined. Surgeries are generally divided into high, intermediate, and low risk for a cardiac event. High-risk procedures are associated with a greater than 5% chance of a perioperative cardiac event, whereas low-risk procedures are associated with a less than 1% chance of a perioperative cardiac event. Intermediate-risk procedures are associated with a risk of a cardiac event between 1% and 5%.

## Surgical Stratification

Patients undergoing low-risk procedures do not require any further cardiac evaluation before surgery. Patients undergoing high-risk or intermediate-risk surgeries need further assessment (Table 6-1). Most orthopedic surgeries fall under the intermediate-risk category and require this next step of cardiac evaluation. The fourth step according to the guidelines of the ACC/AHA is evaluation of the patient's functional capacity. The idea is to try to gauge the patient's cardiac reserve. Cardiac reserve is assessed by determining the highest level of activity a patient can perform without any cardiac signs or symptoms. It is measured in metabolic equivalents. A metabolic equivalent of 1 is the ability to eat, dress, and perform basic self-care; at the other end of the range, 10 metabolic equivalents

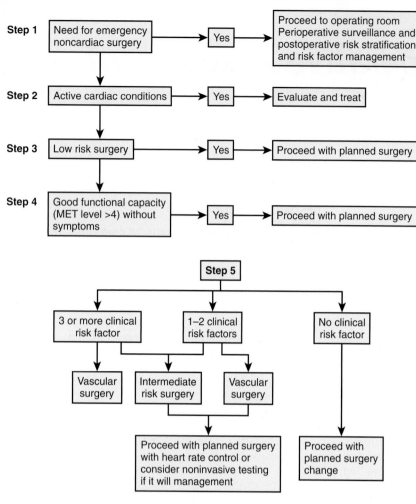

**FIGURE 6-1.** American College of Cardiology/American Heart Association cardiac evaluation and care algorithm for noncardiac surgery based on active clinical conditions, known cardiovascular disease, or cardiac risk factors for patients 50 years of age or older. *(From Fleisher LA, Beckman JA, Brown KA, et al: ACC/AHA 2007 Guidelines on perioperative cardiovascular evaluation and care for noncardiac surgery: executive summary: a report of the American College of Cardiology/American Heart Association Task Force on Practice Guidelines [Writing Committee to Revise the 2002 Guidelines on Perioperative Cardiovascular Evaluation for Noncardiac Surgery]: Developed in Collaboration With the American Society of Echocardiography, American Society of Nuclear Cardiology, Heart Rhythm Society, Society of Cardiovascular Anesthesiologists, Society for Cardiovascular Angiography and Interventions, Society for Vascular Medicine and Biology, and Society for Vascular Surgery. Circulation 116:1971–1996, 2007. © 2007, American Heart Association, Inc.)*

**TABLE 6-1** Surgery Stratification

| | |
|---|---|
| High-risk surgeries | All vascular surgeries except for carotid endarterectomy<br>Surgeries projected to be >3 hours or with large blood loss or fluid shift |
| Intermediate-risk surgeries | All other surgeries including orthopedic surgeries in addition to abdominal and peritoneal, head and neck, and most urologic surgeries |
| Low-risk surgeries | Typically outpatient surgeries such as colonoscopy, endoscopy, skin biopsies, cataract procedures, and breast biopsies |

would be participation in strenuous sports. Most surgeries put a strain on the heart of approximately 4 metabolic equivalents; this is equal to climbing a flight of stairs or walking on level ground at 4 mph. A patient who has a functional capacity greater than 4 metabolic equivalents is thought not to require any further cardiac evaluation and can proceed to surgery.

A patient's functional capacity often is unknown because of dementia, sedation, or other causes of impaired cognition. Patients may have a poor functional capacity because

of a sedentary lifestyle. These patients require step 5 evaluation, which is the determination of their clinical risk factors. Clinical risk factors have been defined differently depending on the source. The ACC/AHA derived the Revised Cardiac Risk Index, which includes the following risk factors:[1]

1. Any history of ischemic heart disease
2. Any history of compensated or prior heart failure
3. Any history of cerebrovascular disease
4. Diabetes mellitus
5. Renal failure

If a patient has none of the above-listed clinical risk factors, the cardiac evaluation is complete. If a patient has one or two risk factors, further cardiac evaluation needs to be considered "if it would change the management of the patient."[1] The physician's knowledge of the patient and a full review of the patient's history, especially a complete review of symptoms and physical examination, are essential for determining which patients need further cardiac assessment.

Patients with three or more risk factors are divided into vascular surgeries and intermediate-risk surgeries. Most elderly patients with trauma fit into this intermediate-risk surgery category. Similar to the previous category of one or two clinical risk factors, initiation of beta blocker therapy providers performing these tests. The actual risk for the development of cancer as a result of in utero exposure to radiation is unknown. Some data suggest that a fetal exposure of 1 to 2 rad may increase the risk of leukemia by a factor of 1.5 to 2.0, increasing the leukemia rate from 1 in 3000 to 1 in 2000.

Abdominal shielding should be used whenever the x-ray procedure allows. The estimated fetal exposure from common radiologic studies is listed in Table 7-1.

## Computed Tomography

The radiation dose to the fetus from a typical CT scan is likely between 1 and 4 rad depending on the study and the gestational age. Although this radiation dose is considerably higher than the radiation dose of a plain x-ray study, it is still below the accepted threshold level for induction of congenital abnormalities. The risk of carcinogenesis is similar to the risk of an x-ray (at a dose of 5 rad, the relative risk of childhood leukemia is 2.0). There is a risk of failed implantation within the first 2 weeks of embryonic life when the dose is greater than 10 rad. At this gestational age (often before the patient is even aware of the pregnancy), there is an "all or none" effect so that should the embryo survive, there are not likely to be any untoward effects.

## Magnetic Resonance Imaging

MRI uses magnets that alter the energy state of hydrogen protons rather than using ionizing radiation. Although a relatively new technique for diagnostic imaging in pregnancy, MRI is thought to be a safer alternative to nuclear imaging. MRI is often used to help diagnose fetal abnormalities. Studies of children up to 9 years of age who were exposed to MRI in utero at 1.5 Tesla did not show negative outcomes. Although a small amount of animal data suggest a potential teratogenic effect of MRI in early pregnancy, no such human studies have been published. According to the American College of Radiology, MRI is recommended in pregnancy if the "risk-benefit ratio to the patient warrants that the study be performed." Results of studies evaluating potential acoustic damage to the fetus from MRI have also shown safety in this area.

Use of the intravenous contrast agent gadolinium in conjunction with MRI has been controversial. Gadolinium crosses the placenta and is excreted by the fetal kidneys into the amniotic fluid. Animal studies of high and repeated doses of gadolinium have been shown to be teratogenic. Although considered a pregnancy category C drug by the U.S. Food and Drug Administration, gadolinium is reserved for cases in pregnancy where the benefits outweigh the potential risks to the fetus.

## Nuclear Imaging

Nuclear studies are performed by combining a chemical agent with a radioisotope. These radiopharmaceuticals, when administered intravenously or orally to the patient,

**TABLE 7-2** Estimated Fetal Exposure from Common Radiologic Procedures

| Procedure | Fetal Exposure |
| --- | --- |
| Chest x-ray (2 views) | 0.02-0.07 mrad |
| Abdominal film (single view) | 100 mrad |
| Intravenous pyelogram | ≥1 rad (depending on number of films) |
| Hip film (single view) | 200 mrad |
| CT scan head/chest | <1 rad |
| CT scan abdomen and lumbar spine | 3.5 rad |

*CT,* Computed tomography.
Data from Williams obstetrics, ed 21, New York, 2001, McGraw-Hill, pp 1143–1158.

can localize to specific organs or cellular receptors, resulting in the ability to image the extent of a disease process in the body. In some diseases, nuclear medicine studies can identify medical problems at an earlier stage than other diagnostic tests. One of the most commonly used isotopes is technetium 99 m (Tc 99 m). The fetal exposure for common nuclear scans such as brain, bone, renal, and cardiovascular scans is small (<0.5 rad).

The American College of Obstetrics and Gynecology published the following guidelines for x-ray examination during pregnancy (Table 7-2):

1. The exposure from a single x-ray procedure does not result in harmful fetal effects. Exposure to less than 5 rad has shown no increase in the rate of fetal anomalies or spontaneous abortion. Patients should be counseled accordingly.
2. The concern regarding fetal effects of high-dose ionizing radiation should not delay or prevent medically indicated diagnostic x-ray procedures from being performed on pregnant women. Imaging procedures such as ultrasound and MRI that are not associated with ionizing radiation should be used in pregnancy in place of x-ray procedures when possible.
3. Radiopaque and paramagnetic contrast agents are unlikely to cause fetal harm; however, they should be used only when medically necessary when the potential benefit outweighs the risk.
4. If multiple x-rays are needed in a pregnant patient, it may be helpful to consult with an expert in radiation dosimetry to calculate a total fetal exposure.
5. MRI and ultrasound are not associated with any harmful fetal effects.

## COMMON MUSCULOSKELETAL COMPLAINTS IN PREGNANCY

Because of the normal physiologic changes that occur in pregnancy, certain musculoskeletal disorders may arise in pregnancy. These disorders may be due to a combination of factors including progesterone-related ligament laxity; peripheral edema of the extremities including the carpal tunnel space; and an altered center of gravity as the pregnancy progresses, which may increase the likelihood of falling.

Common musculoskeletal complaints in pregnancy are summarized as follows:

- Back pain in pregnancy
  - Most common musculoskeletal complaint in pregnancy
  - Often secondary to increasing size of uterus placing pressure on lower spine
  - Exaggerated lordosis of the lumbar spine in pregnancy
  - Sciatic pain very common in pregnancy owing to compression of the sciatic nerve by the uterus
- Carpal tunnel syndrome
  - Common complaint in pregnancy (affects 25% of pregnant women)
  - More common in the third trimester
  - Secondary to edema in the carpal tunnel space compressing the median nerve
  - Usually best treated in pregnancy with wrist splints
  - Surgery not usually necessary during pregnancy because symptoms subside after delivery
- Most common extremity injuries during pregnancy related to falling
  - Ankle sprain (increased laxity of ligaments in pregnancy)
  - Wrist sprain and fracture

In addition to the above-listed complaints, separation of the pubic symphysis is a rare but important musculoskeletal complication of pregnancy. Treatment is usually conservative, with pain medication as needed, physical therapy, and support with abdominal binders to decrease the pressure on the pubic bone.

## FETAL MONITORING DURING NONOBSTETRIC SURGERY

During any surgical procedure in a pregnant woman, there are concerns for both the patient and the fetus. Alterations in maternal blood flow that occur during surgery must be considered first. The circulation to the uteroplacental unit is not autoregulated, and the greatest impact of surgery on the fetus may come from decreased uterine blood flow and decreased oxygen content of the blood.

During the third trimester, uterine circulation represents nearly 10% of maternal cardiac output. Maternal hypotension is likely lead to decreased uterine blood flow and decreased perfusion to the fetus. Although medical therapy with pressors successfully increases the maternal systemic pressure, they have little or no effect on uterine perfusion. Other maneuvers, such as intravenous fluid boluses, changing maternal position to decrease vena caval compression, or leg elevation, are much more effective than medical therapy at increasing uteroplacental blood flow.

## ANESTHESIA DURING PREGNANCY

Concern over the effect of inhalation anesthetic agents mainly arises in the first trimester when exposure can be associated with birth defects. The literature is scant in this area; however, most experts agree that these agents are safe even in the first trimester. Although elective surgery should be postponed until the second trimester or after delivery, orthopedic emergencies requiring surgical correction should proceed because the benefit far outweighs any potential risk.

## PRETERM LABOR

The risk for preterm labor is related to both gestational age and the indication for and type of surgery. Pregnancies in the third trimester are associated with much higher risk for preterm contractions with or without cervical dilation compared with earlier gestational age. Orthopedic surgeries not involving the maternal pelvis are much less likely to stimulate preterm labor than intra-abdominal surgeries.

Postoperative courses complicated by preterm contractions and preterm labor are most likely following abdominal surgeries and disease processes with intraperitoneal inflammation. Both laparoscopic and open techniques have an equal incidence of preterm contractions and labor.

Treatment for preterm contractions, especially in the presence of cervical dilation, is with tocolytics. Studies show that delay of treatment of contractions after surgery can lead to preterm labor and subsequent preterm birth. Although there is no general consensus on the use of prophylactic tocolytics after nonobstetric surgery during pregnancy, most studies suggest that tocolytics be used only if contractions are noted during postoperative monitoring or are appreciated by the patient.

The types of tocolytics used vary widely among medical centers. Options include magnesium sulfate (intravenous), nifedipine (oral), terbutaline (subcutaneous or oral), or indomethacin (oral). These agents generally are equally effective in diminishing contractions when the contractions occur postoperatively, although most studies show that these agents delay delivery by no more than 48 hours.[13,14]

## TRAUMA IN PREGNANCY

Trauma is the leading nonobstetric cause of maternal mortality and affects 7% of pregnancies. The most common form of trauma comes from falls or motor vehicle accidents. Compared with gestational age–matched controls, women who sustained trauma had a higher incidence of spontaneous abortion, preterm labor, fetomaternal hemorrhage, abruptio placentae, and uterine rupture. Approximately 50% of fetal losses in trauma cases are due to placental abruption. Risk of abruption is present with all placental locations, not just when the placenta has an attachment to the anterior uterine wall. Although multiple studies have been unable to predict adverse outcomes such as abruptio placentae and fetal loss adequately, it is accepted that early involvement of an available obstetrician is important to evaluate maternal and fetal well-being.

$Rh_O(D)$ immune globulin (RhoGAM) is indicated in Rh-negative patients who have (1) vaginal bleeding or (2) evidence of fetomaternal hemorrhage as diagnosed by a maternal Kleihauer-Betke stain looking for fetal cells in the maternal circulation. The standard dose of RhoGAM is 300 µg, which is sufficient to cover 30 mL of fetal whole blood in the maternal circulation.

Direct fetal injury secondary to trauma is rare. Most of these cases result from significant maternal injury at later gestational ages (Trauma 22/23). Another rare but life-threatening consequence of trauma is uterine rupture, which occurs most commonly secondary to direct abdominal injuries with substantial force (Trauma 24/25).

Resuscitation of the fetus is best accomplished by resuscitation of the mother. Initial evaluation and treatment of a pregnant injured patient is identical to evaluation and treatment of a nonpregnant injured patient; rapid assessment of the maternal airway, breathing, and circulation and ensuring an adequate airway avoid maternal and fetal hypoxia. In the later stages of pregnancy, the pregnant trauma patient should be placed in the left lateral decubitus position with care to assess the fetus using either ultrasound or an external fetal monitor.

The increased blood volume associated with pregnancy has implications in the trauma patient. Signs of blood loss such as tachycardia and hypotension may not appear until the patient loses nearly 30% of blood volume. The fetus may be experiencing hypoperfusion long before the mother manifests any signs, so early and rapid fluid resuscitation should be administered even in a pregnant patient who is normotensive.

In cases of trauma in which there is isolated extremity injury, imaging with plain x-rays can be safely performed with abdominal shielding. Diagnosis of musculoskeletal trauma should not be delayed because of pregnancy.

Finally, for pregnant patients in minor motor vehicle accidents, clearance of major musculoskeletal injuries should be performed in the same manner as for a nonpregnant patient. Following clearance, it is recommended that all patients beyond 23 weeks' gestation be evaluated in the delivery room for fetal and maternal assessment over the next 4 to 24 hours depending on the severity of the motor vehicle accident because of the risk for placental abruption. Before 23 weeks' gestation, an ultrasound or Doppler auscultation of the fetal heart can be performed in the emergency department by an obstetrician. If the motor vehicle accident is minor, this evaluation should suffice, and the patient can be discharged to follow-up with her obstetrician as an outpatient. For puncture wounds where tetanus may be a concern, vaccination with a tetanus booster is safe throughout pregnancy.

## MEDICATIONS FOR USE IN PREGNANT PATIENTS WITH MUSCULOSKELETAL COMPLAINTS

Nonsteroidal anti-inflammatory drugs (NSAIDs) are the mainstay therapy for many musculoskeletal complaints; however, use of this class of drugs generally should be avoided in pregnancy because of the negative effect on the fetal kidneys leading to decreased fetal urine production and decreased amniotic fluid. In addition, NSAIDs are thought to increase the risk for premature closure of the ductus arteriosus, especially if used for a prolonged period beyond 32 weeks' gestation. We recommend using acetaminophen for minor pain and narcotics for more severe pain. Narcotics are safe in pregnancy because they are not associated with any specific embryopathy or other fetal effects when administered at normal doses for use in the short-term; there is a risk for developing tolerance and increasing the risk of neonatal withdrawal. The use of oral steroids such as prednisone and methylprednisolone is safe in pregnancy because steroids do not cross the placenta in any appreciable amount. Similarly, pain control after orthopedic surgery in pregnant patients can be safely managed with epidural or intravenous patient-controlled anesthesia with no significant effects on the fetus. Local anesthetic blocks for various procedures are also safe and effective in pregnant patients.

## References

1. American College of Obstetricians and Gynecologists: Nonobstetric surgery in pregnancy. ACOG Committee Opinion No. 284, Washington, DC, 2003, ACOG.
2. American College of Obstetricians and Gynecologists: Obstetric aspects of trauma management. ACOG Educational Bulletin No. 251, Washington, DC, 1998, ACOG.
3. American College of Obstetricians and Gynecologists: Critical care in pregnancy. ACOG Practice Bulletin No. 100, Washington, DC, 2009, ACOG.
4. American College of Obstetricians and Gynecologists: Patient safety in the surgical environment. ACOG Committee Opinion No. 328, Washington, DC, 2006, ACOG.
5. Crombleholme W, Sweet RL. Female genital trauma. In McAninch JW, editor: Blaisdell & Trunkey Trauma Management, Volume II, Urogenital Trauma, pp 108–121.
6. American College of Obstetricians and Gynecologists: Guidelines for diagnostic imaging during pregnancy. ACOG Committee Opinion No. 299, Washington, DC, 2004, ACOG.
7. Gray JE: Safety (risk) of diagnostic radiology exposures. In American College of Radiology. Radiation Risk: A Primer, Reston, VA, 1996, American College of Radiology, pp 15–27.
8. Brent RL: The effect of embryonic and fetal exposure to x-ray, microwaves, and ultrasound: counseling the pregnant and nonpregnant patient about these risks. Semin Oncol 16:347–368, 1989.
9. Cunningham FG: General considerations and maternal evaluation. In Williams Obstestrics, ed 21, New York, 2001, McGraw-Hill, pp 1143–1158.
10. Yamazaki JN, Schull WJ: Perinatal loss and neurologic abnormalities among children of the atomic bomb. Nagaski and Hiroshima revisited, 1949 to 1989. JAMA 264:622–623, 1990.
11. Early diagnosis of pregnancy: a symposium. J Reprod Med 26(Suppl 4):149–178, 1981.
12. Chen MM, Coakely FV, Kaimal A, et al: Guidelines for computed tomography and magnetic resonance imaging use during pregnancy and lactation. Obstet Gynecol 112:333–340, 2008.
13. Clements H, Duncan KR, Fielding K, et al: Infants exposed to MRI in utero have a normal pediatric assessment at 9 month of age. Br J Radiol 73:190–194, 2000.
14. Kok RD, de Vries MM, Heerschap A, et al: Absence of harmful effects of magnetic resonance exposure at 1.5T in utero during third trimester of pregnancy: a follow-up study. Magn Reson Imaging 22:851–854, 2004.
15. Heinrichs EL, Fong P, Flannery M, et al: Midgestational exposure of pregnant BALB/c mice to magnetic resonance imaging conditions. Magn Reson Imaging 6:305–313, 1988.
16. Kanal E, Barkovich AJ, Bell C, et al: ACR guidance document for safe MR practices. AJR Am J Roentgenol 188:1447–1474, 2007.
17. Glover P, Hykin J, Gowland P, et al: An assessment of the intrauterine sound intensity level during obstetric echo-planar magnetic resonance imaging. Br J Radiol 68:1090–1094, 1995.
18. Lamont RF: The contemporary use of beta-agonists. Br J Obstet Gynaecol 100:890–892, 1993.
19. Lamont RF, Khan KS, Beattie B, et al: The quality of nifedipine studies used to assess tocolytic efficacy: a systematic review. J Perinat Med 33:287–295, 2005.

# PART II
# Specific Anatomic Regions

## SECTION ONE
## Spine and Upper Extremity

*Spine*
*Shoulder*
*Elbow and Distal Humerus*
*Wrist and Forearm*
*Hand and Digits*

## Chapter 8 *Spine*

Richard Kamin, Paul A. Anderson, Mitchell B. Harris, Jaehon M. Kim, Michael J. Finn, Erin Maslowski, Mark A. Harrast, and Stanley A. Herring

---

**INITIAL EMERGENCY DEPARTMENT TREATMENT**
**PHYSICAL EXAMINATION**
**DIAGNOSTIC IMAGING**
**CERVICAL SPINE**

**THORACIC SPINE**
**LUMBAR SPINE**
**LOW BACK PAIN**
**SPINAL CORD INJURY**

---

Approximately 30% of patients with polytrauma in the United States have a spine injury documented during their evaluation,[1] of which about 13%, or 4% of all polytrauma victims, have spine injuries that require surgical stabilization.[2,3] Spinal cord injury affects approximately 12,000 of these patients a year and is associated with an estimated yearly societal cost of $9.7 billion (in 1998 dollars).[4,5] Although injuries to the thoracolumbar spine outnumber cervical injuries approximately 4 : 1,[6] most spinal cord injuries occur at the cervical level.[4]

## INITIAL EMERGENCY DEPARTMENT TREATMENT

The emergency department evaluation of a patient with concern for injury should include a thorough examination taking into consideration the importance of looking for other injuries (e.g., head, thoracic, abdominal, extremity) and the potential for issues that may have caused the trauma (e.g., hypoglycemia, syncope, seizure) while initiating or maintaining spinal immobilization until the patient can be cleared of spinal cord injury. Initial patient evaluation and trauma management are discussed further in Chapters 1 and 5 respectively. Spinal immobilization should be removed as soon as possible owing to its clear and proven complications. (See discussion of cervical spine clearance later.) Advanced trauma life support and advanced cardiac life support guidelines may provide a good foundation for the evaluation that the patient needs to undergo.

Airway management in a patient with suspected cervical spine injury is fraught with complications, and the importance of minimizing movement while managing the airway must be kept in mind.

## PHYSICAL EXAMINATION

The physical examination should be thorough and include evaluation for other injuries while taking into consideration key points that would be helpful in the patient with a spine injury. In a patient with a spine injury, the level of neurologic injury is best evaluated by a focused motor and sensory examination.

- Motor
  - C3-5—diaphragmatic movement
  - C5—elbow flexion
  - C6—wrist extension
  - C7—wrist flexion
  - C8—finger flexion
  - T1—finger abduction
  - L1-2—hip abduction
  - L3—knee extension
  - L4—ankle dorsiflexion
  - L5—great toe extension
  - S1—great toe flexion, ankle plantar flexion
- Sensory (Fig. 8-1)
  - Injury recording tool (Fig. 8-2)

Spinal cord syndromes are patterns of injuries with associated neurologic findings that are helpful in categorizing spinal cord injuries.

- Cord Syndromes
  - Central cord syndrome
  Central cord syndrome is characterized by motor and sensory impairment in the arms and hands greater than the legs resulting from an injury to the central part of the cervical spinal cord. This syndrome is commonly seen in hyperextension injuries in patients without obvious injuries.
  - Anterior cord syndrome
  Anterior cord syndrome is characterized by loss of motor function and pain and temperature sensation with preservation of fine touch and proprioceptive function below the level of the lesion. This syndrome is often caused by occlusion of the anterior spinal artery.
  - Brown-Séquard syndrome
  Brown-Séquard syndrome is characterized by unilateral loss of motor function, touch, and vibration with contralateral loss of pain and temperature sensation secondary to spinal cord hemisection.
  - SCIWORA
  Spinal cord injury without radiographic abnormality (SCIWORA) is seen in children who may have

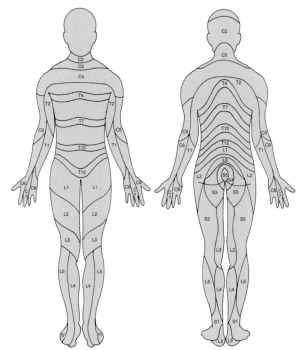

**FIGURE 8-1.** Sensory dermatome chart. C4 includes the upper chest just superior to T2. *(From Browner BD, Jupiter JB, Levine AM, et al, editors: Skeletal trauma: basic science, management, and reconstruction, ed 4, Philadelphia, 2008, Saunders.)*

complete quadriplegia secondary to greater plastic deformation of the spine than tolerated by the neural tissues. SCIWORA can manifest hours after the initial injury.

- Neurogenic shock
  Neurogenic shock syndrome comprising hypotension, bradycardia, and absence of reflexes can manifest in patients with complete or incomplete spinal cord injuries above T6 resulting from a loss of sympathetic tone in the face of maintained vagal tone when the spinal cord is injured. Neurogenic shock should be recognized and treated aggressively with fluid resuscitation and vasopressors.

## DIAGNOSTIC IMAGING

- Plain Radiographs
  The sensitivity of radiographs for identifying cervical spine injury has been estimated at 50% to 80%.[7] Inadequate visualization at the occipitocervical and cervicothoracic junctions is a major limitation of plain x-rays. Although computed tomography (CT) has generally replaced plain radiographs for cervical spine clearance in cases of high-risk patients, plain radiographs can still play an important role in cooperative, neurologically normal patients with minor trauma and a benign cervical spine examination who cannot be cleared clinically. The patient's body habitus and ability to cooperate with the technique needed to get the films should also be taken into consideration.
  The typical set of cervical spine films includes anteroposterior, lateral, and odontoid views. The lateral

view offers the most in regard to injury detection.[8] Disruption of anatomic lines and symmetric joint spaces provides clues to fractures and instability.
  Oblique and swimmer's views improve sensitivity only slightly and generally are not recommended. Flexion and extension views can identify dynamic instability; however, the efficacy, utility, and cost-effectiveness of flexion and extension films in the acute setting has been challenged.[9]

- CT
  Multidetector CT scanning has generally replaced plain radiographs for detecting spine injuries in certain populations. In many trauma centers, CT is the study of choice for patients at moderate to high risk of spine injury; this is especially the case if patients are being scanned to assess for other injuries, which significantly improves cost-effectiveness.[10] More recent studies support the use of CT, which identifies 99.3% of all cervical spine fractures. The missed injuries are typically minor and require minimal to no treatment.[11] However, soft tissue injuries, mainly ligamentous in nature, are poorly detected by CT scan with a negative predictive value of 78%.[7] In a small percentage of patients, ligamentous injuries are significant enough to require surgical intervention and prolonged immobilization.

- Magnetic Resonance Imaging (MRI)
  The indications for acute MRI in the setting of suspicion of acute spine trauma are still being defined. Generally, patients with neurologic or cognitive deficits (i.e., obtunded patients) may undergo MRI, especially in cases where cervical collar clearance or operative stabilization is paramount.[12] However, these are typically patients for whom there is significant difficulty in obtaining MRI because of mechanical ventilation, risk of leaving the intensive care environment, and the need for nursing staff to accompany the patient.[13] Controversy persists regarding the use of multidetector CT only versus additional MRI for cervical spine assessment.[13-16] Based on a meta-analysis yielding 1550 patients with negative multidetector CT, the management of 6% was altered based on the MRI results, and 1% required surgical stabilization.[14]

- CT Angiography and CT Myelography
  There is currently little to support the use of CT angiography or myelography in the emergent evaluation of a patient with suspected spine injury.

- Points to Consider
  - A plain lateral x-ray should be considered in patients with clinically obvious spinal cord injuries so that rapid reduction might be performed if indicated.
  - Most patients who cannot be cleared clinically should have either three-view cervical spine radiographs or cervical CT.
  - If a patient is having CT for another reason, it is often more efficient management to include a cervical CT scan. If possible, scanning down to T4 can ease evaluation of the cervical thoracic junction, a region that is difficult to image with plain radiography, especially in large patients.
  - CT has significantly better sensitivity (>99%) than plain radiographs (55% to 75%) but has 100 times greater radiation dose and an increased risk of cancer.[17]

Patient Name _____

Examiner Name _____ Date/Time of Exam_____

**ASIA**
AMERICAN SPINAL INJURY ASSOCIATION

## STANDARD NEUROLOGICAL CLASSIFICATION OF SPINAL CORD INJURY

**ISC●S**

### MOTOR
KEY MUSCLES
(scoring on reverse side)

| | R | L | |
|---|---|---|---|
| C5 | | | Elbow flexors |
| C6 | | | Wrist extensors |
| C7 | | | Elbow extensors |
| C8 | | | Finger flexors (distal phalanx of middle finger) |
| T1 | | | Finger abductors (little finger) |

UPPER LIMB TOTAL (MAXIMUM)  ☐ + ☐ = ☐
(25)  (25)  (50)

Comments:

| | R | L | |
|---|---|---|---|
| L2 | | | Hip flexors |
| L3 | | | Knee extensors |
| L4 | | | Ankle dorsiflexors |
| L5 | | | Long toe extensors |
| S1 | | | Ankle plantar flexors |

Voluntary anal contraction
(Yes/No) ☐

LOWER LIMB TOTAL (MAXIMUM)  ☐ + ☐ = ☐
(25)  (25)  (50)

### SENSORY
KEY SENSORY POINTS

LIGHT TOUCH    PIN PRICK
R  L          R  L

0 = absent
1 = impaired
2 = normal
NT = not testable

C2, C3, C4, C5, C6, C7, C8, T1, T2, T3, T4, T5, T6, T7, T8, T9, T10, T11, T12, L1, L2, L3, L4, L5, S1, S2, S3, S4-5

Any anal sensation (Yes/No) ☐

TOTALS { ☐ + ☐ = ☐ = ☐
(MAXIMUM) (56) (56)  (56) (56)

☐ + ☐ = ☐ **PIN PRICK SCORE** (max: 112)
= ☐ **LIGHT TOUCH SCORE** (max: 112)

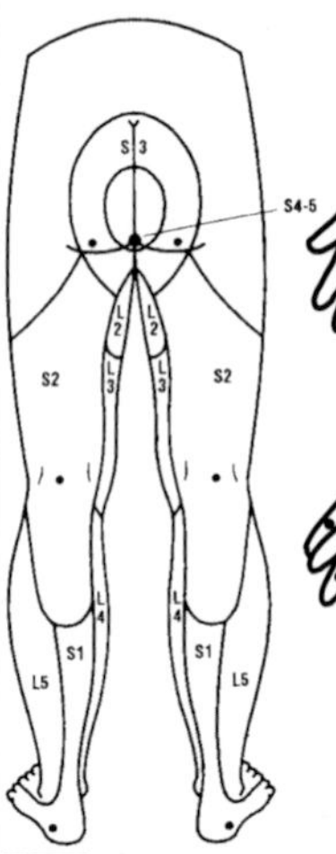

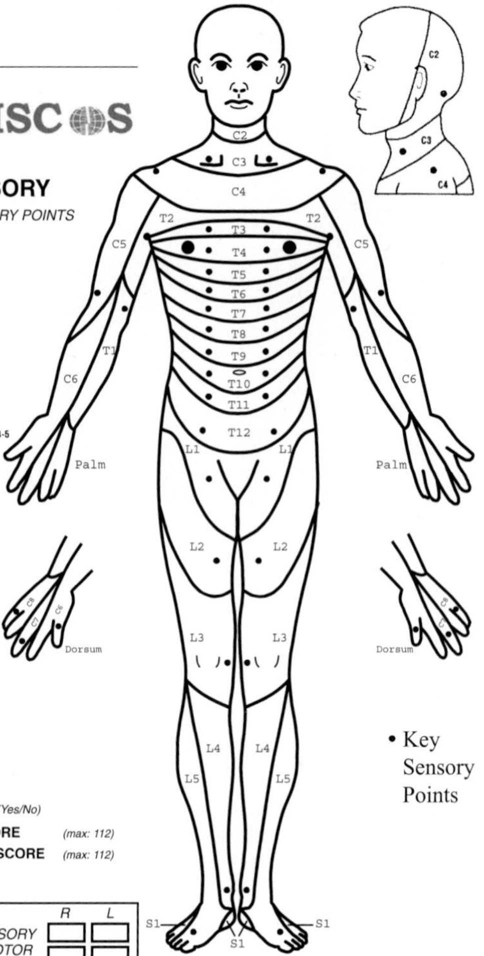

● Key Sensory Points

| NEUROLOGICAL LEVEL | | R | L | | COMPLETE OR INCOMPLETE? ☐ | ZONE OF PARTIAL PRESERVATION | | R | L |
|---|---|---|---|---|---|---|---|---|---|
| The most caudal segment with normal function | SENSORY | ☐ | ☐ | | Incomplete = Any sensory or motor function in S4-S5 | Caudal extent of partially innervated segments | SENSORY | ☐ | ☐ |
| | MOTOR | ☐ | ☐ | | **ASIA IMPAIRMENT SCALE** ☐ | | MOTOR | ☐ | ☐ |

This form may be copied freely but should not be altered without permission from the American Spinal Injury Association.

REV 03/06

### MUSCLE GRADING

0   total paralysis

1   palpable or visible contraction

2   active movement, full range of motion, gravity eliminated

3   active movement, full range of motion, against gravity

4   active movement, full range of motion, against gravity and provides some resistance

5   active movement, full range of motion, against gravity and provides normal resistance

5*  muscle able to exert, in examiner's judgement, sufficient resistance to be considered normal if identifiable inhibiting factors were not present

NT not testable. Patient unable to reliably exert effort or muscle unavailable for testing due to factors such as immobilization, pain on effort or contracture.

### ASIA IMPAIRMENT SCALE

☐ A = Complete : No motor or sensory function is preserved in the sacral segments S4-S5.

☐ B = Incomplete: Sensory but not motor function is preserved below the neurological level and includes the sacral segments S4-S5.

☐ C = Incomplete: Motor function is preserved below the neurological level, and more than half of key muscles below the neurological level have a muscle grade less than 3.

☐ D = Incomplete: Motor function is preserved below the neurological level, and at least half of key muscles below the neurological level have a muscle grade of 3 or more.

☐ E = Normal: Motor and sensory function are normal.

### CLINICAL SYNDROMES
(OPTIONAL)

☐ Central Cord
☐ Brown-Sequard
☐ Anterior Cord
☐ Conus Medullaris
☐ Cauda Equina

### STEPS IN CLASSIFICATION

The following order is recommended in determining the classification of individuals with SCI.

1. Determine sensory levels for right and left sides.

2. Determine motor levels for right and left sides.
   *Note: in regions where there is no myotome to test, the motor level is presumed to be the same as the sensory level.*

3. Determine the single neurological level.
   *This is the lowest segment where motor and sensory function is normal on both sides, and is the most cephalad of the sensory and motor levels determined in steps 1 and 2.*

4. Determine whether the injury is Complete or Incomplete (sacral sparing).
   *If voluntary anal contraction = **No** AND all S4-5 sensory scores = 0 AND any anal sensation = **No**, then injury is COMPLETE. Otherwise injury is incomplete.*

5. Determine ASIA Impairment Scale (AIS) Grade:
   **Is injury Complete?**  If **YES**, AIS=A Record ZPP
   NO ↓  (For ZPP record lowest dermatome or myotome on each side with some [non-zero score] preservation.)

   **Is injury motor incomplete?**  If **NO**, AIS=B
   YES ↓  (Yes=voluntary anal contraction OR motor function more than three levels below the motor level on a given side.)

   **Are at least half of the key muscles below the (single) neurological level graded 3 or better?**
   NO ↓            YES ↓
   AIS=C          AIS=D

   **If sensation and motor function is normal in all segments, AIS=E**
   *Note: AIS E is used in follow up testing when an individual with a documented SCI has recovered normal function. If at initial testing no deficits are found, the individual is neurologically intact; the ASIA Impairment Scale does not apply.*

**FIGURE 8-2.** Injury recording tool. (*Courtesy American Spinal Injury Association, Atlanta, GA.*)

PART II Specific Anatomic Regions

- MRI is not routinely indicated in the evaluation of trauma.[18]

  MRI is indicated in the initial evaluation of suspected or known spine injury in patients with unexplained neurologic deficits, in patients with progressive deterioration, in patients before reduction who are have facet dislocations but are neurologically intact, and in patients for preoperative evaluation.

  MRI should be performed to answer specific questions left unanswered by CT and in the evaluation of a neurologic deficit or when it is considered essential by a consulting expert in formulating a disposition for the patient.

## CERVICAL SPINE

- Anatomy

  The cervical spine is composed of seven vertebrae. The anatomic arrangement of the cervical spine allows for a high degree of mobility in flexion, extension, and rotation. There is significant lateral mobility as well. The high degree of mobility coupled with the burden of supporting the weight of the head leaves the cervical spine vulnerable to injuries. Because spinal cord injuries at the level of the cervical vertebrae are devastating, the stability of the bones and ligaments of the cervical spine is probably the most important in the body.

- History and Mechanism of Injury for Cervical Spine Injuries
  - Significant spine injuries typically involve high-energy trauma.
  - The most common mechanism of injury is motor vehicle accidents followed by falls, violence, and sporting injuries.[19]
  - Detailed information regarding the mechanism of injury is important and should be sought out by the providing physicians.
  - Specifics, such as the height of the fall or the speed of the collision, provide important clues to amount of force involved and the level of suspicion the clinician should have for a spine injury.
  - Intuitively, the speed and magnitude of the impact correlate with the probability of having an injury.[20,21]

- Flexion (http://emedicine.medscape.com/article/824380-overview#aw2aab6b2b3)
  - Simple wedge compression fracture without posterior disruption: Posterior column remains intact—generally a stable fracture (Figure 8-3)
  - Flexion teardrop fracture: Disruption of all three columns—extremely unstable fracture
  - Anterior subluxation: No bony injury but significant displacement can occur with flexion—potentially unstable
  - Bilateral facet dislocation: Extreme form of anterior subluxation—extremely unstable
  - Clay shoveler fracture: Oblique fracture of the base of the spinous process—stable
  - Anterior atlantoaxial dislocation: Unstable

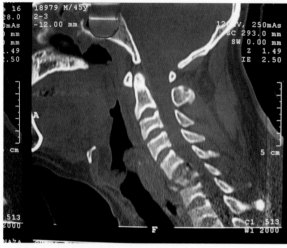

**FIGURE 8-3.** Image showing an injury, which has both bony and ligamentous instability and high risk for spinal cord injury.

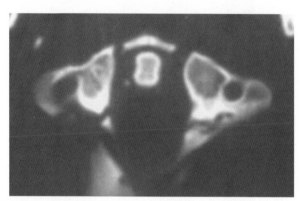

**FIGURE 8-4.** CT scan of a Jefferson burst fracture. Axial image through C1 level shows a five-part fracture of the C1 ring. Fractures are minimally displaced, making plain radiographic diagnosis more difficult. *(From Browner BD, Jupiter JB, Levine AM, et al, editors: Skeletal trauma: basic science, management, and reconstruction, ed 4, Philadelphia, 2008, Saunders.)*

- Flexion-rotation (http://emedicine.medscape.com/article/824380-overview#aw2aab6b2b4)
  - Unilateral facet dislocation: Posterior ligament is disrupted but vertebrae are locked in place—stable
  - Rotary atlantoaxial dislocation: Unstable because of location
- Extension (http://emedicine.medscape.com/article/824380-overview#aw2aab6b2b5)
  - Hangman's fracture: Bilateral fractures through the pedicles of C2—unstable
  - Extension teardrop fracture: Displaced anteroinferior bony fragment—unstable
  - Fracture of the posterior arch of C1: Stable but must be distinguished from Jefferson fracture
  - Posterior atlantoaxial dislocation: Unstable
- Axial Compression (http://emedicine.medscape.com/article/824380-overview#aw2aab6b2b6)
  - Jefferson fracture: Burst fracture of the ring of C1 (Figs. 8-4 and 8-5)—unstable
  - Burst fracture (Fig. 8-6): Disruption of the anterior and middle columns—may be unstable
  - Atlas fracture: Unstable because of location

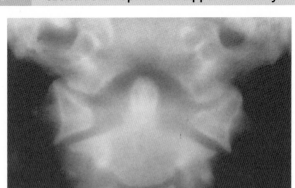

**FIGURE 8-5.** Burst-type, true Jefferson fracture. Anteroposterior tomogram shows splaying of the lateral mass of C1. *(From Levine AM, Edwards CC: Treatment of injuries in the C1-C2 complex. Orthop Clin North Am 17:31-44, 1986.)*

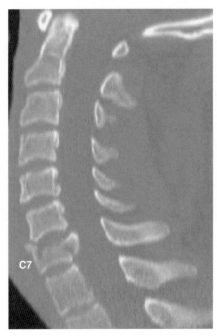

**FIGURE 8-6.** Blunt cervical trauma in this 35-year-old man sustained a C7 compressive flexion injury (burst fracture). *(From Browner BD, Jupiter JB, Levine AM, et al, editors: Skeletal trauma: basic science, management, and reconstruction, ed 4, Philadelphia, 2008, Saunders.)*

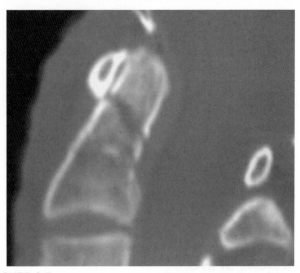

**FIGURE 8-7.** Subtle type II odontoid fracture. Sagittal CT reformation depicts the horizontal fracture plane at the base of the odontoid process. *(From Browner BD, Jupiter JB, Levine AM, et al, editors: Skeletal trauma: basic science, management, and reconstruction, ed 4, Philadelphia, 2008, Saunders.)*

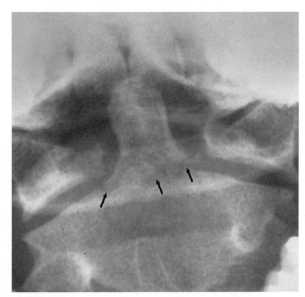

**FIGURE 8-8.** Odontoid fracture with tilt. Open-mouth odontoid view shows a fracture across the base of the odontoid *(arrows)* and lateral tilting of the odontoid process. *(From Browner BD, Jupiter JB, Levine AM, et al, editors: Skeletal trauma: basic science, management, and reconstruction, ed 4, Philadelphia, 2008, Saunders.)*

■ Complex or Multiple Mechanisms (http://emedicine.
  medscape.com/article/824380-overview#aw2aab
  6b2b7)
  ● Odontoid fracture

  Type I: Avulsion of the tip of the dens at the insertion
    site of the alar ligament—mechanically stable but
    can be associated with atlanto-occipital dislocation

  Type II: Base of the dens and most common odontoid
    fractures—unstable (Fig. 8-7)

  Type III: Fracture line into the body of the axis—
    unstable (Fig. 8-8)

  ● Transverse process fracture
  ● Complex fracture or fracture-dislocation (Figs. 8-9
    and 8-10)

■ When to Consult a Specialist
  Consultation is not needed for a patient without radiographic abnormality and a normal neurologic examination.

  Telephone consultation is appropriate for patients with stable injuries seen on radiographic study and a normal neurologic examination.
  ● Isolated single spinous process fractures
  ● Small, minimally displaced avulsion fractures
  ● Compression fractures with minimal height loss
  In-person consultation is indicated for all unstable injures or injuries with associated neurologic deficit.

**TABLE 8-1** Use of Steroids for Spinal Cord Injury

| | Indications | Contraindications | Recommendation | Controversies |
|---|---|---|---|---|
| NASCIS 2[39] | Closed spinal cord injury presenting <8 hr after injury | Nerve root or cauda equina injury only | 30 mg/kg methylprednisolone bolus followed by 5.4 mg/kg maintenance dose over next 23 hr | Significant methodologic flaws |
| | | Gunshot wounds | | Benefit realized in post hoc analysis only |
| | | Life-threatening morbidity | | Effect size small with questionable functional importance |
| | | Pregnant | | Concern for negative effect on wound healing and sepsis |
| | | >8 hr from injury | | |
| NASCIS 3[40] | Closed spinal cord injury presenting <3 hr and between 3 and 8 hr after injury | Nerve root or cauda equina injury only | 30 mg/kg methylprednisolone bolus in all patients | Significant methodologic flaws |
| | | Gunshot wounds | 5.4 mg/kg/hr over next 23 hr if <3 hr from injury | Effect size small with questionable functional importance |
| | | Life-threatening morbidity | 5.4 mg/kg/hr over 47 hr if presenting from 3-8 hr | Increased incidence of pneumonia and sepsis |
| | | Pregnant | | |
| | | >8 hr from injury | | |
| Authors' recommendation | Closed spinal cord injury <8 hr after time of injury | As above | Methylprednisolone can be considered in healthy patients with isolated spinal cord injury | |
| | | Significant medical comorbidities | | |
| | | Evidence of lung injury or pneumonia | | |
| | | Multisystem traumatic injury | | |

Motor vehicle collision with high speed (>100 km/hr or 60 mph), rollover, or ejection

Motorized recreational vehicles

Bicycle collision

• Low-risk mechanisms

Fall from standing

Simple rear-end motor vehicle collision

Assault with minimal head and neck trauma

Many institutions incorporate both sets of clinical guidelines, and physicians can be assured that cervical spine clearance predominantly by a clinical examination is safe, effective, and supported by multiple studies.

For patients who cannot be cleared clinically, further evaluation and imaging of some form are the next steps to rule in or rule out injury.

■ Steroids for Spinal Cord injury

The use of steroids has been called into question more recently because the supporting data show marginal benefit of questionable clinical significance, and their use is associated with a greater incidence of complications, including pulmonary embolism, myopathy, stress ulcers, infections,[22,23] and pneumonia.[24-26]

There is no mandate on the use of a steroid protocol, and use should be based on institutional protocol and the direction of the consulting spine surgeon.

The use of steroids has been recommended in patients who present within 8 hours of injury at an initial bolus of 30 mg/kg given over 15 minutes followed by a 10-20 mL of 1% lidocaine drip administered over the next 23 hours (Table 8-1). Steroids should not be administered more than 8 hours after injury.

■ **Sports-Related Injuries**

In the United States, 10% of all spinal cord injuries occur in sporting endeavors,[30] and most such injuries occur in the cervical spine.

The National Center for Catastrophic Sports Injury Research (NCCSIR) found that the four sports with the highest risk of head and spine injury per 100,000 participants are football, gymnastics, ice hockey, and wrestling.

Although there is no statistically significant difference between the four activities on an incidence per 100,000 basis, the absolute number of injuries is highest in football because 1,800,000 youths play football annually, whereas less than 100,000 participate in each of the other sports.[31]

Although flexion and axial loading forces are associated with most injuries, extension, lateral stretch, and congenital instability have also been implicated.[32]

Immobilization should begin at the time of injury and continue throughout transport and emergency department stabilization and terminate only when cervical spinal cord injury has been either ruled out radiographically or definitively stabilized.[32]

To maintain the airway optimally, the facemask must be removed as quickly as possible any time a player is suspected to have a spinal injury, even if the patient is still conscious (Fig. 8-13).[33]

It is recommended to be prepared for the option of a combined approach to facemask removal, using a cordless screwdriver with a cutting tool (the Trainer's Angel) to capture the time efficiency benefits of the screw driver while offering a contingency for screw removal failure (Fig. 8-14).[34,35]

It is recommended that the helmet (with the facemask removed) and shoulder pads remain in place during the initial clinical and radiographic assessment in the emergency department.[33] When the helmet and shoulder pads are worn together, the spine remains in a relatively neutral position.

To remove the helmet, the cheek pads must be removed and the air padding deflated.[32] The chin strap should stay in place until the helmet is ready to be removed.[7] At the appropriate time, the helmet should be removed by at least two people (Fig. 8-15).[32]

In most cases, shoulder pads can be opened from the front to allow access to the chest for auscultation of breath and heart sounds. The removal of the helmet and shoulder pads is summarized in Boxes 8-1 through 8-3.

CT has been shown to be adequate for initial diagnosis and triage in helmeted athletes.[32]

Toler et al.[36] found that inserting a pocket mask between the chin and facemask (called pocket mask insertion technique) gained an adequate seal for a modified jaw thrust and rescue breathing through the bars of the still-affixed facemask. These investigators found that this technique gained quicker access than removal of the facemask by cordless screwdriver or a quick-release mechanism. However, Toler et al.[36] recommended that in athletes with presumed spinal cord injury without respiratory compromise, the

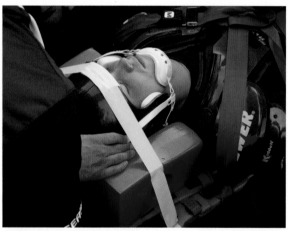

**FIGURE 8-13.** A helmeted athlete with a suspected cervical spine injury arrives in the emergency department with the helmet and shoulder pads still in place on a spine board.

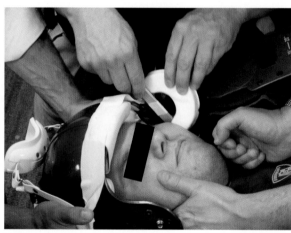

**FIGURE 8-15.** Ear pad removal with a tongue depressor in the emergency department. Note attention to continued cervical spine stabilization.

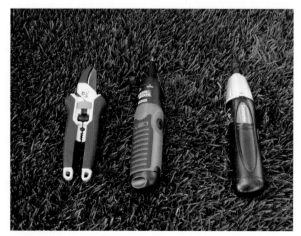

**FIGURE 8-14.** Tool options for facemask removal include a standard cutting tool and two different cordless power screwdrivers.

**Box 8-1 Guidelines for Helmet Removal If Facemask Cannot Be Removed to Gain Access to Airway**

- If design of the helmet and chin strap is such that even after removal of the facemask, the airway cannot be controlled or ventilation provided
- If the helmet and chin straps do not hold the head securely such that immobilization of the helmet does not guarantee immobilization of the head
- If the helmet prevents immobilization for transport in an appropriate position

Adapted from Kleiner DM, Almquist JL: Prehospital care of the spine-injured athlete: a document from the inter-association task force for appropriate care of the spine-injured athlete, Dallas, 2001, National Athletic Trainers' Association.

- When to Consult a Specialist
  Consultation is indicated for patients with open fractures, impending open fractures, floating shoulder injuries, neurovascular compromise, multiple trauma, and scapulothoracic dissociation.
- How and What to Communicate With Specialist
  Information pertaining to an open or closed fracture includes open injury over the fracture site, dimpling of the skin, and tenting or blanching of the skin.
  X-ray description includes amount of displacement, amount of shortening, and whether the fracture is simple or comminuted.
  Important neurovascular findings include strong or feeble pulses and nerve deficit.
  Patient identifying information includes sex and hand dominance.
- Analgesia, Anesthesia Block, and Sedation
  The patient require narcotic pain medications and NSAIDs to control pain in the emergency department.
  If reduction is necessary, the patient usually requires conscious sedation.
- Reduce or Accept Alignment
  Reduction of clavicle fracture is usually not attempted in the emergency department.
- Splint or Immobilize
  Immobilize nondisplaced fractures in a sling.
  Immobilize displaced fractures in a sling or figure-of-eight brace.
- Postreduction Imaging
  X-rays are indicated after reduction only if an attempt at reduction was made.
- Plan for Follow-up Care
  The patient should see an orthopedist for a follow-up examination in 5 to 7 days.
- Outpatient Pain Relief Options
  A short course of NSAIDs and narcotic analgesics may be prescribed until follow-up.
  The patient should apply ice for 48 to 72 hours.

## ACROMIOCLAVICULAR JOINT INJURIES

### *Anatomic Considerations*

The articulation of the acromion and the distal clavicle represents a diarthrodial joint with four planes of motion: anterior/posterior and superior/inferior. The acromioclavicular joint is surrounded by a capsule, has intra-articular synovium, and has an articular cartilage interface. Stability at the acromioclavicular joint is achieved through a combination of both static and dynamic stabilizers. There are four acromioclavicular ligaments: superior, inferior, anterior, and posterior.

### *Classification*

*Type I:* Acromioclavicular ligament sprain with the acromioclavicular joint intact

*Type II:* Acromioclavicular ligament tear, coracoclavicular ligament intact, and acromioclavicular joint subluxed

*Type III:* Acromioclavicular and coracoclavicular ligaments torn and 100% dislocation in joint

*Type IV:* Complete dislocation with posterior displacement of distal clavicle into or through the trapezius muscle

*Type V:* Exaggerated superior dislocation of between 100% and 300% dislocation of the joint increasing the coracoclavicular ligament distance two to three times including disruption of the deltotrapezial fascia

*Type VI:* Complete dislocation with inferior displacement of distal clavicle into a subacromial or subcoracoid position

### *Differential Diagnosis of Traumatic Complaints*

- History
  - Onset of pain or symptoms
  - Location of pain or symptoms
  - Radiation of pain or symptoms
  - Numbness or tingling
  - Loss of function
  - Character of pain (e.g., sharp, dull, ache, burn)
  - Duration of pain or symptoms
  - Intensity of pain (scale 1-10)
  - Exacerbation or remission of pain or symptoms
- Mechanism of Injury
  Direct injury occurs when a person falls onto the acromioclavicular joint with the arm at the side in an adducted position, as is commonly seen in collision sports such as hockey, football, rugby, and karate.
  Indirect injury to the acromioclavicular joint occurs as the result of a fall on an outstretched hand; the fall typically drives the humeral head superiorly into the acromion.
- Timing
  - Acute onset of symptoms related to an injury
  - Symptoms related to acute or specific event
- Pain
  - Pain localized to the anterior shoulder over the acromioclavicular joint
- Dysfunction
  - Patients have discomfort with movement of shoulder
- Physical Examination—Standard Focus Examination
  Examination of a patient with a suspected acromioclavicular injury should be done with the patient standing or sitting, which allows the weight of the arm to stress the acromioclavicular joint and exaggerate any deformity.
  Assess integrity of the skin to rule out an open injury.
  Palpate the acromioclavicular joint and lateral clavicle.
  Palpate mobility of the acromion relative to the lateral clavicle, and check for instability in the vertical and horizontal planes.
  Assess the patient's ability to perform passive and active range of motion of the shoulder.
  Palpate the radial pulse.

Test for sensation in the distribution of axillary, radial, median, and ulnar nerves.

Test for motor function of the anterior interosseous nerve (flexor pollicis longus), posterior interosseous nerve (extensor pollicis longus), and ulnar nerve (interossei).

Examine the entire upper extremity including the clavicle, shoulder, humerus, elbow, forearm, wrist, and hand.

If a patient has more pain than is expected for a simple acromioclavicular joint injury, there should be high suspicion for a coronoid fracture displacement of the clavicle through the trapezial fascia.

■ Diagnostic Testing
Imaging techniques include x-ray, CT, and MRI.

The Zanca view is the most accurate view to visualize the acromioclavicular joint; this view is achieved by tilting the x-ray beam 10 to 15 degrees cephalad and using one half of the standard penetrance (Fig. 9-12).

An axillary view is particularly helpful in visualizing posterior displacement of the distal clavicle.

When there is a normal coracoclavicular interspace but a complete dislocation of the acromioclavicular joint, a coracoid fracture should be suspected. The best view to visualize a suspected coracoid fracture is the Stryker notch view, which is obtained with the patient supine with the palm on the affected side placed on the head; the x-ray beam is tilted 10 degrees cephalad (Fig. 9-13).

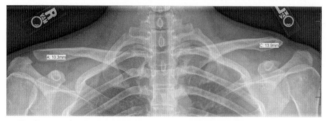

**FIGURE 9-12.** Bilateral Zanca view of the acromioclavicular joints allows for side-to-side comparison measurements.

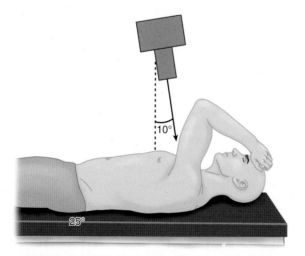

**FIGURE 9-13.** Stryker notch view to assess a suspected coracoid fracture. (*Redrawn from Normal shoulder xrays. eORIF. Available at:* www.eorif.com. *Accessed October 11, 2011.*)

## Treatment of Specific Injuries

■ How and What to Communicate With Specialist
  • Open or closed injury
  • Percent and direction of displacement
  • Neurovascular compromise
  • Patient identifying information
■ Analgesia, Anesthesia Block, and Sedation
The patient frequently requires narcotic pain medications or NSAIDs or both to control pain in the emergency department.
■ Splint or Immobilize
The patient should be immobilized in a sling.
■ Plan for Follow-up Care
The patient should see an orthopedist for a follow-up examination in 7 to 10 days.
■ Outpatient Pain Relief Options
A short course of an NSAID and an opioid analgesic should be prescribed until follow-up.
The patient should apply ice for 48 to 72 hours.
■ Subsequent Management
Type I and II injuries are treated nonsurgically.
Management of type III injuries is controversial. Some orthopedists recommend surgical repair, but most injuries are treated conservatively.
Type IV, V, and VI injuries usually require surgical repair.

## STERNOCLAVICULAR JOINT INJURIES

### Anatomic Considerations

The sternoclavicular joint is the only true joint connecting the axial skeleton to the shoulder girdle. Despite having such an important role, the sternoclavicular joint lacks inherent bony stability and relies solely on ligamentous and capsular attachments. The sternoclavicular joint articulation is held in place by the sternoclavicular capsular ligaments, the costoclavicular ligaments, and the interclavicular ligaments. A relatively large amount of motion is seen at the sternoclavicular joint. Motion at the sternoclavicular joint includes approximately 30 to 35 degrees of upward elevation, 35 degrees of translation in the anterior to posterior plane, and 50 degrees of rotation around the longitudinal axis of the clavicle.

### Differential Diagnosis of Traumatic Complaints

■ History
  • Onset of pain or symptoms
  • Location of pain or symptoms
  • Radiation of pain or symptoms
  • Numbness or tingling
  • Loss of function
  • Character of pain (e.g., sharp, dull, ache, burn)
  • Duration of pain or symptoms
  • Intensity of pain (scale 1-10)
  • Exacerbation or remission of pain or symptoms

- Dyspnea, choking, difficulty swallowing, or a tight feeling in the throat
- Venous congestion in the head or neck
■ Mechanism of Injury
Traumatic injury to the sternoclavicular joint is the most common cause of sternoclavicular joint dislocations.

Motor vehicle collisions and sports participation are the top two causes of traumatic sternoclavicular joint injury.

Posterior dislocations of the sternoclavicular joint typically occur as the result of a direct force to the anteromedial clavicle or the posterolateral shoulder causing the shoulder to roll forward.

Anterior dislocations can occur when an anterolateral force is applied to the clavicle and the shoulder is rolled backward.
■ Timing
Symptoms are usually related to an acute or specific event.
■ Pain
Pain is experienced directly over the sternoclavicular joint.

Movement of the shoulder girdle produces pain.
■ Dysfunction
Posterior dislocations can compress the esophagus, trachea, and subclavian vessels.

Patients may have dyspnea, choking, difficulty swallowing, or a tight feeling in the throat.

Compression of the subclavian vessels may lead to venous congestion in the head or neck.
■ Prehospital Care
If there are any life-threatening symptoms such as dyspnea, venous congestion in the head or neck, difficulty swallowing, or a tight feeling in the throat, the emergency medical services team should be prepared to protect the airway.
■ Physical Examination—Standard Focus Examination
Palpate the sternoclavicular joint to determine if there is a stepoff.

Assess the patient's respiratory status and upper extremity circulation to determine if there is injury or compression to the subclavian vessels, trachea, or esophagus.

Assess the integrity of the skin to rule out an open injury.

Assess the location and amount of swelling, ecchymosis, abrasions, or lacerations.

Assess the patient's ability to move the shoulder through a passive and active range of motion without pain.

Palpate the carotid and radial pulse.

Test for sensation in the distribution of axillary, radial, median, and ulnar nerves.

Test for motor function of the axillary nerve (deltoid), anterior interosseous nerve (flexor pollicis longus), posterior interosseous nerve (extensor pollicis longus), and ulnar nerve (interossei).

Examine the entire upper extremity including the clavicle, shoulder, humerus, elbow, forearm, wrist, and hand.

Patients with mild sprains present with mild to moderate pain associated with movement of the upper extremity. Instability is usually absent, but the sternoclavicular joint may be tender to palpation and slightly swollen.

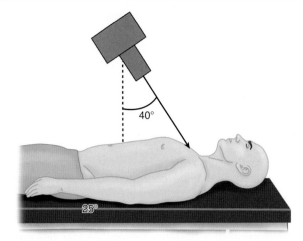

**FIGURE 9-14.** Serendipity view to assess the sternoclavicular joint. *(Redrawn from Normal shoulder xrays. eORIF. Available at: www.eorif.com. Accessed October 11, 2011.)*

Moderate sprains are associated with partial disruption of the sternoclavicular ligaments. The joint may subluxate when manually stressed, but it cannot be visibly dislocated. Patients usually have more swelling and pain than patients with mild sprains, and the sternoclavicular joint is more tender to palpation.

Severe sprains result in complete dislocation, either anterior or posterior, of the sternoclavicular joint. Patients with this injury present with severe pain that is exacerbated by any movement of the upper extremity. The ipsilateral shoulder may appear protracted compared with the contralateral uninjured shoulder. Patients often hold the affected arm across the chest in an adducted position and support it with the contralateral arm. The head may be tilted toward the side of the injured clavicle.
■ Diagnostic Testing
Imaging techniques include x-ray, CT, and MRI.

A standard anteroposterior x-ray of the chest or sternoclavicular joint may suggest an injury to the sternoclavicular joint; however, this is not the best view for visualizing the joint.

The serendipity view is a bilateral view of the sternoclavicular joints achieved by tilting the x-ray tube 40 degrees cephalad and centered on the sternum (Fig. 9-14).

A CT scan performed with the patient supine is the best modality for visualizing and assessing any sternoclavicular joint dislocation.

If a cervical spine injury is considered as part of the injury, a CT scan of the neck can be extended down to include the sternoclavicular joint.

### Treatment of Specific Injuries

■ Develop Plan
Patients with mild and moderate sternoclavicular joint sprains can be safely discharged from the emergency department with a sling for comfort.

Anterior dislocations can be reduced in the emergency department with either an articular block or sedation.

Patients with posterior dislocations need to be taken to the operating room to have surgery performed by an orthopedic surgeon. A cardiothoracic surgeon must be immediately available for rare but serious complications.

Reduction of posterior dislocations should not be attempted in the emergency department.

Patients who have concomitant injuries of the subclavian vessels, esophagus, trachea, or lung need to be appropriately managed by the emergency department physician.

■ When to Consult a Specialist
A specialist should be consulted for nonreducible or unstable anterior dislocations.

All posterior sternoclavicular dislocations require specialist consultation.

Reduction of a posterior sternoclavicular dislocation should be performed in the operating room, unless complications (tracheal compression) necessitate immediate reduction.

An orthopedist may attempt closed reduction in the emergency department with thoracic surgery backup.

■ How and What to Communicate With Specialist
- Open or closed injury
- Anterior or posterior dislocation on x-ray or CT
- Vascular compromise or neurologic deficits
- Patient identifying information

■ Analgesia, Anesthesia Block, and Sedation
The patient requires narcotic pain medications and NSAIDs to control pain in the emergency department.

If reduction is necessary, the patient usually requires conscious sedation.

■ Reduce or Accept Alignment
Anterior dislocations can be reduced closed in the emergency department. Anterior dislocations are often easy to reduce; however, they are usually unstable and dislocate when the pressure is released. However, if the sternoclavicular joint maintains reduction after closed means, the patient should be immobilized in a soft figure-of-eight brace for 6 weeks.

Position the patient supine with a rolled blanket or a sandbag between the scapulae.

The patient's arm on the affected side should be abducted 90 degrees and extended 10 degrees.

The physician applies traction to this arm in line with the clavicle.

The clavicle can be pushed back into position. If necessary, a towel clip can be used to grasp and pull the medial clavicle forward (Fig. 9-15).

■ Splint or Immobilize
The patient should be immobilized in a figure-of-eight clavicle harness or a sling.

■ Postreduction Imaging
If there is an attempt at closed reduction of a sternoclavicular joint, postreduction imaging should be performed.

■ Plan for Follow-up Care
The patient should see an orthopedist for a follow-up examination in 5 to 7 days.

■ Outpatient Pain Relief Options
A short course of NSAIDs and narcotic analgesics can be prescribed until follow-up.

The patient should apply ice for 48 to 72 hours.

## SCAPULA FRACTURES

### Anatomic Considerations

The scapula is a triangular-shaped bone with bony prominences including the coracoid process, acromion, scapular spine, and glenoid. The subscapularis muscle covers most of the anterior surface of the scapula. Posteriorly, the supraspinatus muscle covers the scapula superior to the scapular spine, and the infraspinatus and teres minor cover the scapula inferior to the scapular spine. The glenoid is the articulating surface of the scapula that articulates with the humeral head to form the shoulder joint.

### Differential Diagnosis of Traumatic Complaints

■ History
- Onset of pain or symptoms
- Location of pain or symptoms
- Radiation of pain or symptoms
- Numbness or tingling
- Loss of function
- Character of pain (e.g., sharp, dull, ache, burn)
- Duration of pain or symptoms
- Intensity of pain (scale 1-10)
- Exacerbation or remission of pain or symptoms
- Difficulty breathing

■ Mechanism of Injury
- Motor vehicle collision
- Direct blow
- Fall on outstretched arm
- High-energy blunt trauma
- Shoulder dislocation
- Traction injury to the arm

■ Timing
Symptoms are related to an acute or specific event.

■ Pain
Pain is localized to the shoulder and scapular region.

■ Dysfunction
The patient has difficulty moving the shoulder secondary to pain.

■ Physical Examination—Standard Focus Examination
Inspect the skin for an open injury, ecchymosis, and swelling.

The arm is typically held in an adducted position.

Perform a neurologic examination of the upper extremity to assess for injury.

Check pulses to rule out vascular injury (commonly the axillary artery).

Palpate the clavicle, acromion, coracoid, and spine of the scapula.

Assess active and passive range of motion of the shoulder.

Assess lungs for breath sounds to rule out hemothorax or pneumothorax.

Scapula fractures require a great deal of focused energy directed at the thorax. The emergency department physician should be vigilant to find and manage

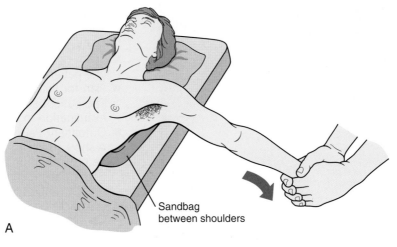

Sandbag
between shoulders

A

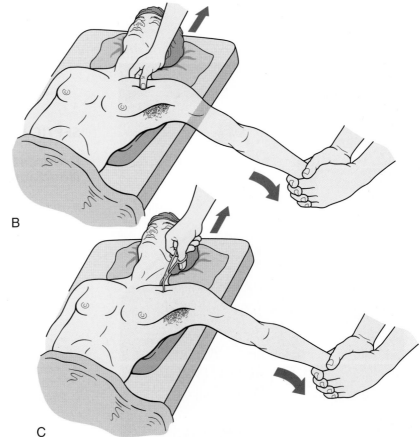

B

C

**FIGURE 9-15.** Manipulative reduction of sternoclavicular dislocation under general anesthesia. **A,** With a support placed between the scapulae, lateral traction is applied. **B,** Direct manipulation of the clavicle. Application of a towel clip **(C)** is occasionally necessary. *(From Browner BD, Levine AM, Jupiter JB, et al: Skeletal trauma, ed 4, Philadelphia, 2009, Saunders.)*

serious associated injuries, including pneumothorax, rib fractures, vertebral fractures, or great vessel injuries.
■ Diagnostic Testing
Imaging techniques include x-ray, CT, and MRI (Fig. 9-16).
Obtain an anteroposterior view of the scapula, supraspinatus outlet view, and axillary view of the shoulder.
If there is uncertainty of the extent of the fracture or if the fracture involves the glenoid, a CT scan should be performed.
MRI is rarely performed in the setting of a scapula fracture.

## Treatment of Specific Injuries

■ When to Consult a Specialist
 • If the humeral head is dislocated or subluxed
 • Associated neurovascular injury or compromise
 • Open injury
■ How and What to Communicate With Specialist
 • Open or closed injury
 • X-ray description
 • Location of fracture on the glenoid
 • Amount of displacement and comminution
 • Neurovascular injury or compromise
 • Patient identifying information—sex, associated injuries, hand dominance

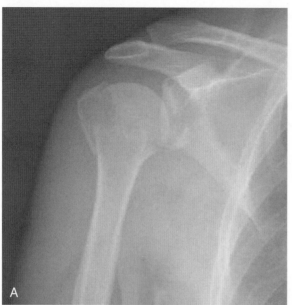

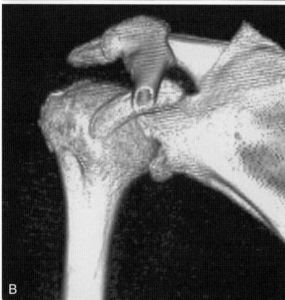

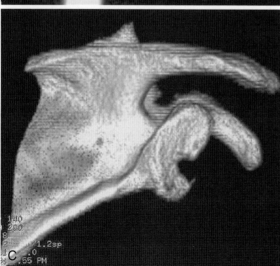

- Analgesia, Anesthesia Block, and Sedation
  The patient requires narcotic pain medications and NSAIDs to control pain in the emergency department.
- Splint or Immobilize
  The patient should be immobilized in a sling.
- Plan for Follow-up Care
  The patient should see an orthopedist for a follow-up examination in 7 to 10 days.
- Outpatient Pain Relief Options
  A short course of an NSAID and narcotic analgesic may be prescribed until follow-up.
    The patient should apply ice for 48 to 72 hours.
    Early range of motion exercises are encouraged.
- Discharge or Admit as Inpatient
  Consider admitting patients with scapula fractures for observation. These fractures are usually associated with significant trauma and intrathoracic injuries.
- Subsequent Management
  Scapula fractures are usually managed nonsurgically.
    Surgical intervention is considered for (1) displaced articular fractures of the glenoid, (2) angulated glenoid neck fractures, (3) acromial fractures associated with a rotator cuff tear, and (4) some coracoid fractures.

## SEPTIC SHOULDER

### Differential Diagnosis of Nontraumatic Complaints

- History
  - Fever
  - Chills
  - Sweats
  - General malaise
  - Reduced appetite
  - Weight loss
  - Redness or skin discoloration
  - Intravenous drug use
  - Penetrating injury to the area
  - Prior surgical intervention
- Timing
  - Chronic or acute infection
- Preexisting illness
  - Immunocompromised status
  - Intravenous drug use
  - History of infection
  - History of recent shoulder surgery
  - Sickle cell disease
- Pain
  - Localized to the shoulder joint
- Dysfunction
  - Pain with minimal movement of the joint

---

**FIGURE 9-16. A,** A 38-year-old man slipped on icy ground and sustained a stable, well-aligned fracture of the proximal end of the humerus and a fracture of the anterior margin of the glenoid. **B,** Three-dimensional CT verified good alignment of the proximal end of the humerus and glenohumeral joint. **C,** Subtraction of the humerus showed that the glenoid fragment was very small. *(From Browner BD, Levine AM, Jupiter JB, et al: Skeletal trauma, ed 4, Philadelphia, 2009, Saunders.)*

- Physical Examination—Standard Focus Examination
Inspect the skin for erythema, penetrating trauma, or needle-stick injuries.
   Palpate the skin for warmth and tenderness.
   Gentle movement of the shoulder joint causes discomfort.
- Diagnostic Testing
Imaging techniques include x-ray, CT, MRI, and ultrasound.
   Standard shoulder x-rays should be obtained but most likely will appear normal in an acute setting.
   MRI or ultrasound is helpful if there is concern for an abscess or to assess for fluid collection in or around the joint.
   CT scan is of little help in the work-up of a patient with suspected septic shoulder.
- Joint Aspiration or Injection
The definitive diagnosis is made via aspiration of the shoulder joint.
   A large area overlying and adjacent to the affected joint is cleaned with povidone-iodine solution. After air drying, the skin is cleaned with an alcohol wipe to remove the povidone-iodine solution from the skin surface. Sterile drapes are placed over the site. Local anesthetic is injected into the overlying skin only.
   A large-bore (18-gauge) needle should be used for aspiration of the joint. A spinal needle may be needed in obese or muscular patients. Remove as much synovial fluid as possible to optimize diagnosis and to relieve pain from joint capsule distention.
   Aspirated fluid should be sent for culture, Gram stain, leukocyte count with differential, and crystal analysis, protein, and glucose
   Joint aspiration is performed via an anterior or posterior approach.
   The posterior approach is usually more effective than the anterior approach. The patient sits upright, and the examiner stands behind the patient. The needle is inserted 2 cm inferior and 2 cm medial to the posterolateral corner of the acromion. The needle is directed toward the coracoid process (anterior and medial) until the tip pierces the capsule.
   For the anterior approach, the patient sits upright, facing the examiner. The needle is inserted midway between the coracoid and the anterolateral corner of the acromion. The needle is directed posterior and slightly inferior. Infection of the overlying skin is a contraindication to joint aspiration.
   Relative contraindications include coagulopathy, hemarthrosis in hemophiliac patients before factor replacement, and the presence of a prosthetic joint.
   It may also be necessary to rule out septic arthritis of the acromioclavicular joint or an infected subacromial bursa.
   The acromioclavicular joint can be aspirated directly from a superior or anterior approach.
   The subacromial bursa is deep to the acromioclavicular joint and extends laterally over the rotator cuff. Aspiration of the bursa should be performed from the site of maximum fluctuance (anterior, posterior, or direct lateral).
   Serum studies including C-reactive protein, sedimentation rate, complete blood count, and blood culture can contribute to the diagnosis. These serum studies are helpful for the orthopedic service in further management and follow-up, but they cannot prove or disprove the diagnosis of septic joint. Aspiration is definitive.
- Joint Fluid Studies
Aspirated joint fluid should be sent for cell count with differential, culture, Gram stain, protein, glucose, and crystals.
- Differential Considerations
It is important to rule out a septic joint based on the results of the joint fluid aspirate. Other considerations include gout, pseudogout, Lyme disease, osteoarthritis, inflammatory arthritis, and traumatic hemarthrosis.

### *Treatment of Specific Problems*

- Develop Plan
The patient should be admitted for pain control and parenteral antibiotics until synovial culture results are available. Broad-spectrum antibiotics should be initiated as soon as a septic joint is suspected.
- Antibiotic Recommendations
  - Neonates and infants: Nafcillin or vancomycin plus aminoglycoside or third-generation cephalosporin, ampicillin/sulbactam
  - Children younger than 5 years: Nafcillin or vancomycin plus cefuroxime, ampicillin/sulbactam
  - Older children and adults: Nafcillin or vancomycin plus third-generation cephalosporin, ampicillin/sulbactam
  - Intravenous drug abusers: Vancomycin plus aminoglycoside, ampicillin/sulbactam
  - Sickle cell patients: Ciprofloxacin, ofloxacin, ceftriaxone
- When to Consult a Specialist
An orthopedist should be consulted any time there is suspicion for a septic joint.
- Analgesia, Anesthesia Block, and Sedation
The patient may require narcotic pain medications and NSAIDs (unless otherwise contraindicated).
- Subsequent Management
Repeat closed needle aspiration, arthroscopy, or open surgical drainage may be required.

## SHOULDER ARTHRITIDES

### *Differential Diagnosis of Nontraumatic Problems*

- History
  - Shoulder pain
  - Swelling
  - Erythema
- Timing
  - Usually insidious onset of pain, may be chronic in nature with flare-ups
- Preexisting Illness
  - Known history of rheumatoid arthritis, osteoarthritis, Lyme disease, gout
  - Sickle cell disease

- Pain
  - Pain localized to shoulder joint
- Dysfunction
  - Discomfort with movement of the shoulder
- Physical Examination—Standard Focus Examination
  Assess active and passive range of motion of the shoulder.
  Palpate the acromioclavicular joint, clavicle, and acromion.
  Perform a neurovascular examination of the involved extremity.
- Diagnostic Testing
  Imaging techniques include x-ray, CT, and MRI.
  X-rays of the shoulder should be the basis for diagnosis.
  With osteoarthritis, there is usually asymmetric joint space narrowing, osteophytes, and subchondral sclerosis.
  With rheumatoid arthritis, there can be symmetric joint space narrowing and periarticular erosions.
- Differential Considerations
  It is important to rule out a septic joint based on history and physical examination. Other potential diagnoses include gout, pseudogout, Lyme disease, osteoarthritis, inflammatory arthritis, and traumatic hemarthrosis.

## Treatment of Specific Problems

### Osteoarthritis

Salicylates or other NSAIDs are the cornerstone of treatment of an acute exacerbation of osteoarthritis. The patient can be immobilized in a sling for comfort. Corticosteroids should not be used in the treatment of osteoarthritis.

- When to Consult an Orthopedist
  Consult with an orthopedist if septic arthritis cannot be ruled out.
- Plan for Follow-up Care
  The patient should see his or her primary care physician or an orthopedist for a follow-up examination in 7 to 10 days.
- Outpatient Pain Relief Options
  A short course of NSAIDs and opioid analgesics should be prescribed until follow-up.
  The patient should apply ice for 48 to 72 hours.

### Rheumatoid Arthritis

Salicylates or other NSAIDs are the cornerstone of treatment of an acute exacerbation of rheumatoid arthritis. The patient can be immobilized in a sling for comfort. A short course of corticosteroids may be considered.

- When to Consult an Orthopedist
  Consult with an orthopedist if septic arthritis cannot be ruled out.
- Plan for Follow-up Care
  The patient should see his or her primary care physician or an orthopedist for a follow-up examination in 7 days.

- Outpatient Pain Relief Options
  A short course of NSAIDs and opioid analgesics should be prescribed until follow-up.
- Subsequent Management
  The patient should see his or her primary care physician for long-term control of rheumatoid arthritis with agents such as antimalarials, gold, and methotrexate.

### Lyme Arthritis

Antibiotics are recommended for 3 to 4 weeks. Antibiotic choices include doxycycline, penicillin G, amoxicillin, and ceftriaxone. Patients with more severe presentations require hospital admission and intravenous antibiotic therapy.

- When to Consult an Orthopedist
  Consult with an orthopedist if septic arthritis cannot be ruled out.
- Plan for Follow-up Care
  The patient should see an orthopedist for a follow-up examination in 7 days.
- Outpatient Pain Relief Options
  A short course of NSAIDs and narcotic analgesics may be prescribed until follow-up.
  The patient should apply ice for 48 to 72 hours.

### Crystal-Induced Synovitis

First-line therapy for gout is an NSAID, such as indomethacin. All NSAID doses should be adjusted for renal function. For patients with normal renal function, the initial dose of indomethacin is 50 mg. Substantial pain relief typically occurs within 2 hours of NSAID administration.

- When to Consult an Orthopedist
  Consult with an orthopedist if septic arthritis cannot be ruled out.
- Plan for Follow-up Care
  The patient should see his or her primary care physician or an orthopedist for a follow-up examination in 7 days.
- Outpatient Pain Relief Options
  Indomethacin is continued three times a day for 3 to 5 days. The patient may be placed in a sling for comfort.
- Subsequent Management
  The patient should see his or her primary care physician for long-term control of gout. Gout-inducing medications (i.e., diuretics, aspirin, or cyclosporine) may need to be eliminated or reduced. Patients may also require prophylactic medications, such as allopurinol or probenecid.

## ROTATOR CUFF INJURIES

### Anatomic Considerations

The rotator cuff consists of four musculotendinous units (supraspinatus, infraspinatus, teres minor, and subscapularis) that arise from the scapula and insert on the proximal humerus (Fig. 9-17). The rotator cuff is a dynamic stabilizer

- When to Consult a Specialist
A telephone consultation should be obtained for glenohumeral capsular injuries or rupture of long head of biceps.

    Bedside consultation is indicated for glenohumeral capsular injuries associated with fracture-dislocation, neurovascular injury, or open injury.
- How and What to Communicate With Specialist
Patient identifying information includes age, gender, hand dominance, mechanism of injury, brief history, and pertinent physical examination findings.

    Findings on x-ray include any incongruity of the glenohumeral joint; fracture of the proximal humerus, clavicle, or scapula; and widening of the acromioclavicular joint.

    Neurovascular status includes specifically the status of the axillary nerve and the suprascapular nerve.
- Outpatient Pain Relief Options
    - Ice application
    - Rest in a sling (short duration only)
    - NSAIDs
    - Acetaminophen (Tylenol)
    - Muscle relaxant
- Further Care Plan Discussion With Patient and Subsequent Management
Complete tears of the long head of the biceps can be treated nonoperatively or operatively depending on multiple factors that include patient demand and activity level, response to physical therapy, presence of coexistent shoulder or elbow pathology, and presence of persistent pain.

    Rupture of the long head of biceps does not result in significant limitation of elbow flexion strength. However, some patients may experience initial fatigue and weakness in supination strength. Popeye's sign, which is a lump in the arm owing to a retracted long head of biceps, may occur in some patients with complete rupture of the long head of biceps and can be a cosmetic concern.

    Patients should be told that grade I and grade II capsular strains do not require surgery. Early range of motion and strengthening exercises when active range of motion has been achieved are elementary for good functional outcome.

- Discharge or Admit as Inpatient
Patients with isolated glenohumeral capsular strains or injury to the long head of biceps can be discharged home on the same day.
- Discharge Care and Instruction for Follow-up
The period of immobilization should be very brief and strictly for pain control. Patients should be encouraged to start moving their shoulder as early as possible to prevent shoulder stiffness.

    Early goals in capsular strains and rupture of the long head of biceps are pain control and early range of motion exercises. Strengthening exercises should be started once active range of motion has been achieved.

    Patients should see an orthopedist for a follow-up examination, and referral to an occupational therapist should be made to ensure active participation of the patient in preventing shoulder stiffness.
- Common Pitfalls
Failure to communicate to the patient the significance of early range of motion exercises leads to capsular stiffness and tightness.

## Bibliography

Della-Giustina D, Harrison B, Hunter DM: Shoulder pain. In Tintinalli JE, Kelen GD, Stapczynski JS, et al, editors: Tintinalli's emergency medicine: A comprehensive study guide, ed 6, New York, 2004, McGraw-Hill.

Green A, Norris TR: Proximal humeral fractures and glenohumeral dislocations. In Browner BD, Jupiter JB, Levine AM, et al, editors: Skeletal trauma: basic science, management, and reconstruction, ed 4, Philadelphia, 2008, Saunders.

Ma OJ, Cline DM, Tintinalli JE, et al: Shoulder and humerus injuries. In: Emergency Medicine Manual, ed 6, New York, 2003, McGraw-Hill.

Ma OJ, Cline DM, Tintinalli JE, et al: Shoulder pain. In Emergency medicine manual, ed 6, New York, 2003, McGraw-Hill.

Ring D, Jupiter JB: Injuries to the shoulder girdle. In Browner BD, Jupiter JB, Levine AM, et al, editors: Skeletal trauma: basic science, management, and reconstruction, ed 4, Philadelphia, 2008, Saunders.

Sweiss N, Millstein ES, Primus GL, et al: Aspiration techniques and indications for surgery, septic arthritis. eMedicine. Available at: http://emedicine.medscape.com. Updated April 1, 2009. Accessed September 13, 2010.

Uehara DT, Rudzinski JP: Injuries to the shoulder complex and humerus. In Tintinalli JE, Kelen GD, Stapczynski JS, et al, editors: Tintinalli's emergency medicine: a comprehensive study guide, ed 6, New York, 2004, McGraw-Hill.

# Chapter 10  *Elbow and Distal Humerus*

Mandeep S. Virk, Nicholas A. Bontempo,
Megan Cummings, and Augustus D. Mazzocca

## HUMERAL SHAFT FRACTURES

### Anatomic Considerations

The shaft of the humerus is circumferentially covered with muscles that provide a rich source of periosteal blood supply. The displacement of fracture fragments in the humerus is determined by the initial velocity of injury and the dynamic action of muscle forces acting across the fracture site. Pectoralis major and deltoid are the two major muscular forces that are responsible for producing characteristic deformities after fractures of the humeral shaft (Fig. 10-1). The most common displacement seen in humerus shaft fractures is shortening, varus angulation, and anterior angulation.

The radial nerve runs in the spiral groove of the shaft of the humerus and then pierces the lateral intermuscular septum to enter the anterior compartment in the distal third of the arm (about 10 to 12 cm above the lateral epicondyle). Consequently, humeral shaft fractures involving the spiral groove or distal third humerus (Holstein-Lewis fracture) are associated with a higher incidence of radial nerve injury (Fig. 10-2).

### Differential Diagnosis of Traumatic Complaints

Humerus shaft fractures account for approximately 3% of all fractures.

- History
  The chief complaints include pain, swelling, and deformity in the affected arm. Other symptoms may include numbness, paresthesia, and inability to extend the wrist and fingers.
  Pathologic fractures can occur spontaneously and may have minimal or no pain.
- Mechanism of Injury
  High-velocity injuries (motor vehicle crash, fall from height) are more common in younger patients.
  Low-velocity injuries (twisting injury, fall from standing height) are more commonly seen in elderly patients.
- Timing of Injury
  Open fractures require immediate irrigation and débridement.
- Preexisting Illness
  • Osteoporosis (older age, steroid use)
  • Metastatic bone disease (in case of pathologic fracture)
- Pain
  • In affected arm
- Dysfunction
  • Inability to use arm
- Prehospital care
  • RICE (rest, ice, compression, and elevation)
  • Splinting with coaptation splint or Sarmiento brace minimizes further soft tissue and neurovascular injury and limits blood loss in open fractures
  • Pressure dressing if open bleeding wound
- Physical Examination
  A complete primary and secondary survey should be performed. Always examine the joint above and below.
  Signs to look for during physical examination include tenderness (most sensitive sign), ecchymosis, swelling, abrasions, open wounds, crepitus, and deformity.

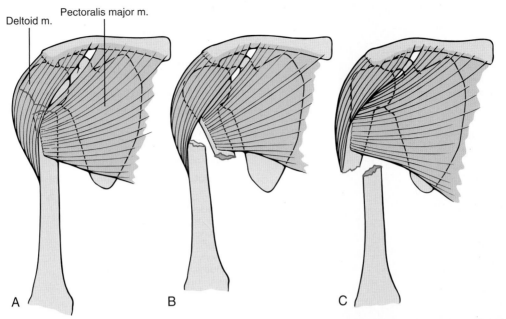

Deltoid m.    Pectoralis major m.

A    B    C

**FIGURE 10-1.** Deforming forces across the fracture site. *(From Browner BD, Levine AM, Jupiter JB, et al: Skeletal trauma, ed 4, Philadelphia, 2009, Saunders.)*

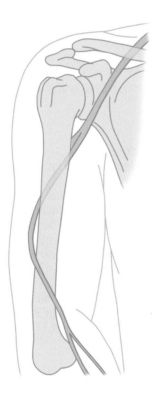

**FIGURE 10-2.** Course of the radial nerve in the arm. The radial nerve is susceptible to injury in the region of the spiral groove (dashed part of the nerve) and distal third.

Perform and document a complete neurovascular examination. The radial nerve is the most common nerve injured in humerus shaft fractures. If a complete neurologic examination cannot be performed in a patient because of altered sensorium (e.g., head injury,

alcohol, drugs) or because of severe pain, it should be documented in the chart.

- Diagnostic Testing
  Imaging techniques include x-ray, bone scan, and computed tomography (CT) scan.

  A minimum of two orthogonal radiographic views (90 degrees to each other) should be obtained, which must include the joint above (shoulder) and the joint below (elbow) (Fig. 10-3).

  Patients with pathologic fracture need more extensive imaging modalities to find the unknown primary or other metastatic lesion (bone scan, CT scan).

  No classification system for humeral shaft fractures has been universally accepted. Fractures are commonly described based on their location in the humerus (Table 10-1). The AO classifies fractures of the humeral shaft into three types based on the fracture line and degree of comminution (Fig. 10-4).

  Measurement of compartment pressure is not indicated unless compartment syndrome is suspected in a patient who is intubated or has altered level of consciousness.

## Treatment of Specific Injuries

- Develop Plan
  Most humeral shaft fractures are managed nonoperatively. Nonoperative management includes performing a closed reduction if initial displacement is unacceptable and immobilization using a splint.

  Nonoperative treatment requires a compliant patient who has no other injuries that would prevent the patient from sitting upright or ambulating. Close supervision and regular follow-up are essential.

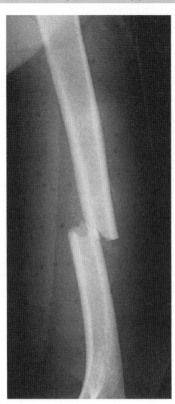

**FIGURE 10-3.** Transverse midshaft humerus fracture. *(From Browner BD, Levine AM, Jupiter JB, et al: Skeletal trauma, ed 4, Philadelphia, 2009, Saunders.)*

**TABLE 10-1** Classification of Humerus Shaft Fracture

**Anatomic Location**

Above pectoralis major insertion
Below pectoralis major insertion, above deltoid insertion
Below deltoid insertion

**Fracture Personality (Direction and Character of Fracture)**

Transverse
Oblique
Spiral
Segmental
Comminuted

**Associated Soft Tissue Injury (Gustilo)**

Open
  Grade 1
  Grade 2
  Grade 3
Periarticular injury
  Glenohumeral
  Elbow joint
Nerve injury
  Radial nerve
  Median nerve
  Ulnar nerve
Vascular injury
  Brachial artery
  Brachial vein
Intrinsic conditions of the bone
  Normal
  Pathologic
  Metabolic
  Metastatic
  Infectious
  Incomplete fractures

From Browner BD, Levine AM, Jupiter JB, et al: Skeletal trauma, ed 4, Philadelphia, 2009, Saunders.

Prolonged recumbence, unstable fracture patterns, and associated injuries may necessitate operative management of humerus shaft fractures (Table 10-2).

Mild deformities are easily concealed by thick musculature around the humerus. Angular and rotational deformities have relatively less functional limitation compared with other parts of the body because of liberal compensation of range of motion at the shoulder joint.

■ Discuss Alternative and Final Care Plan With Patient
All treatment options (operative and nonoperative) with their risks and benefits should be explained to the patient.

If operative treatment is indicated, the orthopedic surgeon should discuss the risks and benefits of operative treatment with the patient. The postoperative course including the weight-bearing status, duration of casting or splinting, physical therapy, time when the patient can start driving, and how long the patient will be out of work should be discussed with the patient.

■ When to Consult a Specialist
Bedside consultation with an orthopedist should be obtained for open humerus shaft fractures or fractures with associated neurovascular deficits.

■ How and What to Communicate With Specialist
  • Patient age, gender, hand dominance, associated musculoskeletal and nonmusculoskeletal injuries
  • Mechanism of injury—low-energy versus high-energy mechanism

  • Open versus closed injury
  • Physical examination findings including neurovascular status of the extremity
  • X-ray description: fracture pattern (transverse, oblique, spiral); fracture location (proximal third, middle third, distal third); degree of comminution (segmental, butterfly fragment)

■ Analgesia, Anesthesia Block, and Sedation
  • Intravenous or oral narcotics for analgesia

■ Reduce or Accept Alignment
The acceptable alignment for humerus shaft fracture includes (1) shortening less than 3 cm, (2) varus deformity less than 30 degrees, and (3) anterior angulation less than 20 degrees.

■ Splint or Immobilize
Methods of immobilizing humerus shaft fractures include functional fracture brace, coaptation splint ("U" splint), hanging cast, Velpeau dressing, abduction splint, and skeletal traction (see Table 10-2).

A functional brace works on the principle of hydraulic compression and active muscle contraction, which bring about fracture reduction (Fig. 10-5). A functional brace allows motion at all joints, is well tolerated by patients, and is lighter compared to a coaptation splint and hanging cast. A hanging cast or coaptation splint is usually exchanged for a functional brace in 1 to 2 weeks.

Essence:  All diaphyseal fractures are divided into three types according to the **contact between the two main fragments after reduction: A** contact >90% = simple fracture, **B** some contact = wedge fracture, **C** no contact = complex fracture.

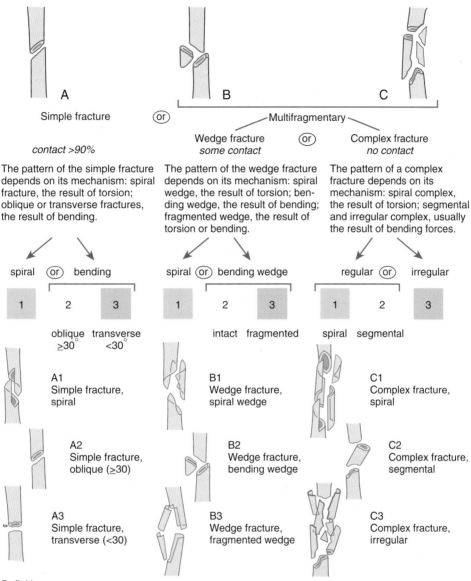

A  Simple fracture

contact >90%

or

B  Multifragmentary  C

Wedge fracture  or  Complex fracture
some contact  no contact

The pattern of the simple fracture depends on its mechanism: spiral fracture, the result of torsion; oblique or transverse fractures, the result of bending.

The pattern of the wedge fracture depends on its mechanism: spiral wedge, the result of torsion; bending wedge, the result of bending; fragmented wedge, the result of torsion or bending.

The pattern of a complex fracture depends on its mechanism: spiral complex, the result of torsion; segmental and irregular complex, usually the result of bending forces.

spiral  or  bending

1    2    3

oblique  transverse
≥30°    <30°

A1  Simple fracture, spiral

A2  Simple fracture, oblique (≥30)

A3  Simple fracture, transverse (<30)

spiral  or  bending wedge

1    2    3

intact  fragmented

B1  Wedge fracture, spiral wedge

B2  Wedge fracture, bending wedge

B3  Wedge fracture, fragmented wedge

regular  or  irregular

1    2    3

spiral  segmental

C1  Complex fracture, spiral

C2  Complex fracture, segmental

C3  Complex fracture, irregular

Definitions

**Simple fracture:** A single circumferential disruption of the diaphysis. Small cortical fragments that represent less than 10% of the circumference are ignored, since they are of no significance for treatment or prognosis.
-**spiral:** A result of torsion.
-**oblique:** The angle of the fracture line with a perpendicular to the long axis of the bone is equal to or greater than 30°.
-**transverse:** The angle of the fracture line with a perpendicular to the long axis of the bone is less than 30°. Usually a small wedge of less than 10% of the circumference can be detected.
**Wedge fracture:** A multifragmentary fracture of the diaphysis with one or more intermediate fragments in which after reduction there is some contact between the main fragments.
-**spiral:** Also called a "butterfly fragment" or a third fragment fracture.
-**bending:** Mostly caused by a direct blow; therefore, the soft tissue lesion is here more severe than in a spiral wedge fracture.
-**fragmented:** A wedge fracture when after reduction the main fragments are still in some contact.
**Complex fracture:** A multifragmentary fracture of the diaphysis with one or more intermediate fragments in which after reduction there is no contact between the main proximal and distal fragments.
-**spiral:** Involving multiple and usually large intermediate fragments of spiral pattern.
-**segmental:** A fracture at two levels (bilocal) or three levels (trilocal). After reduction the intermediate fragments make contact with more than 50% of the circumference of each of the main fragments.
-**irregular:** A diaphyseal fracture with a number of intermediate fragments without any specific pattern usually accompanied by severe soft tissue lesions.

**FIGURE 10-4.** AO classification of humerus shaft fractures. *(From Browner BD, Levine AM, Jupiter JB, et al: Skeletal trauma, ed 4, Philadelphia, 2009, Saunders.)*

**TABLE 10-2** Nonoperative Treatment of Humeral Shaft Fractures

| Treatment Method | Advantages | Disadvantages | Indications |
|---|---|---|---|
| Hanging arm cast | Helps restore length<br><br>Can control angulation through loops at the wrist | Patient must stay erect or semierect<br><br>Distraction can lead to nonunion<br>Limits range of motion of hand, wrist, elbow, and shoulder | Mostly used for initial treatment to obtain reduction in a shortened fracture<br>Usually changed to functional bracing after an initial period of treatment |
| Coaptation splint | Inexpensive<br>Easy to apply<br>Allows motion of hand and wrist | May allow shortening of the fracture<br>Axillary irritation<br>Angular union in obese patients | Initial management of nondisplaced or minimally displaced fractures<br>Usually changed to functional bracing |
| Velpeau dressing/ sling and swathe | Can be useful in uncooperative children or elderly patients | Restricts motion to all joints<br>Potential for skin maceration | Used as initial treatment in uncooperative children or elderly patients |
| Abduction cast/splint | No clear advantages | Poorly tolerated, awkward position with rotator cuff pressure | Always listed as an option in textbooks, but no clear indication for its use |
| Skeletal traction | Can be used in recumbent patients<br>Can be used with large soft tissue defects and allows access to wounds | Requires patient cooperation<br>Risk of infection<br>Requires close supervision<br>Potential for ulnar nerve injury | Rarely used because it has no clear advantage over external fixation |
| Functional fracture bracing | Allows motion of all joints<br>Lightweight and well tolerated<br>Decreased nonunion rate | Is not useful for initial reduction or bringing fracture out to length | Current gold standard for most shaft fractures after an initial period in a hanging cast or coaptation splint |

From Degnan G: In Baratz ME, editor: Orthopaedic surgery: the essentials, New York, 1999, Thieme, p 317.

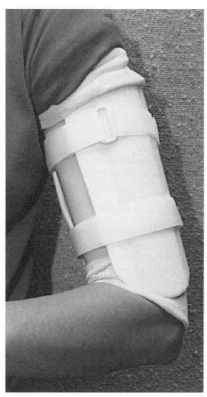

**FIGURE 10-5.** Functional arm brace. *(From Browner BD, Levine AM, Jupiter JB, et al: Skeletal trauma, ed 4, Philadelphia, 2009, Saunders.)*

A coaptation splint is the most widely accepted splint for immobilization of humerus shaft fractures. It is usually applied for 1 to 2 weeks followed by functional bracing of the fracture. A coaptation splint is a U-shaped splint that spans from the axilla running along the medial side of the arm across the elbow and then along the lateral surface of the arm and terminating above the shoulder (Fig. 10-6). The wrist and fingers are free to move, and the forearm is supported with a cuff and collar sling. Axillary irritation and varus deformity in obese women with large breasts are important limitations of the coaptation splint.

A hanging cast relies on traction applied by the weight of the arm, which facilitates fracture reduction (Fig. 10-7). The advantage of a hanging cast is that it can help in restoring length and correct angular deformities via the position of loops at the wrist and length of the suspension straps around the neck. However, for the hanging cast to be effective, patients need to be upright or ambulating. Excessive distraction can lead to nonunion, and immobilization of the elbow and the wrist predisposes to stiffness at these joints. These potential limitations necessitate a more frequent follow-up in patients managed with a hanging cast.

■ Postreduction Imaging

Two orthogonal views of the humerus should be obtained to confirm satisfactory alignment.

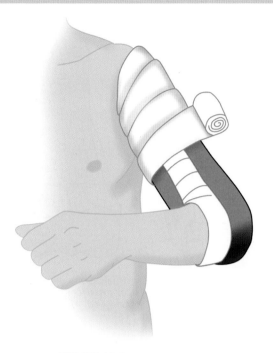

**FIGURE 10-6.** Coaptation splint.

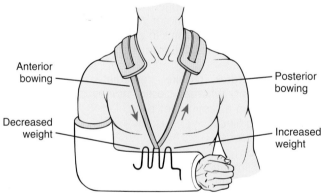

Anterior bowing

Posterior bowing

Decreased weight

Increased weight

**FIGURE 10-7.** Hanging arm cast. *(From Browner BD, Levine AM, Jupiter JB, et al: Skeletal trauma, ed 4, Philadelphia, 2009, Saunders.)*

- Plan for Follow-up Care
  If fracture of the humerus shaft is an isolated injury, the patient can be discharged home the same day.
  The patient should see an orthopedic surgeon for a follow-up examination within 7 to 14 days. At this stage, the coaptation splint is usually replaced with a Sarmiento functional brace.
- Outpatient Pain Relief Options
  - Narcotic pain medications
  - Acetaminophen (Tylenol)
  - Nonsteroidal anti-inflammatory drugs (NSAIDs)
- Further Care Plan Discussion With Patient—How and What to Communicate With Patient
  Keep the splint dry and clean.
  Keep the forearm and wrist elevated. Move the wrist and fingers several times during the day.
  If the fracture is treated nonoperatively, surgery may be required if it does not show signs of healing.

- Discharge or Admit as Inpatient
  If fracture of the humerus shaft is an isolated injury, the patient can be discharged home the same day.
- Subsequent Management
  The patient should see an orthopedic surgeon for a follow-up examination within 7 to 10 days. In patients treated nonoperatively, the coaptation splint is usually replaced with a Sarmiento functional brace at the first visit.
  If the fracture does not show clinical and radiographic progression of healing during follow-up visits, the patient will require surgery.
- Discharge Care and Instruction—Timing for Follow-up
  The patient should see an orthopedic surgeon for a follow-up examination within 7 to 10 days.
- Common Pitfalls
  - Communication failure with the patient
  - Axillary irritation from the coaptation splint—ensure good padding of the axilla
  - Swelling of the hand and fingers—keep the wrist elevated, and move wrist and fingers several times during the day.
- Special Considerations
  Open fracture of the humerus is an orthopedic emergency. Management should include the following:
  - Immediate orthopedic consultation
  - Antibiotics and tetanus prophylaxis after discussion with the orthopedic team
  - Preparation of the patient for surgery (emergent irrigation and débridement)
  Vascular injuries with fractures of the humerus shaft are uncommon. However, the following general approach should be employed when managing such injuries.
  External hemorrhage should be controlled with direct pressure in the emergency department.
  Any deformity should be corrected by grossly aligning the extremity and splinting the fracture.
  Consultation with a vascular surgeon should be sought immediately.
  Avoid placing clips, forceps, or clamps in the emergency department because of risk of damaging vascular structures and surrounding nerves.
  In patients with open fractures with absent pulses, the fracture should be reduced, irrigated, dressed, and temporarily splinted, and the patient should receive antibiotics and tetanus prophylaxis in the emergency department before going directly to the operating room.
  Patients with closed fracture with indirect signs of vascular injury (bruit, thrill, expanding hematoma, signs of ischemia and compartment syndrome [pulselessness, pallor, paresthesia, pain on extension, and paralysis]) should preferably undergo further imaging (angiography) to delineate the extent of vascular injury.
  Patients with closed fractures of the humerus shaft with radial nerve injury are best managed expectantly. Most radial nerve injuries recover spontaneously. Immediate nerve exploration is warranted in the following situations:
  - Open fracture
  - High-velocity gunshot wounds

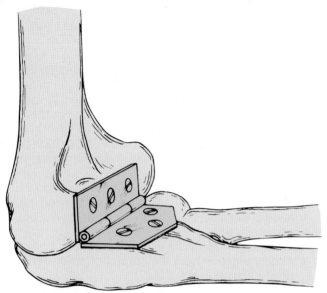

**FIGURE 10-8.** The distal end of humerus flattens anteroposteriorly into two columns (medial and lateral) that connect with the trochlea similar to the ends of a spool held between the thumb and the index finger. *(From Browner BD, Levine AM, Jupiter JB, et al: Skeletal trauma, ed 4, Philadelphia, 2009, Saunders.)*

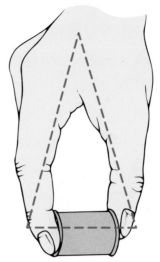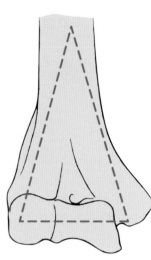

**FIGURE 10-9.** Diagrammatic representation of anterior and posterior view of the columns of the distal humerus. *(From Browner BD, Levine AM, Jupiter JB, et al: Skeletal trauma, ed 4, Philadelphia, 2009, Saunders.)*

- Injury with sharp object
- Associated vascular injury
  In secondary nerve palsies, it has not been convincingly established that early exploration results in significantly better recovery compared with expectant management or delayed exploration.

## DISTAL HUMERAL FRACTURES

### Anatomic Considerations

The distal humerus articulates with the radial head and proximal ulna to form a hinge synovial joint (Fig. 10-8). The radial head articulates with the capitellum to form the radiocapitellar joint. The radial head also articulates with the lesser sigmoid notch of the ulna to form the superior radioulnar joint. The articular surfaces of the olecranon and the coronoid form the greater sigmoid notch, which articulates with the trochlea of the humerus to form the ulnohumeral joint. The distal humerus is triangular-shaped and splits terminally in a wishbone fashion to form the two columns that connect the trochlea to the shaft (Figs. 10-9 and 10-10).

### Differential Diagnosis of Traumatic Complaints

Distal humerus fractures are among the most challenging fractures to manage.

- History
  Pain and swelling in the elbow and inability to move the elbow are the most common complaints.
  Other symptoms include numbness, paresthesia, and muscle weakness in the forearm and hand.

- Mechanism of Injury
  Fractures have a bimodal age distribution of occurrence. Fractures in younger patients are usually due to high-velocity trauma (motor vehicle accidents, fall from height), whereas fractures in elderly patients are due to low-velocity injuries (fall from standing height).
- Timing
  Open fractures require immediate irrigation and débridement, whereas closed injuries can be treated surgically on a semiurgent basis.
- Preexisting Illness
  - Osteoporosis
- Dysfunction
  - Painful limitation of range of motion of the elbow
- Prehospital Care
  - RICE (rest, ice, compression, and elevation)
  - Splinting with long arm posterior splint improves pain, minimizes further soft tissue and neurovascular injury, and limits blood loss in open fractures
  - Pressure dressing if there are open bleeding wounds
- Physical Examination
  A complete primary and secondary survey should be performed.
  Signs to look for during physical examination include tenderness (lateral epicondyle, medial epicondyle), deformity at the elbow, ecchymosis (around the elbow region), swelling, crepitus, and open wounds.
  Assess for painful limitation of elbow motion (flexion and extension and supination and pronation).
  A complete vascular and neurologic examination should be performed and documented. If a complete neurologic examination cannot be performed in a patient because of altered sensorium (e.g., head injury, alcohol, drugs) or because of severe pain, the most complete examination possible should be performed and documented.
  Examination of the joint above and below should be performed to rule out associated injuries.

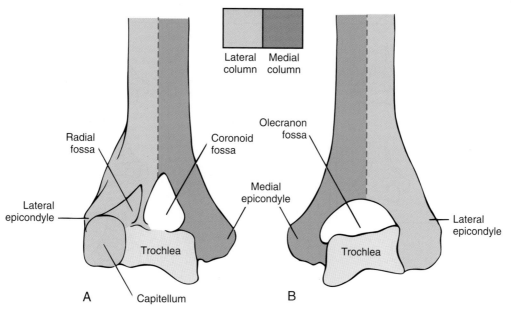

FIGURE 10-10. The elbow joint: hinge synovial joint. *(From Browner BD, Levine AM, Jupiter JB, et al: Skeletal trauma, ed 4, Philadelphia, 2009, Saunders.)*

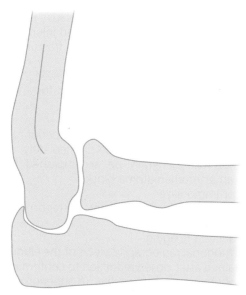

FIGURE 10-11. Radial head–capitellum view is a modified lateral view of the elbow that is obtained by angling the tube 45 degrees toward the radial head, which eliminates any overlap by the surrounding bones.

■ Diagnostic Testing
Imaging techniques include x-ray and CT scan.
　Standard anteroposterior and lateral views of the elbow joint should be obtained. Oblique views are helpful in defining the fracture anatomy. A radial head–capitellum view shows the radiocapitellar joint without any superimposition from surrounding bones (Fig. 10-11).
　Traction views are helpful to delineate fracture pattern if CT is unavailable.
　A CT scan of the elbow (with three-dimensional reconstruction) should be considered for preoperative planning in patients with comminuted fractures.

　Davies et al. classified distal humerus fractures into three subtypes based on location of the primary fracture line (Fig. 10-12): (1) extra-articular, (2) predominantly intra-articular, and (3) predominantly articular.
■ Joint Aspiration and Injection
The elbow joint should be injected with 1% methylene blue (1:10 diluted with normal saline) if there is any suspicion of a surrounding wound communicating with the fracture site. Extravasation of the blue-colored fluid from the wound would confirm it as an open fracture, which is an orthopedic emergency and requires emergent irrigation and débridement in the operating room (Fig. 10-13).
　Compartment pressure usually is not measured unless compartment syndrome is suspected in a unconscious or intubated patient.

## Treatment of Specific Injuries

■ Develop Plan
Undisplaced fractures can be managed nonoperatively with a long arm posterior splint.
　All displaced fractures are best managed surgically with anatomic reduction and stable internal fixation that allows early range of motion.
■ Discuss Alternative and Final Care Plan With Patient
If the patient is being treated nonoperatively, a posterior long arm splint is applied for 6 weeks. If the fracture displaces during the follow-up period, the patient will need operative intervention. The patient should be told that elbow stiffness and some loss of elbow motion are common with nonoperative treatment.
　If operative treatment is indicated, the orthopedic surgeon should discuss the risks and benefits of operative treatment with the patient. The postoperative course including the activity status, duration of casting

1. Extra-articular     2. Predominantly intra-articular     3. Predominantly articular

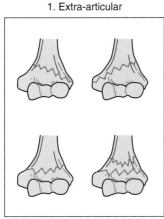 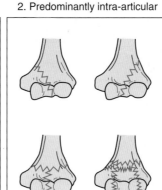 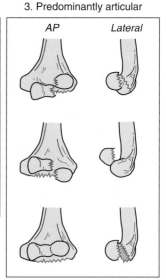

**FIGURE 10-12.** Classification of distal humerus fractures. *(From Browner BD, Levine AM, Jupiter JB, et al: Skeletal trauma, ed 4, Philadelphia, 2009, Saunders.)*

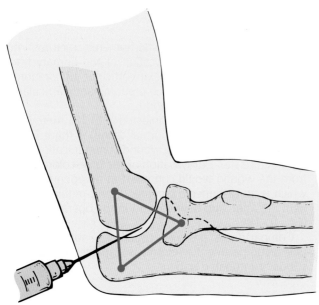

**FIGURE 10-13.** Landmarks for diagnostic injection into the elbow. *(From Browner BD, Levine AM, Jupiter JB, et al: Skeletal trauma, ed 4, Philadelphia, 2009, Saunders.)*

or splinting, physical therapy, time when the patient can start driving, and how long the patient will be out of work should be discussed with the patient.

■ When to Consult a Specialist
Bedside or telephone consultation with an orthopedic specialist should be obtained for all distal humerus fractures.

■ How and What to Communicate With Specialist
- Patient age, gender, hand dominance, associated musculoskeletal and nonmusculoskeletal injuries
- Mechanism of injury—low-energy versus high-energy mechanism
- Open versus closed injury

- Physical examination findings including neurovascular status of the extremity
- X-ray description: displaced versus undisplaced; severity of comminution; associated injuries (dislocation of the elbow joint, forearm fracture, floating elbow)

■ Analgesia, Anesthesia Block, and Sedation
Intravenous narcotics are administered for analgesia. Nerve block is not usually performed.

■ Reduce or Accept Alignment
The ulnohumeral, radiocapitellar, or superior radioulnar joint if dislocated should be immediately reduced. Reduction can generally be accomplished with the aid of an arthro/hematoma block.

■ Splint or Immobilize
Apply a well-padded long arm posterior splint (Fig. 10-14) or coaptation splint

■ Postreduction Imaging
Two orthogonal radiographic views of the elbow should be obtained after closed reduction to confirm reduction of ulnohumeral, radiocapitellar, or superior radioulnar dislocation.

■ Plan for Follow-up Care
Patients with an undisplaced fracture should see an orthopedic surgeon for a follow-up examination in 7 to 10 days. If the fracture displaces during the follow-up period, the patient will require operative intervention.

In patients treated operatively by an orthopedic surgeon, follow-up is dictated by the operating surgeon. Surgical timing varies depending on the fracture, associated symptoms, and other concerns.

■ Outpatient Pain Relief Options
- Low-potency narcotics
- Acetaminophen (Tylenol)
- NSAIDs

■ Further Care Plan Discussion With Patient—How and What to Communicate With Patient
If the patient is being treated nonoperatively, a posterior long arm splint is applied for 6 weeks. If the fracture

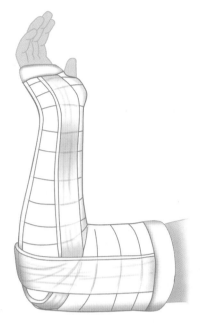

**FIGURE 10-14.** Long arm posterior splint.

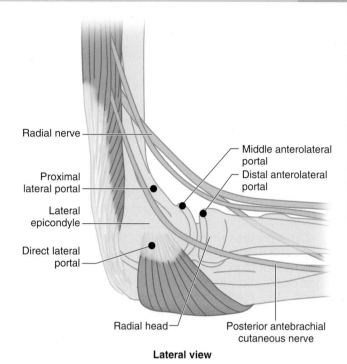

**Lateral view**

**FIGURE 10-15.** Radiocapitellar joint. *(Redrawn from Baker CL, Jones GL: Arthroscopy of the elbow. Am J Sports Med 27:251–264, 1999.)*

displaces during the follow-up period, the patient will need operative intervention. The patient should be told that elbow stiffness and that some loss of range of motion can occur with nonoperative treatment.

If operative treatment is indicated, risks and benefits should be discussed with the patient, including, but not limited to, infection, nerve injury (ulnar and radial), nonunion, hardware prominence, and loss of terminal extension.

- Discharge or Admit as Inpatient
  A patient who has an isolated closed undisplaced distal humerus fracture can be discharged home after application of a long arm posterior splint.

  A patient with a displaced closed distal humerus fracture should have surgery during the same admission or electively (if neurovascular and skin conditions are good) as an outpatient on an urgent basis.

- Subsequent Management
  Undisplaced fractures can be managed nonoperatively in a long arm posterior splint, although there is a trend toward operative fixation to allow early mobilization.

  Patients who are not candidates for surgery because of their medical comorbidities can be managed with the "bag of bones" technique. These patients are immobilized for 2 to 3 weeks in a splint and mobilized thereafter.

  Displaced fractures are invariably treated with open reduction and internal fixation. Patients with compromised skin can be operated on when swelling subsides.

- Discharge Care and Instruction—Timing for Follow-up
  Patients with an undisplaced fracture managed conservatively should see an orthopedic surgeon for a follow-up examination in 7 to 10 days.

  In patients treated operatively by an orthopedic surgeon, follow-up is dictated by the operating surgeon.

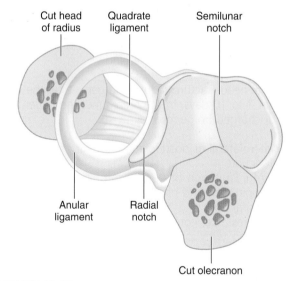

**FIGURE 10-16.** Ligaments supporting the superior radioulnar joint.

## RADIAL HEAD FRACTURES

### Anatomic Considerations

The upper concave surface of the radial head articulates superiorly with the capitellum to form the radiocapitellar joint. The radial head also articulates medially with the lesser sigmoid notch of ulna to form the proximal radioulnar joint (Figs. 10-15 and 10-16).

The radial head is a secondary stabilizer of the elbow to valgus stress and contributes to anteroposterior instability. The radiocapitellar joint transmits approximately 60% of the force across the elbow joint.

## Differential Diagnosis of Traumatic Complaints

Radial head fractures constitute 10% of all fractures around the elbow. Radial head fracture is the most common fracture of the elbow.

■ History
The patient reports pain on the lateral or anterolateral aspect of the elbow, swelling, and difficulty in moving the elbow.
  Other possible symptoms include paresthesia, numbness, and motor weakness in the forearm or hand.
■ Mechanism of Injury
The classic injury described is a fall on an outstretched hand. The mechanism of injury involves an axially directed force transmitted up from the wrist with the elbow in flexion and the forearm in pronation. This mechanism of injury necessitates a search for other injuries with a similar mechanism (carpal injuries, distal radioulnar joint disruption, interosseous membrane disruption [Essex-Lopresti fracture] and distal radius fractures).
  Another mechanism described for failure of the radial head is the posterolateral rotatory instability pattern, in which subluxation of radial head results in shear fracture.
  The radial head can fail in compression if severe valgus force is applied to the elbow.
■ Timing
If radial head fracture requires surgery, it can be done within 7 to 10 days. In the meantime, the patient can be discharged home in a splint.
■ Pain
  • Anterolateral or posterolateral aspect of elbow
■ Dysfunction
  • Painful limitation of flexion and extension of elbow or supination and pronation of forearm, or both
■ Prehospital care
  • RICE (rest, ice, compression, and elevation)
  • Splinting with long arm posterior splint minimizes further soft tissue and neurovascular injury and limits blood loss in open fractures.
  • Pressure dressing if there are open bleeding wounds
■ Physical Examination
A complete primary and secondary survey should be performed.
  Signs to look for during physical examination include tenderness (at radial head), ecchymosis (overlying the anterolateral aspect of elbow), swelling, and open wounds.
  Assess for painful limitation of elbow motion (flexion and extension and supination and pronation). Patient cooperation and good pain control are required to conduct this part of the examination successfully. Aspiration of the elbow joint and instillation of lidocaine may be required if there is block to the range of motion.

Pain in the distal radioulnar joint and along the interosseous membrane of the forearm is suggestive of Essex-Lopresti fracture.
  Ecchymosis, swelling, and tenderness along the imaginary line drawn from the medial epicondyle to the coronoid process are suggestive of injury to the medial collateral ligament.
  A complete vascular and neurologic examination should be performed and documented. If a complete neurologic examination cannot be performed in a patient because of altered sensorium (e.g., head injury, alcohol, drugs) or because of severe pain, it should be documented in the chart.
  Examine the joint above and below to rule out associated injuries (coronoid fractures, distal humerus fracture, and Monteggia fracture-dislocation).
■ Diagnostic Testing
Imaging techniques include x-ray and CT scan.
  A minimum of two orthogonal views of the elbow (anteroposterior and lateral) must be obtained. A radial head–capitellum view is a special projection for the radial head and provides a nonsuperimposed image of the radial head (see Fig. 10-11).
  A posteroanterior radiograph of wrist in neutral rotation should be obtained when the clinical examination reveals forearm or ulnar-sided wrist pain, which is suggestive of injury to the interosseous ligament.
  CT scanning is a useful tool for preoperative planning for open reduction and internal fixation of complex fractures and is helpful in diagnosing associated injuries.
■ Fracture Classification
The Mason classification is the most widely used classification system for radial head fractures (Fig. 10-17).
  • Type I—nondisplaced or minimally displaced
  • Type II—displaced two-part fracture of the head or neck
  • Type III—comminuted fractures of three or more parts with the head either attached or detached from the neck.
  • Type IV—radial head fractures associated with elbow dislocation
■ Joint Aspiration and Injection
Aspiration of the elbow joint and injection of lidocaine can be performed to help determine if the lack of range of motion or appropriate range of motion is due to pain versus a mechanical block secondary to incongruency of the radiocapitellar joint or an osteochondral fragment.
  The elbow joint should be injected with 1% methylene blue (1 : 10 diluted with normal saline) if there is any suspicion of a surrounding wound communicating with the fracture site. Extravasation of the blue-colored fluid from the wound would confirm it as an open fracture, which is an orthopedic emergency and requires emergent irrigation and débridement (see Fig. 10-13).
  Undisplaced or minimally displaced fractures (<2 mm; Mason type I) are managed nonoperatively. Nonoperative treatment consists of a posterior splint in supination or a sling for a week or so followed by early mobilization. In young and active patients, the period of immobilization is usually extended for about 2 weeks

Type I

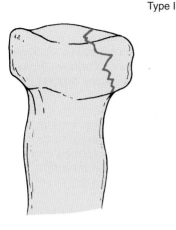

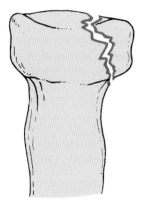

Type II

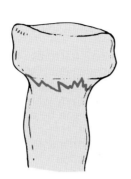

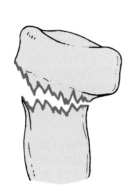

Type III

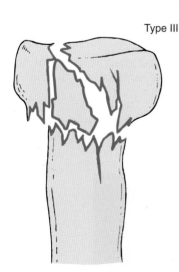

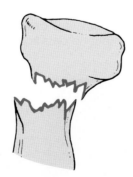

**FIGURE 10-17.** Mason classification. *(From Browner BD, Levine AM, Jupiter JB, et al: Skeletal trauma, ed 4, Philadelphia, 2009, Saunders.)*

followed by protected functional mobilization for another 2 weeks.

Type II and type III fractures are best managed with surgery (open reduction and internal fixation, excision, or radial head arthroplasty).

## Treatment of Specific Injuries

■ Discuss Alternative and Final Care Plan With Patient
If the patient is being treated nonoperatively, a sling is provided for comfort only. In the outpatient follow-up period, if the fracture displaces or the patient is unable to perform flexion and extension range of motion, surgical intervention may be needed.

If operative treatment is contemplated, the orthopedic surgeon should discuss the risks and benefits of operative treatment with the patient. The postoperative course including duration of casting or splinting, physical therapy, time when the patient can start driving, and how long the patient will be out of work should be discussed with the patient. Surgery can be safely performed within 7 to 10 days.

■ When to Consult a Specialist
Bedside consultation is indicated for Mason type II, III, and IV fractures, which are likely to require surgical care.

Follow-up arrangements only are indicated for undisplaced radial head fracture without any limitation of range of motion and no wrist pain or tenderness.

■ How and What to Communicate With Specialist
• Patient age, gender, hand dominance, associated other musculoskeletal and nonmusculoskeletal injuries
• Mechanism of injury—low-energy versus high-energy mechanism
• Open versus closed injury
• Physical examination findings including neurovascular status of the extremity
• X-ray description: displaced versus undisplaced; degree of comminution; associated injuries (dislocation of the elbow joint, Essex-Lopresti fracture, distal radius fracture)

■ Analgesia
Intravenous or oral narcotics are given in the emergency department.

Oral over-the-counter medications are prescribed for pain at home, with oral narcotic medications added for more severe pain.

■ Splint or Immobilize
• Arm sling
• Posterior splint

■ Postsplint Imaging
Imaging after splinting usually is not required.

Further radiographic examination is performed at the follow-up office visit with the orthopedic surgeon.

■ Plan for Follow-up Care
Patients treated nonoperatively should see an orthopedic surgeon for a follow-up examination in 7 to 14 days. If the fracture does not displace, nonoperative treatment is continued, and early range of motion exercises are initiated.

In patients treated operatively by an orthopedic surgeon, follow-up is dictated by the operating surgeon.

■ Outpatient Pain Relief Options
  • Low-potency oral narcotics
  • Acetaminophen (Tylenol)
  • NSAIDs

■ Further Care Plan Discussion With Patient—How and What to Communicate With Patient

The patient should be warned about elbow stiffness and that some loss of terminal extension can occur.

If the patient is being treated nonoperatively, it should be clearly stated to the patient that the sling is for comfort only. The patient must begin early mobilization (within 7 to 10 days) with range of motion exercises. If the patient is not progressing appropriately with respect to range of motion of the elbow, physical therapy referral should be sought.

Inform the patient that surgery may be required if the fracture displaces or does not heal or if there is block to range of motion.

■ Common Pitfalls
  • Missing associated injuries

## OLECRANON FRACTURES

### *Anatomic Considerations*

The triceps tendon inserts onto the dorsal surface of the olecranon and is the major deforming muscular force in fracture of the olecranon. The ulnar nerve runs medial to the olecranon in the cubital tunnel.

### *Differential Diagnosis of Traumatic Complaints*

Approximately 10% of fractures of the elbow in adults are fractures of the olecranon process.

■ History

The patient usually presents with pain and swelling predominantly on the posterior aspect of the elbow and inability to use the elbow.

■ Mechanism of Injury

Direct trauma involves a blunt force to the olecranon or a direct fall on the point of the elbow.

An indirect mechanism of injury involves muscular pull of the triceps in the presence of elbow flexion, which results in avulsion of the olecranon process from the rest of the ulna.

■ Timing

Open fractures require immediate irrigation and débridement. Open reduction and internal fixation of closed olecranon fractures can be performed urgently or electively within 7 to 10 days. In the meantime, the patient can be discharged home in a splint.

■ Pain
  • Predominantly on the posterior aspect of the elbow

■ Dysfunction
  • Inability to flex or extend the elbow

■ Prehospital Care
  • RICE (rest, ice, compression, and elevation)
  • Splinting with long arm posterior splint minimizes further soft tissue and neurovascular injury and limits blood loss in open fractures
  • Pressure dressing if there are open bleeding wounds

■ Physical Examination—Standard Focus Examination

A complete primary and secondary survey should be performed.

Signs to look for during physical examination include tenderness (at the olecranon posteriorly), ecchymosis and swelling (overlying the posterior aspect of elbow), open wounds, palpable defect at the fracture site, crepitus, and painful limitation of elbow range of motion.

Always examine the joint above and below.

A complete vascular and neurologic examination should be performed and documented. If a complete neurologic examination cannot be performed in a patient because of altered sensorium (e.g., head injury, alcohol, drugs) or because of severe pain, it should be documented in the chart.

■ Diagnostic Testing

At least two orthogonal radiographic views of the elbow joint (anteroposterior and lateral) should be obtained (Fig. 10-18).

■ Fracture Classification

Numerous classification systems have been described, but no classification system is universally accepted.

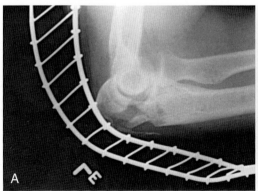
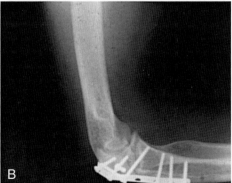

**FIGURE 10-18.** Olecranon fracture. *(From Browner BD, Levine AM, Jupiter JB, et al: Skeletal trauma, ed 4, Philadelphia, 2009, Saunders.)*

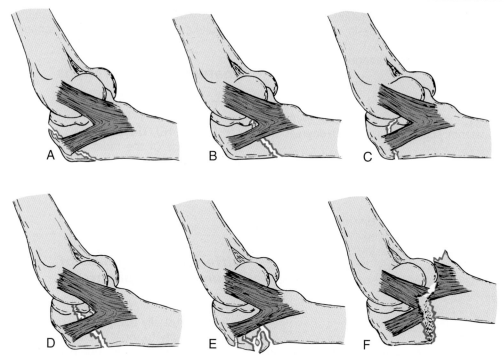

**FIGURE 10-19.** Olecranon fracture classification of Colton. *(From Browner BD, Levine AM, Jupiter JB, et al: Skeletal trauma, ed 4, Philadelphia, 2009, Saunders.)*

Classifications are based on the orientation of the fracture line, the degree of displacement, the amount of comminution, and the stability of the ulnohumeral joint. Colton classified olecranon fractures into four categories and proposed the mechanism of injury for each subtype (Fig. 10-19).

Fractures are described as nondisplaced and stable if they are displaced less than 2 mm and exhibit no change in position with gentle flexion to 90 degrees or with extension against gravity.

Displaced fractures are divided further into avulsion fractures, transverse or oblique fractures, isolated comminuted fractures, or fractures with associated dislocations.

■ Joint Aspiration and Injection
The elbow joint should be injected with 1% methylene blue (1 : 10 diluted with normal saline) if there is any suspicion of a surrounding wound communicating with the fracture site. Extravasation of the blue-colored fluid from the wound would confirm it as an open fracture, which is an orthopedic emergency and requires emergent irrigation and débridement (see Fig. 10-13).

## Treatment of Specific Injuries

■ Develop Plan
Olecranon fractures are intra-articular fractures and warrant early anatomic reduction, stable fixation, and early motion.

Undisplaced and stable fractures with intact extensor apparatus are uncommon and are treated by nonoperative methods. All other fractures are managed by open reduction and internal fixation.

■ Discuss Alternative and Final Care Plan With Patient
If the patient is being treated nonoperatively, a posterior long arm splint is applied for 4 weeks. If the fracture displaces during the follow-up period, the patient will need operative intervention.

If operative treatment is indicated, the orthopedic surgeon should discuss the risks and benefits of operative treatment. Surgery is commonly performed on the same admission. The postoperative course including the weight-bearing status, duration of casting or splinting, physical therapy, time when the patient can start driving, and how long the patient will be out of work should be discussed with the patient.

■ When to Consult a Specialist
A telephone consultation with an orthopedist should be obtained for olecranon fracture.

A bedside consultation with an orthopedist should be obtained for Monteggia fracture-dislocations.

Follow-up arrangements only are indicated for undisplaced olecranon fracture without any associated injuries (uncommon).

■ How and What to Communicate With Specialist
  • Patient age, gender, hand dominance, associated other musculoskeletal and nonmusculoskeletal injuries
  • Mechanism of injury—low-energy versus high-energy mechanism
  • Open versus closed injury
  • Physical examination findings including neurovascular status of the extremity
  • X-ray description: orientation of fracture line (transverse, oblique); displaced versus nondisplaced; degree of comminution; any dislocation of elbow joint

- Analgesia, Anesthesia Block, and Sedation
  - Intravenous or oral narcotic analgesia
- Reduce or Accept Alignment
  Nondisplaced fractures can be managed with nonoperative treatment.
- Splint or Immobilize
  A long arm posterior splint should be applied in all cases. Nonoperative management consists of immobilization in a posterior splint or cast in 90 degrees of flexion for 4 weeks.
- Postreduction Imaging
  Postreduction imaging usually is unnecessary for olecranon fractures.
- Plan for Follow-up Care
  Patients with an undisplaced fracture managed conservatively should see an orthopedic surgeon for a follow-up examination in 7 to 10 days.
  In patients treated operatively by an orthopedic surgeon, follow-up is dictated by the operating surgeon.
- Outpatient Pain Relief Options
  - Low-potency oral narcotics
  - Acetaminophen (Tylenol)
  - NSAIDs
- Further Care Plan Discussion With Patient—How and What to Communicate With Patient
  The injury and the different treatment options available with attendant risks and benefits should be discussed with the patient.
  The patient should be advised to keep the splint dry and clean.
  The patient should be directed to keep the forearm and wrist elevated and to move the fingers and shoulder several times during the day.
  The patient should see an orthopedist for a follow-up examination and definitive care of the fracture.
- Discharge or Admit as Inpatient
  A patient who has an isolated undisplaced olecranon fracture can be discharged home after application of a long arm posterior splint.
  All patients with displaced isolated olecranon fracture should have surgery in the same admission or electively as an outpatient on an urgent basis.
- Subsequent Management
  All patients with a displaced isolated olecranon fracture should have surgery in the same admission or electively as an outpatient on an urgent basis.
- Discharge Care and Instruction—Timing for Follow-up
  The patient should be directed to keep the splint dry and to elevate the upper extremity to minimize swelling. The patient should be encouraged to move the fingers and shoulder joint actively to prevent stiffness.
  If the patient is being treated nonoperatively, a follow-up examination with an orthopedic surgeon should be scheduled in 7 to 10 days.
  Follow-up for patients treated operatively is dictated by the operating surgeon.

## MONTEGGIA LESIONS

Dislocation of the proximal radioulnar joint in association with proximal forearm fracture is termed a *Monteggia* *lesion* or *Monteggia fracture*. These injuries are infrequent in adults and are challenging to manage.

### Anatomic Considerations

The proximal radioulnar joint is supported by two ligaments, the annular ligament and the quadrate ligament (see Fig. 10-16). The annular ligament wraps around the circumference of the radial head and is attached to the anterior and posterior margins of the lesser sigmoid notch. The quadrate ligament extends from the inferior margin of the lesser sigmoid notch to the neck of the proximal radius.

### Differential Diagnosis of Traumatic Complaints

- History
  Patients usually complain of pain, swelling, deformity, and inability to move the elbow after the injury.
  Other symptoms include paresthesia, numbness, and motor weakness in the distal forearm and hand.
- Mechanism of Injury
  Multiple mechanisms in the setting of high-energy and low-energy injuries have been described, which involve (1) extension and hyperpronation of the forearm, (2) blunt force on the posterior forearm, and (3) fall on the flexed elbow or outstretched arm.
- Timing
  Open fractures require immediate irrigation and débridement.
  The dislocated radial head should be immediately reduced by closed reduction. If reduction is successful, the final surgery can be performed within 7 to 10 days. If the radial head cannot be reduced, the patient will require emergent open reduction and internal fixation of the fracture and reduction of dislocation.
- Pain
  - Elbow pain
- Dysfunction
  - Limitation of elbow motion
- Prehospital care
  - RICE (rest, ice, compression, and elevation)
  - Splinting with long arm posterior splint minimizes further soft tissue and neurovascular injury and limits blood loss in open fractures
  - Pressure dressing if there are open bleeding wounds
- Physical Examination—Standard Focus Examination
  A complete primary and secondary survey should be performed.
  Signs to look for during physical examination include tenderness (along the proximal ulna and radius), ecchymosis (around the elbow), swelling, palpable radial head (anteriorly in the cubital fossa, posteriorly or laterally), and open wounds.
  Assess for painful limitation of elbow motion (flexion and extension and supination and pronation).
  Examination of the joint above and below should be performed to rule out associated injuries.

A complete vascular and neurologic examination should be performed and documented. If a complete neurologic examination cannot be performed in a patient because of altered sensorium (e.g., head injury, alcohol, drugs) or because of severe pain, it should be documented in the chart. The posterior interosseous nerve is the most common nerve injured in Monteggia fractures.

- Diagnostic Testing

A minimum of two orthogonal radiographic views of the elbow joint (anteroposterior and lateral) should be obtained.

A forearm posteroanterior and lateral view should be obtained.

- Fracture Classification

Bado's classification (Fig. 10-20 and Table 10-3) is the widely accepted classification system for Monteggia fractures. Bado classified these fractures based on the direction in which the radial head dislocates during this injury.

- Joint Aspiration and Injection

The elbow joint should be injected with 1% methylene blue (1:10 diluted with normal saline) if there is any suspicion of a surrounding wound communicating with the fracture site. Extravasation of the blue-colored fluid from the wound would confirm it as an open fracture, which is an orthopedic emergency and requires emergent irrigation and débridement (see Fig. 10-13).

**TABLE 10-3** Bado's Classification

| Fracture Type | Description |
|---|---|
| I | Fracture of the ulnar diaphysis at any level with anterior angulation at the fracture site and associated anterior dislocation of the radial head |
| II | Fracture of the ulnar diaphysis with posterior angulation at the fracture site and posterolateral dislocation of the radial head |
| III | Fracture of the ulnar metaphysis with lateral or anterolateral dislocation of the radial head |
| IV | Fracture of the proximal third of the radius and ulna at the same level with anterior dislocation of the radial head |

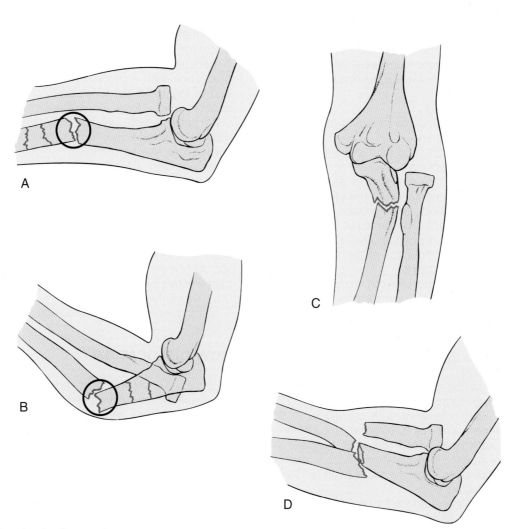

**FIGURE 10-20.** Bado's classification of Monteggia lesions. *(From Browner BD, Levine AM, Jupiter JB, et al: Skeletal trauma, ed 4, Philadelphia, 2009, Saunders.)*

Compartment pressure is measured if compartment syndrome is suspected in patients who are intubated or have altered level of consciousness.

Serum studies

No specific laboratory studies

## Treatment of Specific Injuries

■ Develop Plan
Nonoperative management in adults should be considered only if the medical health of the patient is a contraindication to surgery.

Monteggia fracture-dislocations are best managed with open reduction and internal fixation.

■ Discuss Alternative and Final Care Plan With Patient
The orthopedic surgeon should discuss the risks and benefits of operative treatment with the patient. The postoperative course including the weight-bearing status, duration of casting or splinting, physical therapy, time when the patient can start driving, and how long the patient will be out of work should be discussed with the patient.

■ When to Consult a Specialist
A bedside consultation with an orthopedist should be obtained for Monteggia fracture-dislocation.

■ How and What to Communicate With Specialist
• Patient age, gender, hand dominance, associated musculoskeletal and nonmusculoskeletal injuries
• Mechanism of injury—low-energy versus high-energy mechanism
• Open versus closed injury
• Physical examination findings including neurovascular status of the extremity
• X-ray description: orientation of fracture line (transverse, oblique); displaced versus nondisplaced; degree of comminution; direction of dislocation of the radial head and angulation of the ulna fracture

■ Analgesia, Anesthesia Block, and Sedation
Intravenous sedation and intra-articular injection of lidocaine aid in achieving good analgesia and muscle relaxation during closed reduction of the radial head.

■ Reduce or Accept Alignment
The radial head should be reduced early. Reduction is achieved by the combination of traction and supination of the forearm and direct gentle pressure on the radial head.

Inability to reduce the radial head is an indication for emergent operative treatment.

■ Splint or Immobilize
After reduction of the radial head, the arc of stability in flexion and extension should be assessed.

A posterior long arm splint with the elbow in 90 degrees of flexion and full supination is commonly used. If the radial head is unstable in 90 degrees of flexion (usually in posterior dislocations), a lesser degree of flexion is required to keep the radial head reduced.

■ Postreduction Imaging
At least two orthogonal radiographic views of the elbow joint (anteroposterior and lateral) should be obtained.

A reduced radial head would be aligned under the capitellum on the anteroposterior view of the elbow.

On a true lateral view of the elbow, the radiocapitellar line (drawn through the center of neck and head of the radius) should pass through the center of the capitellum.

■ Plan for Follow-up Care
In patients treated operatively by an orthopedic surgeon, follow-up is dictated by the operating surgeon.

Patients managed with successful closed reduction of the radial head should see an orthopedic specialist for a follow-up examination and elective definitive fracture care.

■ Outpatient Pain Relief Options
• Acetaminophen (Tylenol)
• Narcotic analgesic
• NSAIDs

■ Further Care Plan Discussion With Patient—How and What to Communicate With Patient
The injury and the different treatment options available with attendant risks and benefits should be discussed with the patient.

The patient should be advised to keep the splint dry and clean.

The patient should be directed to keep the forearm and wrist elevated. The patient should move the fingers and shoulder several times during the day.

The patient should see an orthopedist for a follow-up examination and definitive care of the fracture.

■ Discharge or Admit as Inpatient
A patient who has an isolated Monteggia fracture-dislocation with a successful closed and stable reduction of the radial head can be discharged home after application of a long arm posterior splint.

All patients with an open or unstable radial head dislocation should undergo emergency surgery.

■ Subsequent Management
A patient with a Monteggia fracture-dislocation with a successful closed and stable reduction of the radial head requires elective open reduction and internal fixation by an orthopedist.

■ Discharge Care and Instruction—Timing for Follow-up
A patient with a Monteggia fracture-dislocation with a successful closed and stable reduction of radial head should see an orthopedist in the follow-up period to plan elective surgery.

■ Common Pitfalls
• Missing a radial head dislocation

## ELBOW DISLOCATION

The elbow is the second most common joint to be dislocated. A fall on an outstretched hand and sports-related injury are the two most common causes of elbow dislocation.

### Anatomic Considerations

The elbow joint is a highly congruent hinge synovial joint. Stability is provided by bony and soft tissue structures. The coronoid, radial head, and anterior capsule constitute primary restraint to posterior displacement, and the

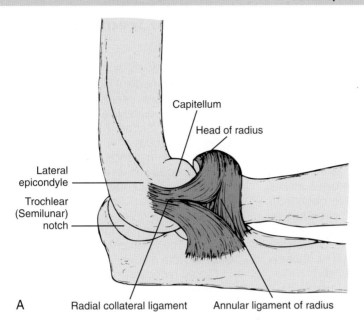

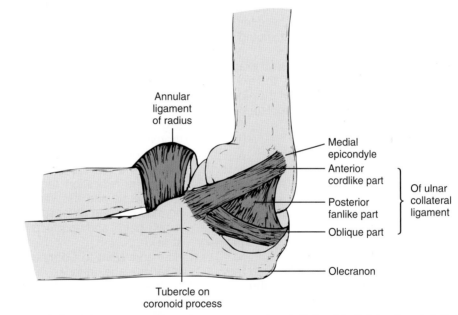

**FIGURE 10-21.** Ligament support of elbow. *(From Browner BD, Levine AM, MD, Jupiter JB, Trafton PG, Christian Krettek C. Skeletal trauma, ed 4, Philadelphia, 2009, Saunders.)*

olecranon process provides restraint to anterior translation. The medial collateral ligament is the primary restraint to valgus stress, and the radial head is a secondary restraint to valgus stress (Fig. 10-21). The lateral collateral ligament complex provides primary restraint to varus stress. The anteromedial part of the coronoid provides restraint to the varus stress.

## Differential Diagnosis of Traumatic Complaints

- History
  Pain, deformity, and inability to use the elbow after injury (most commonly a fall on an outstretched hand) are the most common presenting symptoms.

- Mechanism of Injury
  Two theories have been proposed for elbow dislocations.
  - Axial compression with elbow hyperextended leading to the olecranon impinging on the fossa and levering the proximal forearm out of the capsular constraints.
  - Axial loading of a flexed elbow in combination with a rotational force on the forearm
- Timing
  Elbow dislocation is an orthopedic emergency and mandates emergent reduction.
- Pain
  - In the elbow region
- Dysfunction
  - Inability to flex and extend elbow

- Prehospital Care
  - RICE (rest, ice, compression, and elevation)
  - Splinting with long arm posterior splint minimizes further soft tissue and neurovascular injury and limits blood loss in open fractures
  - Pressure dressing if there are open bleeding wounds
- Physical Examination—Standard Focus Examination
  A complete primary and secondary survey should be performed.

  Signs to look for during physical examination include tenderness, ecchymosis and swelling (around the elbow), deformity (prominent olecranon process makes this diagnosis clear before radiographs are obtained), open wounds, and painful limitation of elbow range of motion.

  The relationship between the tip of the olecranon, lateral epicondyle, and medial epicondyle is inverse (normally form a triangle with base proximally).

  Examine the joint above and below.

  A complete vascular and neurologic examination should be performed and documented. If a complete neurologic examination cannot be performed in a patient because of altered sensorium (e.g., head injury, alcohol, drugs) or because of severe pain, it should be documented in the chart.

  After closed reduction of the elbow, physical examination should be repeated and documented; this examination must include assessing the stability of the elbow joint in varying degrees of flexion and a complete neurovascular examination.
- Diagnostic Testing
  Imaging techniques include x-ray and CT scan.

  A minimum of two orthogonal radiographic views of the elbow joint (anteroposterior and lateral) should be obtained.

  Oblique views are helpful in diagnosing occult fractures.

  CT scan is indicated if there is associated intra-articular fracture or incongruent reduction.

  Elbow dislocations are classified as simple when they are not associated with fractures around the elbow.

  Complicated elbow dislocations have periarticular fractures.

  Based on the direction in which the forearm displaces with respect to the distal humerus, elbow dislocations are classified as posterior (subclassified as posterolateral or posteromedial), anterior, and divergent (Fig. 10-22). Posterior dislocations constitute more than 90% of dislocations, and posterolateral is the most common subtype.
- Joint Aspiration and Injection
  The elbow joint should be injected with 1% methylene blue (1 : 10 diluted with normal saline) if there is any suspicion of a surrounding wound communicating with the fracture site. Extravasation of the blue-colored fluid from the wound confirms it as an open fracture, which is an orthopedic emergency and requires emergent irrigation and débridement (see Fig. 10-13).

  Joint injection with lidocaine can provide almost complete relief of pain and render joint reduction easy and comfortable. A careful neurologic examination should be performed before injecting lidocaine.

## Treatment of Specific Injuries

- Develop Plan
  Elbow dislocation is an orthopedic emergency and mandates immediate closed reduction. Clinically apparent dislocations can have a hematoma/arthro block placed immediately after documentation of distal sensory examination. Many patients allow gentle relocation techniques after this block is placed. The authors generally try to relocate the elbow immediately when clinically apparent, even before obtaining plain radiographs, to reduce the patient's discomfort and risk to neurovascular structures.

  Open elbow dislocations, unstable fracture patterns, or compartment syndrome requires operative intervention. The open dislocation should be reduced while awaiting the availability of a operating room.

  Closed reduction can be achieved by techniques performed in the prone position (Fig. 10-23) and in the supine position (Fig. 10-24).
- Discuss Alternative and Final Care Plan With Patient
  The patient should be informed that if closed reduction fails, open reduction would be required to reduce the dislocation.
- When to Consult a Specialist
  A bedside consultation should be obtained with an orthopedist for complex elbow dislocations that cannot be reduced, simple dislocations that cannot be reduced (rare), and complicated elbow dislocations (e.g., open, neurovascular deficit, compartment syndrome). Delaying reduction attempts for any reason for a prolonged period results in unnecessary discomfort to the patient and risk to neurovascular structures. The relocation technique is easy, requires very little energy, and has very little risk. An anatomically normal, reduced dislocation of the elbow nearly eliminates pain and protects neurovascular structures at risk.
- How and What to Communicate With Specialist
  - Patient age, gender, hand dominance, associated other musculoskeletal and nonmusculoskeletal injuries
  - Mechanism of injury—low-energy versus high-energy mechanism
  - Duration of injury, presence of compartment syndrome
  - Open versus closed injury
  - Physical examination findings including neurovascular status of the extremity
  - X-ray description: type of dislocation (anterior, posterior or divergent), associated fractures
- Analgesia, Anesthesia Block, and Sedation
  Arthro/hematoma block has been generally adequate for elbow reductions in the emergency department.

  Conscious sedation is indicated to provide adequate muscle relaxation and analgesia if arthroblock is insufficient.
- Reduce or Accept Alignment
  The elbow joint (ulnohumeral and radiocapitellar) should be concentric and symmetric after the reduction. Nonconcentric reduction is usually due to soft tissue interposition or chondral fragments. Patients

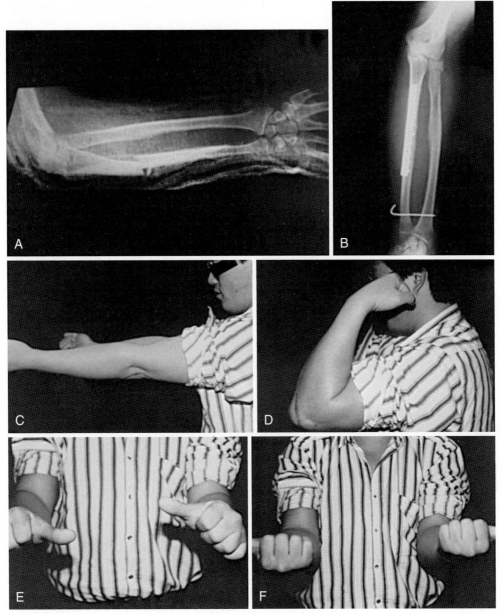

**FIGURE 10-22.** Elbow dislocations are classified as posterior (subclassified as posterolateral or posteromedial), anterior, and divergent. *(From Browner BD, Levine AM, Jupiter JB, et al: Skeletal trauma, ed 4, Philadelphia, 2009, Saunders.)*

complain of persisting limitations of range of motion and pressure in the joint.
■ Splint or Immobilize
Apply a posterior long arm splint in flexion.
■ Postreduction Imaging
Two orthogonal radiographic views of the elbow joint (anteroposterior and lateral) should be obtained and assessed for congruent of reduction and presence of fractures.
■ Plan for Follow-up Care
After open or closed reduction of dislocation, patients should see an orthopedist for a follow-up examination and referral to a physical therapist.
■ Outpatient Pain Relief Options
  • Acetaminophen (Tylenol)
  • Narcotic analgesic
  • NSAIDs

■ Further Care Plan Discussion With Patient—How and What to Communicate With Patient
The injury, the different treatment options available with attendant risks and benefits, complications, and future prognosis should be discussed with the patient. Patients should be warned about the risk of elbow stiffness, elbow instability, myositis ossificans and chronic elbow pain, and osteoarthritis.
Patients should be informed about the symptoms and signs of compartment syndrome and that they should return immediately to the emergency department if any of the symptoms are present.
The patient should be advised to keep the splint dry and clean.
The patient should be directed to keep the forearm and wrist elevated. The patient should move the fingers and shoulder several times during the day.

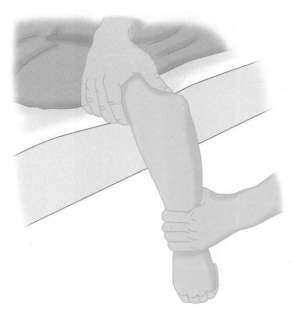

**FIGURE 10-23.** Reduction of elbow dislocation in prone position: one-person technique (**A** and **B**) and two-person technique (**C**).

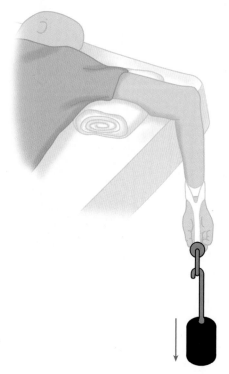

**FIGURE 10-24.** Reduction of elbow dislocation in the supine position.

The patient should see an orthopedist for a follow-up examination definitive management.

■ Discharge or Admit as Inpatient
Patients with isolated simple dislocations without significant swelling can be discharged home, provided that they understand the symptoms of compartment syndrome and have an adult with them at home for next few days.

---

**Box 10-1 Common Causes of Lateral Elbow Pain**

1. Lateral epicondylitis
2. Radial tunnel syndrome
3. Radiocapitellar osteochondrosis
4. Posterolateral elbow plica
5. Posterolateral elbow instability
6. Cervical radiculopathy (C5-6)

Patients with open elbow dislocations, vascular injury, multiple attempts at closed reduction, open reduction, or any suspicion of compartment syndrome should be admitted.
■ Subsequent Management
Patients with elbow dislocations have high risk for elbow stiffness and should be immobilized for a short period only (<3 weeks).
Patients with associated fractures or an unstable elbow may require surgery.
■ Discharge Care and Instruction—Timing for Follow-up
Patients should see an orthopedist in less than 1 week to formulate the plan for physical therapy and rehabilitation.

## SUPRACONDYLAR HUMERUS FRACTURES

Supracondylar humerus fractures are the most common elbow fractures in children. Children 5 to 7 years old are most commonly affected. This injury is discussed in detail in Chapter 21.

## SOFT TISSUE INJURIES—ANNULAR RADIAL LIGAMENT DISPLACEMENT

Displacement of the annular ligament into the radio-capitellar space is also termed *nursemaid's elbow, pulled elbow,* or *radial head subluxation.* It is a common childhood condition seen in children 1 to 4 years old. This injury is discussed in detail in Chapter 21.

## PAINFUL ATRAUMATIC ELBOW

### Differential Diagnosis of Traumatic Complaints

An infective or inflammatory etiology of elbow pain is the most common nontraumatic cause of elbow pain. An infective etiology should always be ruled out during the work-up of elbow pain of atraumatic etiology. The source of pain in and around the elbow can be localized to distinct anatomic structures with a thorough history and physical examination. Pain radiating from other anatomic regions such as the neck, shoulder, and wrist should also be in the differential diagnosis of elbow pain (Boxes 10-1 through 10-4).

1. Medial epicondylitis
2. Ulnar neuritis
3. Cervical radiculopathy (C7-8)
4. Ulnar collateral ligament instability

### Box 10-3 Common Causes of Posterior Elbow Pain

1. Olecranon bursitis
2. Crystal arthropathy
3. Triceps tendinitis

### Box 10-4 Common Causes of Painful, Hot, and Swollen Elbow

- Septic arthritis—unless proved otherwise
- Inflammatory—rheumatoid arthritis, Reiter syndrome, ankylosing spondyloarthropathy
- Crystal arthropathy—gout, CPPD, pseudogout
- Neoplastic—synovial osteochondromatosis, pigmented villonodular synovitis, metastatic lesion
- Subcutaneous abscess—diabetic, intravenous drug user
- Cellulitis

*CPPD,* Calcium pyrophosphate dihydrate deposition.

- History
  - Elbow pain, swelling, and limitation of motion without any history of trauma
- Preexisting Illness
  - Chronic medical conditions (e.g., diabetes, chronic renal failure, liver failure, terminal illness)
  - Rheumatologic disease (e.g., rheumatoid arthritis, systemic lupus erythematosus)
  - Immunosuppressive drugs (e.g., chemotherapy, steroids)
  - Immunosuppressive states (e.g., acquired immunodeficiency syndrome [AIDS])
  - Intravenous drug use
  - Sexually transmitted disease (e.g., gonorrhea)
  - Total elbow arthroplasty
- Pain
  - Elbow pain, especially pain with range of motion
- Dysfunction
  - Reduced ability to move the elbow
- Prehospital Care
  - RICE (rest, ice, compression, and elevation)
- Physical Examination—Standard Focus Examination
  Signs to look for during physical examination include tenderness, old scars, open or draining wounds, fullness in the paraolecranon region, ecchymosis (around

the elbow), palpable fibrous cord in subcutaneous tissue, or injection marks from intravenous drug use.

Painful limitation of the elbow motion (flexion and extension and supination and pronation) is a very sensitive sign for intra-articular pathology.

Painful swelling over the olecranon bursa without significant elbow range of motion pain indicates bursitis without intra-articular pathology.

A complete vascular and neurologic examination should be performed and documented.

Examination of the joint above and below and other joints in the body should be performed to rule out polyarticular involvement.

- Diagnostic Testing
  Imaging techniques include x-ray, ultrasound, CT scan, and magnetic resonance imaging (MRI).

  At least two orthogonal radiographic views of the elbow joint (anteroposterior and lateral) should be obtained.

  Ultrasound is useful in diagnosing infection in a chronically deformed or inflamed joint.

  CT scan and MRI are more sensitive for imaging of suspected periarticular abscess or osteomyelitis.
- Joint Aspiration and Injection
  Aspiration of the elbow is the most definitive procedure to establish the diagnosis of intra-articular pathology (see Fig. 10-13).

  Compartment pressure should be measured if clinically indicated.

  There are no serum studies that can prove or disprove the presence of a serious intra-articular process.

  Erythrocyte sedimentation rate, C-reactive protein, and complete blood count with differential (infective etiology has a high erythrocyte sedimentation rate or C-reactive protein and elevated white blood cell count with a left shift; cell counts >50,000/mm$^3$ are highly suggestive of infection) should be performed.

  Blood culture

  Lyme disease serology

  Screening for rheumatic diseases (rheumatoid factor, antinuclear antibody, serum uric acid)

  Fluid analysis is the most sensitive and specific test for most serious causes of acute atraumatic arthritis and should include gross inspection, string test, cell count, Gram stain, culture (aerobic, anaerobic, fungal, mycobacterial), polarized microscopy for crystals, protein, and glucose.

## Treatment of Specific Injuries

- Develop Plan
  Septic arthritis can be treated with emergent elbow arthrotomy and irrigation and débridement, or serial aspiration with close observation can be considered.

  Infected olecranon bursitis can be treated with bedside aspiration or incision and drainage.

  Noninfected elbow bursitis can be treated with rest, elevation, and NSAIDs.

  Options for treatment of gout include NSAIDs, colchicine, and corticosteroids. Colchicine is most effective in the first 24 to 48 hours.

■ Discuss Alternative and Final Care Plan With Patient
Infective processes may require prolonged antibiotic treatment.

Long-term sequelae of septic arthritis include arthritis, chronic infection, and stiffness.

■ When to Consult a Specialist
Bedside consultation

A bedside consultation with an orthopedist should be obtained for a patient with suspected elbow septic arthritis and other infective elbow pathology that may require urgent operative irrigation.

A telephone consultation or final follow-up examination with a rheumatologist is recommended for a patient with a suspected inflammatory, noninfective etiology of elbow pain.

■ How and What to Communicate With Specialist
  • Physical examination findings including the limitation of range of motion and neurovascular examination
  • X-ray description: periarticular effusion, fat pad sign, foreign body (needle tips) pseudogout deposits in the joint capsule, osteoarthritis
  • Patient age, hand dominance, presence of elbow arthroplasty

■ Splint or Immobilize
Apply an arm sling for comfort.

■ Outpatient Pain Relief Options
  • Acetaminophen (Tylenol) and NSAIDs for elbow pain of noninfective etiology
  • Oral antibiotics
  • Patients with inflammatory arthritis can use NSAIDs.
  • If the patient has renal insufficiency or severe pain, oral narcotics can be considered for pain control.

■ Further Care Plan Discussion With Patient—How and What to Communicate With Patient
Septic arthritis and significant infected olecranon bursitis require admission and surgical drainage. Infective processes require antibiotics (intravenous and oral).

Long-term sequelae of septic arthritis (arthritis, chronic infection, stiffness) should be explained to the patient.

■ Discharge or Admit as Inpatient
Patients with septic arthritis of the elbow should be admitted.

Patients with infective olecranon bursitis should be admitted or have close follow-up.

■ Subsequent Management
  • Septic arthritis—elbow arthrotomy (open or arthroscopic) and irrigation and débridement
  • Infective olecranon bursa—incision and drainage

■ Discharge Care and Instruction—Timing for Follow-up
For patients with septic arthritis and infected olecranon bursitis, follow-up is dictated by the operating surgeon.

Patients with a noninfectious etiology can be discharged home with pain control, rest, and follow-up with the patient's primary physician.

## Bibliography

Colton CL: Fractures of the olecranon in adults: classification and management. Injury 5:121–129, 1973.

Eathiraju S, Mudgal CS, Jupiter JB: Monteggia fracture-dislocation. Hand Clin 23:165–177, 2007.

Ekholm R, Ponzer S, Törnkvist H, et al: The Holstein-Lewis humeral shaft fracture: aspects of radial nerve injury, primary treatment, and outcome. J Orthop Trauma 22:693–697, 2008.

Galano GJ, Ahmad CS, Levine WN: Current treatment strategies for bicolumnar distal humerus fractures. J Am Acad Orthop Surg 18:20–30, 2010.

Keith MP, Gilliland WR: Updates in the management of gout. Am J Med 120:221–224, 2007.

Kuhn MA, Ross G: Acute elbow dislocations. Orthop Clin North Am 39:155–161, 2008.

Li SF, Cassidy C, Chang C, et al: Diagnostic utility of laboratory tests in septic arthritis. Emerg Med J 24:75–77, 2007.

Margaretten ME, Kohlwes J, Moore D, et al: Does this adult patient have septic arthritis? JAMA 297:1478–1488, 2007.

Martin BD, Johansen JA, Edwards SG: Complications related to simple dislocations of elbow. Hand Clin 24:9–25, 2008.

Mason ML: Some observations on fractures of the head of the radius with a review of one hundred cases. Br J Surg 42:123–132, 1954.

Mathews CJ, Coakley G: Septic arthritis: current diagnostic and therapeutic algorithm. Curr Opin Rheumatol 20:457–462, 2008.

Mckee MD, Jupiter JD: Trauma to the adult elbow and fractures to the distal humerus. In Browner BD, editor: Skeletal trauma, ed 4, Philadelphia, 2008, Saunders.

Newman SD, Mauffrey C, Krikler S: Olecranon fractures. Injury 40:575–581, 2009.

Nork SE, Jones CB, Henley MB: Surgical treatment of olecranon fractures. Am J Orthop 30:577–586, 2001.

Pollock JW, Faber KJ, Athwal GS: Distal humerus fractures. Orthop Clin North Am 39:187–200, 2008.

Rosenblatt Y, Athwal GS, Faber KJ: Current recommendations for the treatment of radial head fractures. Orthop Clin North Am 39:173–185, 2008.

Sarmiento A, Zagorski JB, Zych GA, et al: Functional bracing for the treatment of fractures of the humeral diaphysis. J Bone Joint Surg Am 82:478–486, 2000.

Shao YC, Harwood P, Grotz MR, et al: Radial nerve palsy associated with fractures of the shaft of the humerus: a systematic review. J Bone Joint Surg Br 87:1647–1652, 2005.

Sotereanos DG, Darlis NA, Wright TW, et al: Unstable fracture dislocation of the elbow. Instr Course Lect 56:369–376, 2007.

Tejwani NC, Mehta H: Fractures of the radial head and neck: current concepts in management. J Am Acad Orthop Surg 15:380–387, 2007.

Veillette CJ, Steinmann SP: Olecranon fractures. Orthop Clin North Am 39:229–236, 2008.

# Chapter 11

# Wrist and Forearm

Craig M. Rodner, Adam Fleit,
and John Grady

## CARPAL FRACTURES AND CARPAL INSTABILITY

### Scaphoid Fractures

■ Anatomy
The scaphoid resides in the proximal carpal row at its radialmost extent articulating with the radius, lunate, capitate, and trapezium. It plays a key role in wrist biomechanics, serving as a link between the proximal and distal carpal rows and preventing excessive wrist extension. The proximal pole of the scaphoid is almost completely covered in cartilage with a negligible direct blood supply. The two major nutrient arteries, the dorsal and volar scaphoid arteries, enter the bone at its distal pole and branch proximally (Fig. 11-1). This retrograde blood supply results in a propensity for nonunions to develop with fractures of the middle and proximal aspects of the scaphoid, particularly when they are displaced.

■ Mechanism of Injury
Scaphoid fractures are traumatic injuries that can occur after a high-energy fall onto an outstretched hand. During impact, the individual's arm is usually in a pronated and extended position. The thenar aspect of the hand makes impact with the ground, leading to the scaphoid fracture. The mechanism of many scaphoid fractures lies in dorsal compression of the scaphoid by the radius and volar compression of the scaphoid by the ground. These forces place a significant amount of tension on the scaphoid, leading to fracture. Stress fractures of the scaphoid can be seen in individuals who place repetitive stress on the bone, such as gymnasts.

In many situations, patients do not experience significant pain and dysfunction after the fracture, so they do not immediately seek clinical care. These patients believe they experienced a "wrist sprain" that will resolve on its own. Other patients with higher energy mechanisms have significant pain and swelling in the thenar area that is more suspicious of a fracture.

The management of scaphoid fractures varies depending on the location of the fracture and the mechanism of the fracture, so it is very important to elicit a thorough history in all patients with pain around the hand and wrist. Because of the negative impact on wrist mechanics from a scaphoid fracture nonunion, identification of these injuries is very important in any patient who presents with traumatic wrist pain so that appropriate care can be administered. Compartment syndrome can rarely occur in association with scaphoid fractures (owing to severe localized swelling), so patients should be assessed for pain with passive extension of the fingers and the strength of their pulses, and compartment pressure should be determined if necessary.

■ Physical Examination
Physical examination should start with inspection of the affected areas looking for tenderness, ecchymosis, abrasions, and edema. A thorough neurovascular examination is essential. Palpation of all bones of the affected limb can help to identify fractures.

Some patients with scaphoid fractures can have obvious swelling around the radial aspect of the wrist. However, swelling is not a reliable physical examination finding. The scaphoid can be easily palpated in the floor of the anatomic snuffbox between the extensor pollicis longus and brevis at the level of the wrist joint. Also, the scaphoid tubercle, located on the volar aspect of the radial proximal wrist, is a reliable landmark to elicit pain specific to scaphoid injury.

■ Clinical Testing for Scaphoid Fracture
  • Anatomic snuffbox tenderness
  • Scaphoid tubercle tenderness
  • Pain with longitudinal compression of the thumb
■ Diagnostic Testing
  • Four-view scaphoid series
  Given the high degree of variation in the initial presentation of scaphoid fractures and the unreliability of

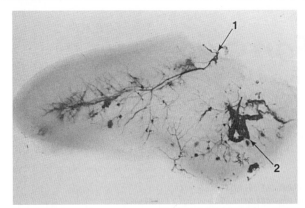

**FIGURE 11-1.** Sagittal section of the scaphoid with the proximal pole oriented to the left. *1,* Dorsal scaphoid branch of the radial artery; *2,* volar scaphoid arterial branch. *(From Gelberman RH, Menon J: The vascularity of the scaphoid bone. J Hand Surg Am 5:508–513, 1980.)*

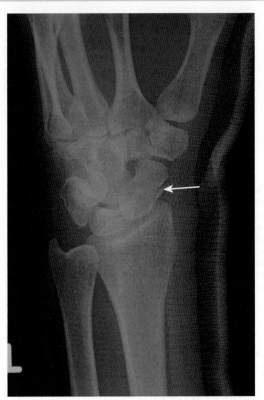

**FIGURE 11-2.** Oblique radiograph of an obvious displaced fracture of the scaphoid waist.

individual clinical examination findings, radiography is very important in making the diagnosis of a scaphoid fracture. At least four radiographic views should be obtained in all patients with a suspected scaphoid fracture: a posteroanterior view of the wrist (the hand should be in a fist to improve visualization of the scaphoid), a true lateral view of the wrist, an ulnar oblique view in which the wrist is semipronated and held in ulnar deviation, and a radial oblique view. The same set of radiographs can be performed on the nonaffected hand so that necessary comparisons can be made if the diagnosis of a scaphoid fracture is in question. Additional views can be obtained as necessary, but most scaphoid fractures can be seen with the combination of the above-mentioned four radiographs. Although the diagnosis of an acute scaphoid fracture may be obvious on a single view if the fracture is displaced (Fig. 11-2), sometimes additional projections, such as a posteroanterior ulnar deviation view, are required to elucidate more subtle fracture lines (Fig. 11-3).

Scaphoid fractures are usually visualized as a clear line but can sometimes appear opaque if segments of bone overlie each other. Fractures of the distal pole and tubercle and small, incomplete fractures of the scaphoid can be difficult to detect on radiographs. Angulated fractures of the scaphoid are particularly dangerous because they have a high incidence of poor healing, with the consequent development of nonunion, malunion, and osteoarthritis.

Finally, given the vague history often described by patients with scaphoid fractures, it is important to differentiate radiographically between acute fractures and chronic fractures that have gone on to nonunion. These two entities have distinct radiographic features. An acute fracture has a single clear fracture line in the scaphoid, as noted previously. However, in a scaphoid with nonunion, one sees bony resorption at the fracture site (Fig. 11-4) and possibly the development of degenerative changes at the radioscaphoid articulation (Fig. 11-5).

Often, the history and physical examination suggest a scaphoid fracture, but x-rays do not reveal any

scaphoid pathology. In this situation, the clinician should protect the injured wrist with a thumb spica splint or cast and repeat plain radiographs in 2 weeks. Alternatively, the clinician could use other imaging modalities, including magnetic resonance imaging (MRI) and computed tomography (CT) scans. MRI can be performed 48 hours after the acute injury to identify occult fractures. CT scan is useful for operative planning.

■ Treatment

All patients with a suspected scaphoid fracture should be placed in a thumb spica splint or cast. The interphalangeal joint of the thumb may be left free, but the thumb metacarpophalangeal (MCP), carpometacarpal, and wrist joints all should be included. Whether to extend the splint or cast proximally to immobilize the elbow joint is a matter of debate. In patients who have only clinical snuffbox tenderness and no radiographic evidence of a scaphoid fracture, a short-arm thumb spica splint or cast is sufficient. However, the most conservative approach in the emergency department in patients who have an obvious fracture of the scaphoid waist or proximal pole on x-ray is to immobilize the elbow, although clinical data supporting this practice are mixed. Most patients with scaphoid fractures are treated as outpatients, with follow-up within 2 weeks with an orthopedic surgeon to discuss surgical and nonsurgical treatment options.

In all cases, the patient should leave the emergency department with the scaphoid fracture immobilized with a splint in as close to a reduced position as possible

shortened owing to its flexed posture relative to the rest of the proximal carpal row. The "cortical ring" or "signet ring" sign, referring to the dense, circular cortex of the scaphoid tubercle, which is made more prominent as the scaphoid assumes a flexed position, can be seen on anteroposterior or posteroanterior radiographs. This foreshortened posture of the scaphoid produces more of an end-on view of the scaphoid tubercle than normal (Fig. 11-9). A distance of less than 7 mm from this cortical ring to the proximal pole of the scaphoid is indicative of scapholunate instability. On the lateral radiograph, the scapholunate angle can be determined by the intersection of the longitudinal axes of the scaphoid and lunate (Fig. 11-10). Normally, this angle is between 30 degrees and 60 degrees.

When the scapholunate ligamentous complex is rendered incompetent, the scapholunate angle increases as the lunate assumes an extended position relative to the scaphoid, which has a tendency to flex. A scapholunate angle greater than 60 degrees is consistent with a DISI pattern and suggestive of scapholunate dissociation (Fig. 11-11).

■ Treatment

Patients with acute SLIL injury can be placed in a removable wrist splint for comfort. Patients should have follow-up arranged with a wrist specialist so that appropriate care can be administered. Pain can be managed after emergency department discharge, in patients for whom such medications are not contraindicated, with analgesics and, if warranted, with combination products, such as hydrocodone with acetaminophen. Active motion of the uninjured digits should be encouraged.

### Midcarpal Dislocations

■ Anatomy

The carpal bones are bound together by two sets of ligaments: the intrinsic carpal ligaments and the extrinsic carpal ligaments. The intrinsic carpal ligaments connect the carpal bones to each other, whereas the extrinsic carpal ligaments connect the carpal bones to the radius and ulna proximally and the metacarpals distally. In midcarpal dislocations, a substantial amount of ligamentous damage occurs, enabling dislocation of the carpus.

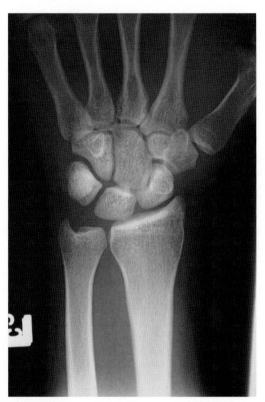

**FIGURE 11-9.** "Cortical ring" or "signet ring" sign refers to the end-on view of the scaphoid tubercle as the scaphoid assumes a flexed, foreshortened posture relative to the rest of the proximal carpal row.

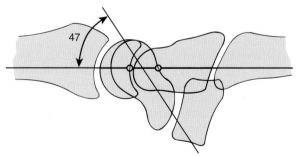

**FIGURE 11-10.** Normal scapholunate angle as represented in the original drawings from Linscheid et al. *(From Linscheid RL, Dobyns JH, Beabout JW, et al. Traumatic instability of the wrist. J Bone Joint Surg Am 54:1612–1632, 1972.)*

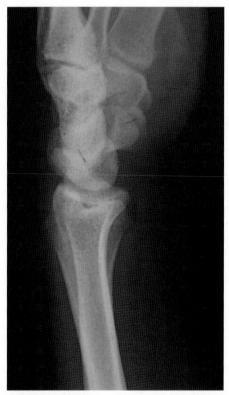

**FIGURE 11-11.** Scapholunate angle of greater than 60 degrees on a lateral radiograph is indicative of scapholunate dissociation and a DISI pattern.

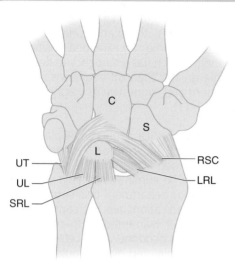

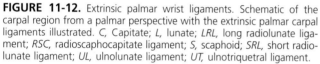

**FIGURE 11-12.** Extrinsic palmar wrist ligaments. Schematic of the carpal region from a palmar perspective with the extrinsic palmar carpal ligaments illustrated. *C,* Capitate; *L,* lunate; *LRL,* long radiolunate ligament; *RSC,* radioscaphocapitate ligament; *S,* scaphoid; *SRL,* short radiolunate ligament; *UL,* ulnolunate ligament; *UT,* ulnotriquetral ligament.

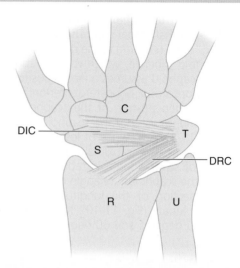

**FIGURE 11-13.** Extrinsic dorsal wrist ligaments. Schematic of the carpal region from a dorsal perspective with the extrinsic dorsal carpal ligaments illustrated. *C,* Capitate; *DIC,* dorsal intercarpal ligament; *DRC,* dorsal radiocarpal ligament; *R,* radius; *S,* scaphoid; *T,* triquetrum; *U,* ulna.

The most important and frequently injured intrinsic ligaments are the scapholunate and lunotriquetral ligaments. Each ligament has a dorsal and a volar component. The dorsal portion of the SLIL is stronger than the volar portion. The converse is true of the lunotriquetral ligament with the volar segment being the stronger of the two.

The palmar (or volar) extrinsic wrist ligaments include the radioscaphocapitate, short radiolunate, and long radiolunate ligaments (Fig. 11-12). These ligaments connect and stabilize the radiocarpal joint palmarly. Maintaining the ulna in its typical relationship to the carpus are the ulnotriquetral and ulnolunate ligaments. Important dorsal extrinsic ligaments are the dorsal radiocarpal and dorsal intercarpal ligaments (Fig. 11-13).

■ Mechanism of Injury

Midcarpal dislocations are injuries that occur secondary to high-energy trauma, such as falling from a great height or a motor vehicle accident. The history usually involves a young person who sustains a high-energy fall in which an axial load is applied to a hyperextended, ulnarly deviated wrist. With this mechanism, the capitate is driven dorsally, while the lunate remains located within the lunate fossa of the radius, creating a midcarpal, or perilunate, dislocation (Fig. 11-14). Alternatively, the patient can have a flexed wrist at the time of injury resulting in anterior displacement of the carpus in relation to the lunate, described as a volarly displaced perilunate dislocation. If the scaphoid remains in articulation with the radius, shear forces can cause it to fracture, leading to a trans-scaphoid perilunate dislocation, which is the most common type of carpal fracture-dislocation. Occasionally, the distal carpal row snaps back into place after the fall, and the lunate is forced anteriorly into the carpal tunnel. This injury

pattern results in a lunate seemingly floating in the volar soft tissues of the wrist on a lateral x-ray and is termed a lunate dislocation.

The key in early management of these injuries is prompt recognition. Perilunate dislocations are easily missed on initial x-rays. Late treatment of a dislocation usually results in a more difficult treatment and a much less successful outcome. As with any dislocated joint, treatment outcomes are optimized with acute reduction and potentially operative stabilization to maintain the reduction.

■ Physical Examination

Findings on physical examination of these injuries include wrist edema, deformity, ecchymosis, and pain with palpation or motion of the carpus. Identification of open wounds is important. A sensory and motor examination of the hand should also be performed. For carpal dislocations, compartment syndrome manifests early on as acute carpal tunnel syndrome; this is especially true of volar lunate dislocations. The patient has decreased sensation in the median nerve distribution of the hand and excruciating pain. Persistence of severe pain despite reduction and immobilization differentiates the symptoms of acute carpal tunnel syndrome from the initial wrist trauma.

Often patients with these types of injuries have sustained a high-energy trauma, which can complicate the physical examination. Distracting and more impressive injuries can take the focus of the patient and health care provider away from other small bone injuries. Swelling or ecchymosis around the wrist in a patient with a high-energy trauma and distracting injuries should prompt x-ray investigation.

■ Diagnostic Testing

Radiographic examination is essential for diagnosis of midcarpal dislocation. Posteroanterior, lateral, and

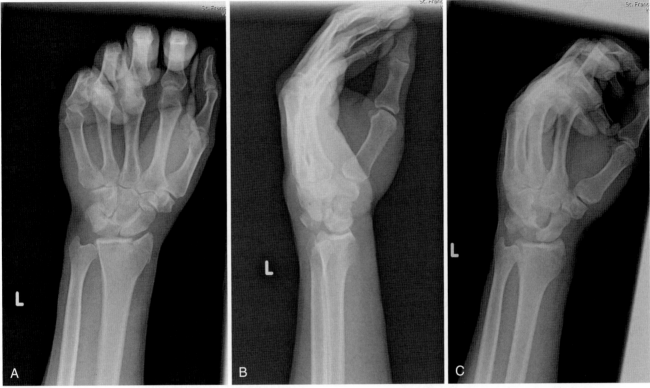

**FIGURE 11-14.** Posteroanterior **(A),** lateral **(B),** and oblique **(C)** plain radiographs of a midcarpal dislocation show the capitate lying dorsal to the lunate on the lateral projection. An intra-articular radial styloid fracture is also present.

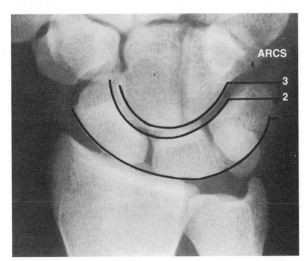

**FIGURE 11-15.** In a normal wrist, three smooth arcs can be drawn on an anteroposterior or posteroanterior radiograph. If there is a break in any of these lines, an intracarpal malalignment should be suspected. *(From Bellinghausen HW, Gilula LA, Young LV, et al: Posttraumatic palmar carpal subluxation: report of two cases. J Bone Joint Surg Am 65:999, 1983.)*

oblique wrist x-rays are necessary. A normal posteroanterior view of the wrist allows for assessment of three arcs, termed Gilula lines, which can be superimposed on the proximal and distal carpal rows (Fig. 11-15). In midcarpal dislocations, these normally smooth lines are interrupted. The shape of the lunate can also be assessed on posteroanterior views of the wrist. Normally, the lunate appears quadrilateral in shape, but the lunate is rotated in perilunate dislocations and may appear more triangular.

Lateral views of the wrist are important for differentiating between lunate dislocation and perilunate dislocation. In a perilunate dislocation, the capitate and distal carpal row is usually displaced dorsally (less commonly, it may be volar), while the lunate remains in articulation with the radius. In a dislocation of the lunate, the distal carpal row sits in its normal position, while the lunate is shifted volarly. Normally, the lunate articulates with the head of the capitate, but this articulation is disrupted in perilunate and lunate dislocations owing to volar rotation of the lunate.

Although CT scan is rarely needed in the emergency department setting for these injuries, when the clinician is unsure of the midcarpal alignment after radiographic examination, advanced imaging studies can be obtained to confirm congruity.

■ Treatment

After recognition of a midcarpal dislocation, closed reduction should be attempted. Before any attempt at closed reduction, it is helpful to apply 10 minutes of continuous axial traction via finger traps. Often conscious sedation is needed, but occasionally an effective hematoma block can provide adequate analgesia to allow for manipulation. For dorsal perilunate and lunate dislocations, a similar reduction maneuver is performed. The arm is suspended from finger traps, and 10 lb of traction is applied to the limb, which allows for relaxation of the forearm musculature. After approximately 10 minutes of traction time, the reduction maneuver can be performed. The elbow is placed at 90 degrees. An assistant may apply countertraction by pushing down on the anterior aspect of the arm. With the wrist slightly extended, gentle axial traction is placed on the wrist (Fig. 11-16). Without releasing this traction and with the lunate stabilized volarly by the practitioner's thumb, the wrist is flexed to bring the capitate back into its anatomic articulation with the lunate. A snap may indicate that the proximal pole of the capitate has overcome the dorsal rim of the lunate, at which point traction can be released and the wrist brought back to neutral. A similar procedure, albeit reversed, should be

performed for volarly displaced perilunate dislocations. The patient should be placed in a sugar-tong splint after reduction. If the closed reduction is unsuccessful, open reduction is necessary as soon as possible.

In all cases of midcarpal dislocation, the patient should leave the emergency department only after his or her wrist has been reduced and splinted, with post-reduction radiographs confirming adequate intercarpal alignment. Pain can be managed after emergency department discharge, in patients for whom such medications are not contraindicated, with analgesics and, if warranted, with combination products, such as hydrocodone with acetaminophen. Active motion of the uninjured digits should be encouraged.

## COMPARTMENT SYNDROME

- Anatomy
  There are three distinct compartments in the forearm: the volar compartment, the dorsal compartment and the mobile wad (Fig. 11-17). The hand contains 10 compartments: thenar compartment, hypothenar compartment, four dorsal interosseous compartments, three volar interosseous compartments, and adductor compartment (Fig. 11-18). An unyielding fascial sleeve surrounds each compartment.

  Compartment syndrome may occur when an inflammatory response to an injury causes high intracompartmental pressure to develop. This increased pressure leads to a reduction in venous outflow, increased tissue pressure, more tissue damage, and ultimately an interruption in arterial blood flow. As a result, tissues with a high oxygen requirement, such as skeletal muscle, become ischemic, and necrosis eventually ensues. Nerves that course through the compartment are also susceptible to injury secondary to interruption in blood flow and pressure. The outcome is a limb with significant and sometimes complete loss of function.

- Mechanism of Injury
  Compartment syndrome can develop as a consequence of distal radius fractures, diaphyseal forearm

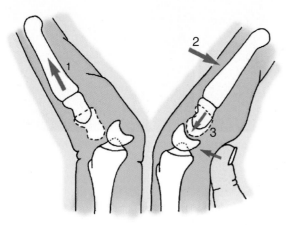

**FIGURE 11-16.** Schematic representation of the reduction maneuver for dorsal perilunate dislocations. Before any closed reduction attempt, it is helpful to apply 10 minutes of continuous axial traction via finger traps. *1,* With the wrist slightly extended, gentle manual traction is applied. *2,* Without releasing this traction, and with the lunate stabilized volarly by the practitioner's thumb, the wrist is flexed. If a snap occurs, this might indicate that the proximal pole of the capitate has overcome the dorsal rim of the lunate. *3,* At this juncture, traction is released, and the wrist is brought back to a neutral position. *(From Wolfe SW, Hotchkiss RN, Pederson WC, et al, editors: Green's operative hand surgery, ed 6, Philadelphia, 2011, Churchill Livingstone.)*

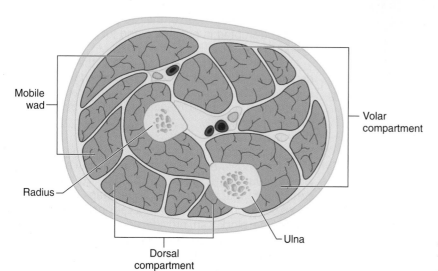

**FIGURE 11-17.** Cross section through the upper third of the forearm. The three compartments of the forearm, in contrast to the compartments of the leg, are interconnected.

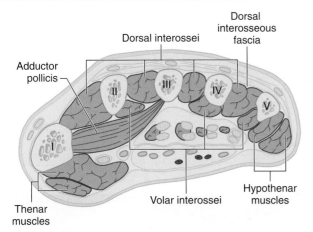

**FIGURE 11-18.** Cross section through the palm shows the 10 compartments of the hand.

Labels on figure: Dorsal interossei, Dorsal interosseous fascia, Adductor pollicis, Hypothenar muscles, Volar interossei, Thenar muscles

fractures, or soft tissue crush injuries. Several rarer conditions are also associated with compartment syndrome, including injection injuries, bites, lower velocity gunshot wounds, toxic shock syndrome, leukemic infiltration, viral myositis, arthroscopic infusion of fluid into a joint space, and nephrotic syndrome. An open fracture does not eliminate the risk of compartment syndrome developing. In patients with compartment syndrome, it is crucial that clinicians make the diagnosis as early as possible. Delayed diagnosis may lead to severe complications, including permanent loss of motor and sensory function of the extremity. The most reliable indicator of compartment syndrome is pain. Patients classically experience pain that is constant and severe. In lower energy injuries, the pain may seem out of proportion to the injury. Nerve dysfunction in the affected compartment may lead to paresthetic pain such as burning, numbness, and tingling, which can progress to hypoesthesia. In patients with fractures, pain persists and worsens despite reduction and immobilization. When compartment syndrome occurs in the forearm, patients experience excruciating pain when they move their fingers actively or passively.

■ Physical Examination

Compartment syndrome is marked early in its course by patient distress secondary to tense muscular compartments and excruciating pain with passive stretch of the digits. Also, decreased sensation in peripheral nerve distributions and edema are often present. Later findings include hypoesthesia, loss of pulses, and pallor of the affected extremity.

Although pain is the best clinical indicator of compartment syndrome, some individuals with compartment syndrome do not complain of pain. If the individual has received a large amount of analgesia; is unconscious, obtunded, or sedated; has loss of nerve function in the affected compartment; or is a child, he or she might not be able to express clearly the sensation of pain. In these situations, measurement of compartment pressures is indicated if compartment syndrome is suspected.

■ Diagnostic Testing

If the clinician is unsure of whether the patient has compartment syndrome after a thorough physical examination, the intracompartmental pressure should be measured. The intracompartmental pressure serves as an indirect proxy for the amount of blood flow and oxygen saturation received by skeletal muscle. Although the exact intracompartmental pressure value that constitutes compartment syndrome is not agreed on, a value greater than 30 mm Hg is concerning. The value of 30 mm Hg is commonly used because this is the capillary blood pressure, so an intracompartmental pressure near this value would result in minimal blood flow through that compartment. Many clinicians subtract the intracompartmental pressure from the patient's diastolic blood pressure (to get the $\Delta P$) as an alternative measurement because it accounts for differences in blood pressure between individuals. A $\Delta P$ of less than 30 mm Hg supports the diagnosis of compartment syndrome.

■ Treatment

If compartment syndrome is suspected, emergent orthopedic or vascular surgery consultation is needed. When the diagnosis of compartment syndrome is established, compartment fasciotomies should be performed as soon as possible.

## DISTAL RADIUS FRACTURES

■ Anatomy

The radius is the more lateral forearm bone, and it articulates with the scaphoid, lunate, and ulna at its distal aspect. The distal radioulnar joint (DRUJ) consists of an articulation between the head of the ulna and the sigmoid notch of the distal radius. The sigmoid notch is quite shallow, so stable articulation with the head of the ulna is contingent on soft tissue support. The main soft tissue stabilizer of the DRUJ is the triangular fibrocartilage complex. The DRUJ is essential for forearm pronation and supination.

Specific radiographic landmarks are seen in patients with normal distal radius anatomy (Fig. 11-19). The angle at which the articular surface of the distal radius slopes, called the radial inclination, is normally 23 degrees. The radial height, which is the difference in length between the radial styloid and the distalmost aspect of the ulna, is normally 12 mm. The radius normally has a palmar or volar tilt of 11 degrees. These radiographic measurements may be disrupted in distal radius fractures.

In distal radius fractures, the extensor pollicus longus tendon is vulnerable to injury in both the acute and the subacute setting. The extensor pollicus longus resides in the third dorsal extensor compartment of the forearm. It allows for extension of the interphalangeal joint of the thumb and moves from ulnar to radial in a very sharp fashion over the distal radius hinging around the dorsally palpable landmark of Lister tubercle. It can be injured during the initial trauma or rupture late secondary to attrition (a phenomenon most commonly seen with nondisplaced fractures).

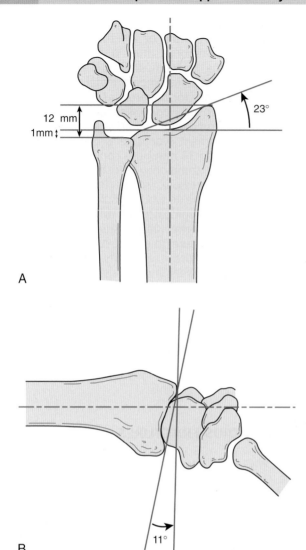

A

B

**FIGURE 11-19. A,** Measurements of normal radiographic parameters of the distal radius and ulna. Radial inclination is measured off the perpendicular to the radial shaft (average 23 degrees). Radial length is the difference in length between the ulnar head and the tip of the radial styloid (average 12 mm). Ulnar variance is the difference in length between the ulnar head and the ulnar aspect of the distal radius (depicted as 1 mm ulnar-negative here). **B,** Palmar or volar tilt is measured off the lateral radiograph (average 11 degrees). *(From Browner BD, Jupiter JB, Levine AM, et al, editors: Skeletal trauma: basic science, management, and reconstruction, ed 4, Philadelphia, 2008, Saunders.)*

The median nerve is also susceptible to injury during distal radius fractures both acutely and subacutely. The median nerve runs in the carpal tunnel, which is bordered volarly by the transverse carpal ligament, dorsally by the carpal bones, ulnarly by the hamate and pisiform, and radially by the scaphoid and trapezium. The proximal aspect of the carpal tunnel is defined by the pisiform and scaphoid tubercles, whereas the distal aspect is defined by hook of hamate and tubercle of trapezium. In dorsally displaced distal radius fractures, the proximal radial shaft occupies a volar position where it can intrude into the carpal tunnel and compress the median nerve. Simple swelling secondary to distal radius fractures may also cause compression of the median nerve.

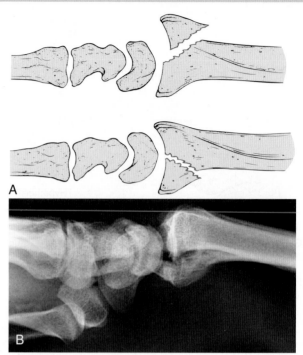

A

B

**FIGURE 11-20. A,** Two-part intra-articular Barton fracture-subluxation is inherently unstable and may occur in either a dorsal or a volar direction. **B,** Lateral radiograph of a volar Barton fracture-subluxation. *(From Browner BD, Jupiter JB, Levine AM, et al, editors: Skeletal trauma: basic science, management, and reconstruction, ed 4, Philadelphia, 2008, Saunders.)*

■ Mechanism of Injury

Fractures of the distal radius occur in three distinct groups. Women older than 40 years most commonly sustain fractures of the distal radius. The other two groups that sustain fractures are adults younger than 50 years and children 5 to 14 years old.

In women older than 40 years, the most common history is a fall onto an outstretched hand from a standing position. The fall is often low energy in nature. The biggest risk factor for distal radius fracture in this population is underlying osteoporosis or osteopenia. When individuals with low bone density fall on an outstretched hand, the compromised trabecular latticework of the distal radius cannot withstand the force of the fall as well as normal bone can, and a fracture often results. Patients with distal radius fractures that occur with this mechanism should be referred by their primary care physician for bone density evaluation. Distal radius fractures that occur in younger adults may be the result of high-energy trauma. These distal radius fractures are more likely to be intra-articular and comminuted, reflecting their high-energy nature. Distal radius fractures occur in various patterns. In the literature, they have often been described as extra-articular and dorsally displaced (Colles fracture) occurring after a fall onto an extended wrist. If the wrist is flexed on impact, the fracture may instead be displaced volarly (Smith fracture). Two-part intra-articular volar or dorsal shear (Barton) fractures are inherently unstable and may lead to volar or dorsal subluxation of the carpus depending on the size of the radius fracture fragment (Fig. 11-20).

In practice, many distal radius fractures do not fall into the simple extra-articular patterns described by Colles and Smith or the intra-articular shear pattern of Barton. Intra-articular fractures of the distal radius often are not easily characterized and may involve several fracture lines that do not readily fit into historical eponyms.

■ Physical Examination

Several findings on physical examination are commonly seen in displaced distal radius fractures. Dorsal displacement of the distal fragment may occur because the fracture often occurs after a fall on the palmar aspect of the hand, producing a characteristic deformity. Radial deviation of the distal radius fragment with shortening often occurs secondary to the radial and proximal pull of the brachioradialis insertion on the radial styloid. As with any injury, edema and pain occur at the site of trauma. Evaluation of both the volar and the dorsal surfaces of the wrist for soft tissue injuries and exposed bone is important. A thorough examination of hand function and sensation should also be performed to evaluate for tendon rupture or neurologic injury. Of particular concern is the development of acute carpal tunnel syndrome. Traumatic inflammation can increase the pressure in the carpal tunnel resulting in compression of the median nerve within the fibro-osseous borders of the carpal tunnel. In cases of acute carpal tunnel syndrome, patients experience exquisite burning pain and paresthesias in the median nerve distribution despite closed reduction and immobilization of the fracture. This presentation requires urgent orthopedic consultation for transverse carpal ligament release to relieve pressure on a compromised median nerve.

If a patient is suspected to have a distal radius fracture, the ipsilateral shoulder, elbow, and carpus should also be thoroughly inspected to ensure that the patient does not have any other associated fractures of the upper extremity.

■ Diagnostic Testing

If a distal radius fracture is suspected, posteroanterior, oblique, and lateral wrist radiographs should be obtained to determine whether the fracture is intra-articular or extra-articular, the extent of metaphyseal extension and comminution, and the presence of concomitant injuries such as a scaphoid fracture. The distal radius radiographic parameters of radial inclination and length, the congruity of the DRUJ, and involvement of the ulnar styloid all can be evaluated on the postero-anterior view (Fig. 11-21). The lateral projection allows determination of the volar tilt, relative alignment of the distal radius and ulna (an indicator of DRUJ stability), and whether there is any instability of the carpal bones relative to the radius, each other, and the metacarpals. On a normal lateral wrist film, a straight line can be drawn from the radial shaft through the lunate, the capitate, and the longitudinal axis of the metacarpals to ensure that no concomitant radiocarpal, intercarpal (perilunate), or carpometacarpal subluxation or dislocation is present. Oblique wrist films provide perhaps the best view of more subtle radial styloid fractures. If a distal radius fracture is particularly complex, a CT scan may provide detailed information about the orientation of intra-articular fracture lines and delineate more

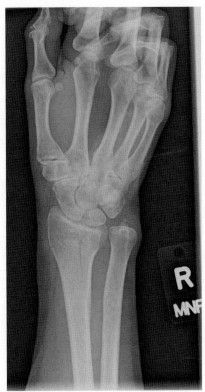

**FIGURE 11-21.** Posteroanterior radiograph of a 60-year-old woman who sustained a distal radius and ulnar styloid fracture after a fall on ice. Although her radial inclination seems normal, there is dramatic incongruity of the DRUJ with resultant ulnar positivity.

precisely fracture fragments that involve the scaphoid facet, lunate facet, or DRUJ. Although informative in certain circumstances, CT scans are not typically a part of emergency care of a patient and are really helpful only after reduction, when the fracture is out to length, to facilitate preoperative planning.

■ Treatment

After appropriate clinical and radiographic evaluation, distal radius fractures should be reduced and immobilized. To facilitate reduction, adequate pain control and muscle relaxation should be obtained. A hematoma block with or without intravenous administration of a benzodiazepine is often effective in relieving pain and relaxing patients.

Reduction of distal radius fractures can be assisted by hanging the upper extremity by the fingers with the elbow at 90 degrees (Fig. 11-22). This maneuver is thought to fatigue the deforming muscles making reduction of the displaced distal fragment easier. (Hanging the extremity has not been shown to be associated with a superior reduction quality or success rate compared with reductions without suspension.) After the arm is allowed to hang from the gauze wrap or finger traps for 5 to 10 minutes, the fracture is reduced. An assistant may provide countertraction by placing force on the anterior aspect of the arm; alternatively, if no assistant is available, gauze wrap can be tied into a loop and placed around the arm. The practitioner's foot can be placed through the loop and used

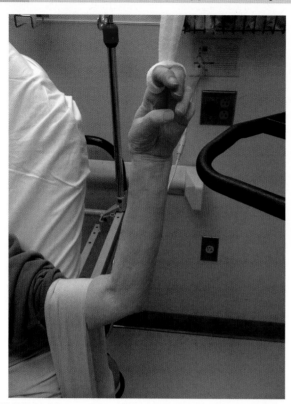

**FIGURE 11-22.** Reduction of distal radius fractures starts with hanging the upper extremity by the fingers using finger traps with the elbow at 90 degrees. This maneuver fatigues the deforming muscles making reduction of the displaced distal fragment easier. After several minutes, the fracture is reduced.

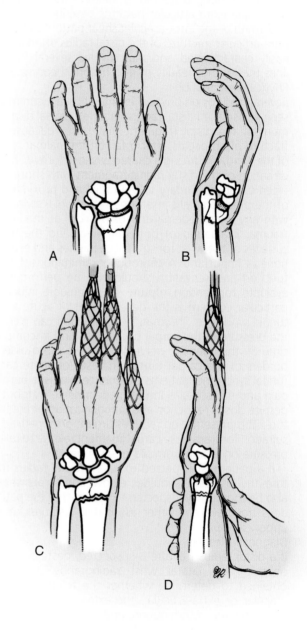

**FIGURE 11-23. A** and **B,** Distal radius (Colles type) fracture. **C** and **D,** After suspending the arm from finger traps or gauze wrap and allowing for fracture disimpaction, pressure can be applied with the thumb over the distal fragment. *(From Wolfe SW, Hotchkiss RN, Pederson WC, et al, editors: Green's operative hand surgery, ed 6, Philadelphia, 2011, Churchill Livingstone. Copyright Elizabeth Martin.)*

to provide countertraction during the reduction maneuver. For some dorsally displaced (Colles type) fractures, the suspension of the arm from finger traps for several minutes may be enough to allow for fracture disimpaction, and all that may be required for fracture reduction is pressure applied with the thumb over the distal fragment (Fig. 11-23). Classically, the reduction of distal radius fractures has been obtained by increasing the initial deformity until one cortex engages; this contact point is used as a fulcrum to realign the distal fracture fragment with the shaft. For dorsally displaced (Colles type) fractures, manual traction is applied and maintained while the distal fracture fragment is hyperextended to unlock the fracture and then flexed or volarly translated to realign the distal fragment with the proximal shaft (Fig. 11-24). The principle of this manual reduction maneuver is based on the application of tension to the soft tissue hinge (i.e., periosteum and overlying tendons that reside on the concavity of the angulation). After reduction, the wrist is immobilized in a well-padded sugar-tong splint or valved cast molded to the contours of the wrist in slight ulnar deviation (to try to restore radial inclination and length) and volar translation (to try to restore palmar tilt). Immobilizing the wrist in excessive forearm pronation, wrist flexion, and ulnar deviation (the Cotton-Loder position) should be avoided so as not to cause or exacerbate median nerve compression. If DRUJ instability is detected on

lateral radiographs, supination of the forearm may help to reduce a dorsally subluxed distal ulna, whereas pronation of the forearm may help to reduce the rarer situation of a volarly subluxed distal ulna. The splint or cast should not be extended distal to the metacarpal heads so as to allow for full range of motion of the digits and thumb (Fig. 11-25). Splints that are extended distal to the MCP joints limit the patient's ability to move his or her fingers and may lead unnecessarily to digital

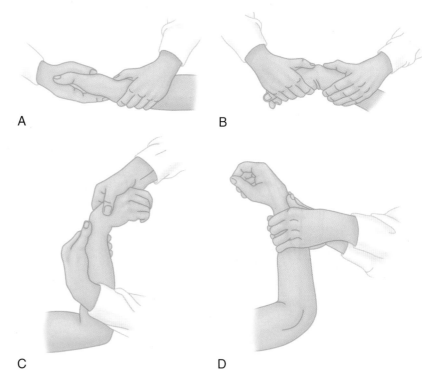

**FIGURE 11-24.** Manual reduction of a distal radius (Colles type) fracture. **A,** Disimpaction with longitudinal traction and extension of the wrist. **B,** Reduction with flexion of the wrist to restore palmar tilt and ulnar deviation to restore radial inclination. **C-D,** Stabilization with double-thumb pressure on the distal fracture fragment in neutral forearm rotation, with slight wrist flexion and ulnar deviation. Extreme pronation, flexion, and ulnar deviation (Cotton-Loder position) should be avoided because of problems encountered with median nerve compression.

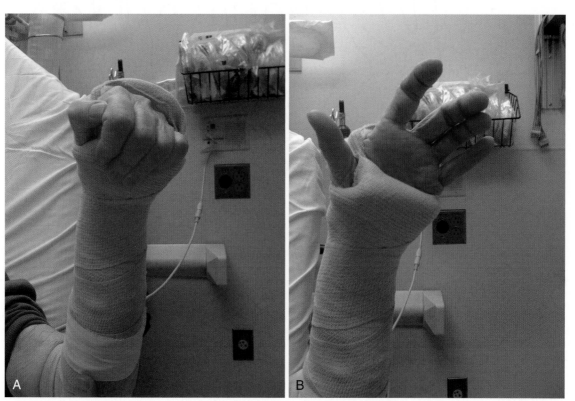

**FIGURE 11-25.** The splint applied after reduction of a distal radius fracture should not extend distal to the metacarpal heads so as to allow for full flexion **(A)** and extension **(B)** of the digits. Splints that are extended distal to the MCP joints limit the patient's ability to move the fingers and may lead unnecessarily to digital stiffness.

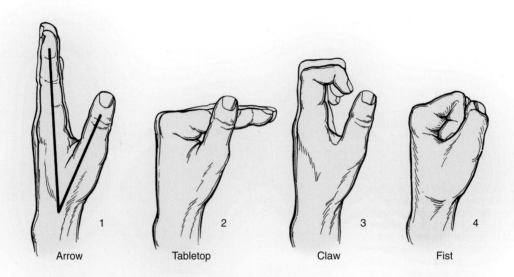

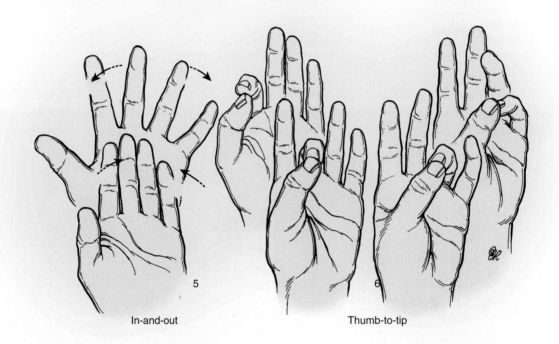

**FIGURE 11-26.** "Six-pack" exercises to promote digital motion after a patient's wrist is immobilized because of a fracture. Artist's depiction of the position that the patient's hand should assume when performing these exercises. It is helpful to show the patient how full MCP joint extension makes the hand look like an arrow, whereas full MCP joint flexion makes the hand look like a tabletop. Full MCP joint extension combined with proximal and distal interphalangeal (IP) joint flexion looks like a claw, whereas complete MCP and IP joint flexion creates a fist. Abduction and adduction of the fingers create an in-and-out motion. In the last of the exercises, the patient tries to touch the tip of his or her thumb to the tip of each finger. *(From Wolfe SW, Hotchkiss RN, Pederson WC, et al, editors: Green's operative hand surgery, ed 6, Philadelphia, 2011, Churchill Livingstone. Copyright Elizabeth Martin.)*

stiffness. Unnecessary immobilization of joints prolongs rehabilitation and adversely affects outcomes. During the period of fracture immobilization, digital motion should be encouraged. The "six-pack" finger exercises popularized by Dobyns are easy for patients to remember and perform (Fig. 11-26).

The goal of reduction is to realign the distal radius within acceptable radiographic parameters to allow for optimal function of the wrist. After reduction, a clinical examination should be performed to see if the patient's pain or neurovascular examination is stabilizing or worsening. In addition, plain radiographs should be

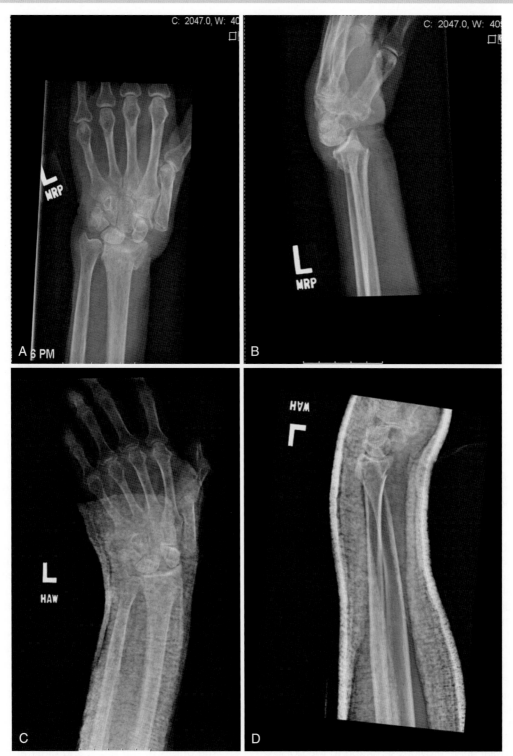

**FIGURE 11-27.** Plain radiographs of an osteopenic 80-year-old woman after a fall on an outstretched hand (same patient is depicted in Figures 11-22 and 11-23). Posteroanterior **(A)** and lateral **(B)** plain radiographs before reduction reveal a dorsally angulated and shortened distal radius fracture. Posteroanterior **(C)** and lateral **(D)** radiographs after reduction and splinting show dramatic improvement in radial inclination, length, and volar tilt. Note the incidental findings of a static scapholunate gap (unknown acuity) and prior trapeziectomy procedure with thumb metacarpal subsidence.

obtained and compared with images obtained before reduction to look for improved coronal and sagittal alignment and to inspect the carpus again for any concomitant injuries that may have been overlooked (Fig. 11-27). If the patient's clinical status is stable and an

adequate reduction is obtained and held in place with a properly molded splint, no other urgent intervention is required. If the emergency department physician feels comfortable performing and evaluating a distal radius reduction, he or she should attempt the procedure and arrange for prompt orthopedic aftercare. If the fracture cannot be adequately reduced or the fracture is open with contamination, orthopedic consultation should be obtained.

In all cases, the patient should leave the emergency department with the distal radius fracture immobilized with a splint in as close to a reduced position as possible as confirmed by adequate postreduction radiographs. Pain can be managed after emergency department discharge, in patients for whom such medications are not contraindicated, with analgesics and, if warranted, with combination products, such as hydrocodone with acetaminophen. Active motion of the uninjured digits should be encouraged.

## FOREARM FRACTURES

■ Anatomy

The radius and ulna are connected via the proximal radioulnar joint, the interosseous membrane, and the DRUJ. The ulna and the distal third of the radius lie in subcutaneous tissue, making them vulnerable to injury at these locations.

The proximal radioulnar joint consists of an articulation between the head of the radius and ulna. Stable articulation depends on soft tissue stabilization from the annular ligament, which completely surrounds the joint.

The interosseous membrane runs along almost the entire length of the forearm with fibers originating on the radius and running distally at an oblique angle before inserting on the ulna. When a force is exerted onto an individual's hand, the force is sequentially transmitted from the carpus to the radius, from the radius to the interosseous membrane, from the interosseous membrane to the ulna, and finally from the ulna to the humerus. The interosseous membrane is important for absorbing forces that are directed to the hand.

The radial nerve enters the proximal forearm radially and anterior to the elbow. It promptly splits into the superficial and deep radial nerve. The deep radial nerve is renamed the posterior interosseous nerve once it dives under the proximal edge of the supinator muscle (at the arcade of Fröhse). With fractures of the radial neck and head, the posterior interosseous nerve can be injured, resulting in an inability to extend the digits. Usually wrist extension is spared because of the dual innervation of the wrist extensors by both the radial nerve proper and the posterior interosseous nerve. The superficial radial nerve provides sensation to the dorsoradial aspect of the hand and wrist. It courses along the undersurface of the brachioradialis along with the radial artery before traveling subcutaneously in the distal one third of the forearm, where it can be injured by both penetrating and closed trauma.

The ulnar nerve passes posterior and medial to the elbow as it enters the forearm. It courses deep to the flexor carpi ulnaris. Injury can occur via laceration from penetrating trauma or from sharp bone ends resulting in sensory changes in the ulnar aspect of the hand and weakness of little finger abduction. The anterior interosseous nerve is a pure motor branch of the median nerve that, as its name suggests, travels along the volar (anterior) aspect of the interosseous membrane. It innervates the deep extrinsic flexor layer of the forearm—the pronator quadratus, the flexor pollicis longus, and the lateral half of the flexor digitorum profundus tendons (index and middle fingers).

The forearm receives dual circulation from the radial and ulnar arteries. The ulnar artery runs with the ulnar nerve while the radial artery travels with the superficial radial nerve along the undersurface of the brachioradialis in the proximal forearm. Vascular injury occurs in a similar manner as injuries to the ulnar and radial nerve.

■ Mechanism of Injury

Fractures to both bones of the forearm usually result from either a direct blow or high-energy trauma. Examples of high-energy trauma include motor vehicle accidents, gunshot wounds, and falls from a great height. Athletic injuries are rarely responsible for forearm fractures because these types of injuries usually do not possess the requisite amount of energy needed to cause these fractures. Isolated fractures to the radius and ulna may occur and are often associated with concomitant ligamentous injuries (i.e., Monteggia and Galeazzi fractures, which are discussed later).

■ Physical Examination

Because fractures to the shafts of both the ulna and the radius are most commonly displaced, they are quite apparent on inspection. If the fracture is not obvious, a swollen and tender forearm might indicate a nondisplaced fracture of either of the forearm bones. In this case, the entire forearm should be imaged with plain radiographs, including the elbow and wrist, to ensure a fracture is not missed.

The radial, ulnar, and median nerves all are susceptible to injury as they course through the forearm and must be assessed in the emergency department after forearm trauma. A neurologic assessment of the motor (and mixed sensory and motor) nerves coursing through the forearm can be accomplished in a matter of seconds by testing a few key motor functions:

• Making a fist (median and ulnar nerves)
• Wrist and finger extension (radial nerve)
• Abduction of small finger and index finger away from midline (ulnar nerve)
• Extension of the interphalangeal joint of the thumb (posterior interosseous nerve)
• Flexion of the interphalangeal joint of the thumb (anterior interosseous nerve)

The pulses of the radial and ulnar arteries should be evaluated. If pulses feel abnormal or the patient sustained penetrating trauma to the forearm, the physician should consider further imaging to evaluate the vascular tree of the forearm. Given the subcutaneous location of the radius and ulna, open fractures are common and vigilance for pinhole soft tissue defects is necessary.

As always, the remainder of the limb should be palpated to ensure other injuries of the upper extremity are not missed. Plain radiographs should be ordered as necessary based on physical examination findings.

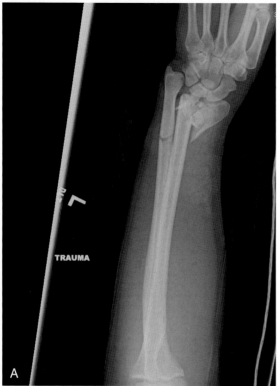

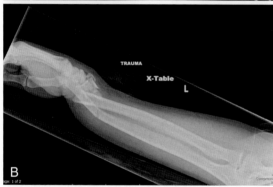

**FIGURE 11-28.** Anteroposterior **(A)** and lateral **(B)** forearm radiographs of a distal third fracture of the radius that extends into the articular surface, with a concomitant fracture of the ulnar shaft, which represents a Galeazzi variant because the DRUJ has been rendered unstable and has dislocated.

- Diagnostic Testing

  Imaging should consist of anteroposterior and lateral views of the forearm that include the elbow and the wrist. If an isolated ulna fracture is diagnosed, dedicated elbow images should be ordered to evaluate for a Monteggia variant in which there is radial head subluxation or dislocation. If an isolated radius shaft fracture is present, dedicated images of the wrist should be ordered to evaluate for DRUJ disruption. Fractures of the distal third of the radius that extend into the articular surface or involve a fracture of the ulnar shaft may represent a Galeazzi variant if the DRUJ is also rendered unstable and dislocates (Fig. 11-28).

- Treatment

  Untreated fractures of the shafts of the radius or ulna result in a significant amount of dysfunction. If the bow of the radius and ulna are not recreated in an anatomic way, supination and pronation of the forearm are limited. Most of these fractures require open reduction and internal fixation to restore function. However, a gentle closed reduction should be performed and a sugar-tong splint should be applied to take pressure off surrounding neurovascular structures, reduce pain, and relieve any tented skin. Often, hanging the arm from the fingers, as with distal radius fractures, and placing an interosseous mold on the splint aid in better aligning the fractures. The orthopedic specialist on call should be contacted by telephone because sometimes these patients may be admitted to the hospital and operated on the next day. However, it is also reasonable to discharge a patient with a properly molded splint to be treated as an outpatient with close follow-up. If the patient is discharged, the signs and symptoms of compartment syndrome should be discussed because of the relatively high incidence of compartment syndrome with this injury. The patient should be instructed to return to the emergency department for prompt evaluation and treatment if symptoms develop over the next several days.

### Galeazzi and Monteggia Fractures

- Anatomy

  In Galeazzi fractures, the radial shaft is fractured at a point between the middle and distal one third of the bone, with concomitant subluxation or dislocation of the DRUJ. Monteggia fractures are fractures of the proximal one third of the ulna in which the proximal radioulnar joint is also injured with resultant subluxation, dislocation, or fracture of the radial head. The proximal radioulnar joint consists of an articulation between the head of the radius and the radial notch of the ulna. Stable articulation depends on soft tissue stabilization from the annular ligament that completely surrounds the joint. In Bado type I and type II Monteggia lesions, the direction of the radial head dislocation anteriorly or posteriorly is predicted by the apex, either anterior or posterior, of the ulna shaft fracture (Fig. 11-29).

- Mechanism of Injury

  Galeazzi fractures and Monteggia fractures are traumatic injuries. The main mechanisms by which these injuries occur include high-energy trauma such as motor vehicle accidents, direct blows to the forearm, and penetrating trauma.

- Physical Examination

  On inspection, patients with Galeazzi fractures usually have pain, soft tissue swelling, and tenderness to palpation over the distal one third of the radius and the wrist. The large distal radius fragment is usually angulated leading to a grossly apparent deformity. Dislocation of the DRUJ can be appreciated on inspection via an abnormally prominent ulnar head.

  Patients with Monteggia fractures have tenderness, swelling, and perhaps ecchymosis over the ulna shaft and deformity around the elbow if the radial head is dislocated. If the elbow is not deformed, tenderness

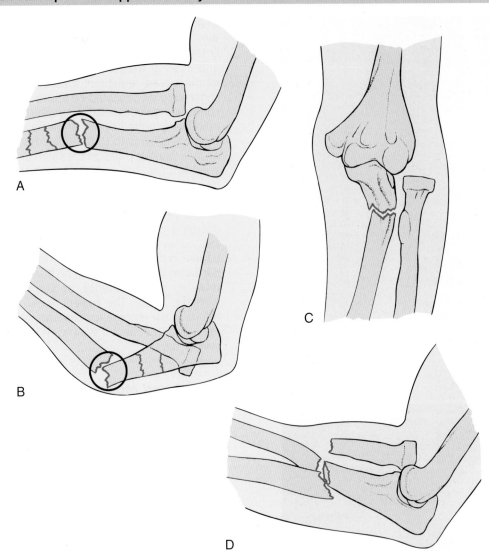

**FIGURE 11-29.** Classification of Monteggia lesions by Bado. **A,** Type I—anterior angulation of the ulnar fracture and anterior dislocation of the radial head. **B,** Type II—posterior angulation of the ulnar fracture and posterior dislocation of the radial head. **C,** Type III—fracture of the proximal ulna metaphysis and lateral dislocation of the radial head. **D,** Type IV—anterior dislocation of the radial head and fracture of the radial and ulnar shafts. *(From Browner BD, Jupiter JB, Levine AM, et al, editors: Skeletal trauma: basic science, management, and reconstruction, ed 4, Philadelphia, 2008, Saunders.)*

over the radial head may indicate injury to the radio-capitellar joint.

■ Diagnostic Testing

The diagnosis of Galeazzi and Monteggia fractures should be confirmed with anteroposterior and lateral radiographs of the forearm, wrist, and elbow. Radiographic findings indicative of DRUJ injury include fractures at the base of the ulnar styloid or widening of the distance between the distal ulna and sigmoid notch of the distal radius on a posteroanterior radiograph. On a lateral view of the wrist, incongruity between the sagittal profiles of the distal radius and ulna is indicative of DRUJ injury. In Monteggia fractures, the important landmarks to assess when inspecting plain radiographs are the radiocapitellar joint, proximal radioulnar joint, and articulation between the ulna and humerus. A commonly noted radiographic feature of Monteggia fractures is that the head of the radius is usually dislocated in the same direction as the apex of the ulnar

fracture. Radiographic evaluation of the radiocapitellar joint is important to determine if the radial head is in its normal position. A line is drawn through the radius parallel to the long axis of this bone. This line should aim toward the capitellum on all radiographs of the elbow. If it does not, the radial head should be considered malaligned.

■ Treatment

Galeazzi and Monteggia injuries almost always require operative management, so discussing the case with the orthopedic surgeon on call is helpful for operative planning. Galeazzi fractures should be reduced and splinted similar to all distal radius fractures. Reducing the distal radius often brings the DRUJ into better alignment, taking pressure off surrounding soft tissues. Monteggia fracture-dislocations should also be reduced in the emergency department. Conscious sedation is usually required for reduction because the muscle forces acting to deform the bones are significant, and manipulation is quite painful. The affected arm should be hung by the fingertips in a similar fashion as described with distal radius fractures. Reducing the proximal ulna fracture often allows the subluxed or dislocated radial head to fall into its normal articulation with the capitellum by restoring the normal length of the forearm. After the fracture is reduced and the radial head is located, a well-padded sugar-tong splint should be placed to maintain the reduction.

In all cases, the patient should leave the emergency department with the forearm fracture immobilized with a splint in as close to a reduced position as possible as confirmed by adequate postreduction radiographs. Patients generally leave with a plan for follow-up that includes surgical intervention. Pain can be managed after emergency department discharge, in patients for whom such medications are not contraindicated, with analgesics and, if warranted, with combination products, such as hydrocodone with acetaminophen. Active motion of the uninjured digits should be encouraged.

## PAINFUL ATRAUMATIC WRIST

### Septic Wrist

■ Anatomy
The articular cartilage of joints is avascular, so infections of the joint space can quickly degrade the cartilage, leading to permanent joint damage. As a result, septic arthritis is a surgical emergency.

■ History
Several histories are consistent with septic arthritis of the wrist. Direct penetrating trauma to the wrist joint space is the most common cause of septic arthritis. Another common history involves an infection of the tissue adjacent to the wrist (e.g., flexor tenosynovitis) spreading directly into the wrist, causing a septic wrist. A septic wrist can also occur secondary to hematogenous seeding of the joint.

Numerous risk factors increase an individual's chance of developing septic arthritis. Intravenous drug use, endocarditis, and underlying infections all increase an individual's risk for bacteremia, which increases the risk of hematogenous seeding of the wrist. Orthopedic implants in a person's wrist, rheumatoid arthritis (RA), immunocompromised disease states, and compromised skin (i.e., ulcers, eczema) all increase a person's risk for developing a septic wrist.

The main bacterial pathogens responsible for septic arthritis in adults are methicillin-sensitive *Staphylococcus aureus,* methicillin-resistant *S. aureus,* group B streptococci, *Escherichia coli, Neisseria gonorrheae,* and *Pseudomonas aeruginosa.* Patients with a septic wrist usually present with severe pain, redness, tenderness, and swelling in the affected wrist.

Septic joints are surgical emergencies because infection rapidly leads to irreversible damage of the articular cartilage and joint functioning. Patients with septic wrist pain generally have a slowly increasing syndrome of pain, immobility, and swelling over several days. These patients generally present to emergency departments or their primary care offices. Arthrocentesis, Gram stain, and an orthopedic surgery consultation all can be performed in the emergency department. Empiric antibiotic administration should be held until after the arthrocentesis has been performed unless the patient has signs of systemic illness. The arthrocentesis may help to identify an organism so that antibiotic treatment can be tailored specifically.

■ Physical Examination
The patient's vital signs should be monitored because patients with septic arthritis could theoretically become hemodynamically unstable. On inspection, the affected wrist usually appears red and swollen. On palpation, the wrist usually is markedly tender, and an effusion within the joint is commonly detected. Patients usually have limited range of motion of the affected joint secondary to exquisite pain. A neurovascular examination should be performed to ensure that no damage to these structures has occurred.

■ Diagnostic Testing
Radiographs should be obtained in patients with suspected septic arthritis. Imaging allows identification of any bony abnormalities or foreign bodies. MRI is helpful for showing intra-articular fluid when the diagnosis is in question or initial arthrocentesis yields no fluid. MRI does not need to be performed for routine diagnosis of a septic wrist.

Joint aspiration is essential for the diagnosis of septic arthritis of the wrist and should be performed in all patients who present with risk factors for septic wrist or fever associated with an atraumatic, painful, and swollen wrist. In acute bacterial septic arthritis, the aspirated synovial fluid should contain at least 50,000 neutrophils/μL (usually >100,000/μL). An elevated neutrophil count in the absence of crystals is concerning enough to bring the patient urgently to the operating room for irrigation and débridement. Synovial fluid should be obtained for culture before antibiotics are started because this allows for antibiotic therapy to be targeted to specific pathogens. A Gram stain of the synovial fluid should be done. The synovial fluid should also be studied for protein and glucose concentrations; glucose is commonly low, and protein is high. Evaluation for crystals is also essential because the cell count can be elevated greater than 50,000/μL in patients with crystalline arthropathies (i.e., gout and pseudogout). Wrist arthrocentesis is a relatively straightforward procedure. The most reliable location on the wrist for successful aspiration is dorsally, in the soft spot just distal to Lister tubercle at the radiocarpal joint. This spot is located between the third (extensor pollicis longus tendon) and fourth (extensor digitorum communis tendon to the index finger) dorsal compartments of the wrist.

A complete blood count should be done because patients with septic arthritis usually have leukocytosis with a left shift. The clinician may also draw serum levels of erythrocyte sedimentation rate and C-reactive protein because these markers of inflammation are usually elevated in septic arthritis. Normal results of the complete blood count, erythrocyte sedimentation rate, and C-reactive protein do not exclude septic arthritis as the cause for the symptoms. Blood cultures should be done as well in the case of hematogenous seeding of the wrist joint.

- Treatment

If septic arthritis is diagnosed, urgent irrigation and débridement should be undertaken in the operating room. The surgical consultant can make the determination with respect to the timing of the operation.

## Osteoarthritis

- Anatomy

Osteoarthritis is a noninflammatory disease in which the hyaline cartilage that lines the articular surface of a joint gradually deteriorates. As a result, the affected joint is subject to secondary changes that include subchondral sclerosis and the development of osteophytes at the periphery of the affected joint. In the hand, the osteophytic outcroppings that develop at the proximal interphalangeal joint are called Bouchard nodes, and the osteophytic outcroppings that develop at the distal interphalangeal joint are called Heberden nodes.

- History

Primary osteoarthritis usually manifests in the larger, weight-bearing joints of the body but can also manifest in the wrist joint. Primary osteoarthritis has an idiopathic etiology. Patients with osteoarthritis of the hands generally are older than 40 years. There is usually no association with specific underlying illnesses.

Secondary osteoarthritis can occur in the wrist. Usually patients with secondary wrist osteoarthritis have a history of trauma to the distal radius or to the carpus. Traumatic injuries that commonly lead to secondary osteoarthritis of the wrist include fracture of a carpal bone (e.g., scaphoid), intercarpal instability secondary to carpal fracture or intercarpal ligamentous injury (e.g., SLIL tear), intra-articular fractures of the distal radius, and Kienbock disease. These injuries alter intercarpal and radiocarpal articulations and cause changes in the distribution of joint forces. As a result, degeneration of the articular cartilage of the wrist occurs.

The main clinical feature of osteoarthritis is pain. Initially, patients experience pain in the affected joint that is worse with activity and alleviated by rest. However, patients may eventually experience pain at night and while resting. The pain associated with osteoarthritis causes significant dysfunction of the wrist during later stages of the disease because the wrist is unable to function normally. Patients often experience a significant loss in grip strength and in hand dexterity.

Patients with wrist osteoarthritis can present acutely with loss of function in the flexors or extensors of the hand. This event is usually painless, but pain occasionally is present. The osteophytes that develop with osteoarthritis provide a jagged, uneven surface for flexor and extensor tendons to move over during muscle contraction. As wrist osteoarthritis worsens, flexor and extensor tendons can rupture. The flexor pollicis longus tendon runs along the distal pole of the scaphoid as it courses toward the thumb and is particularly prone to rupture.

- Physical Examination

The patient's wrist should be examined for gross deformity, which is more common in RA than in osteoarthritis. On palpation, the clinician might feel osteophytic outcroppings around the wrist. Range of motion testing is important for diagnosing secondary osteoarthritis of the wrist. Early in the disease course, patients experience pain at the extremes of an arc of motion. As osteoarthritis progresses, the patient experiences pain with smaller and smaller arcs of motion. Patients with late-stage disease often have almost no ability to move their wrists and have tremendous wrist stiffness. As noted earlier, patients with significant secondary wrist osteoarthritis develop impaired grip strength and hand dexterity, both of which should be tested. Because patients with secondary wrist osteoarthritis can have tendon rupture, flexion and extension of the MCP, proximal interphalangeal, and distal interphalangeal joints of each finger should be carefully evaluated.

- Diagnostic Testing

Posteroanterior and lateral radiographs of the wrist should be obtained to confirm the diagnosis of wrist osteoarthritis. The clinician should examine each of the carpal articulations for the degenerative changes seen with osteoarthritis (osteophytes, joint space narrowing, subchondral sclerosis, and cysts). No other imaging modalities should be needed to diagnose wrist osteoarthritis.

Patients occasionally present with a swollen and painful wrist. In these situations, arthrocentesis should be performed to rule out septic joint.

- Treatment

Wrist osteoarthritis is usually treated on a symptomatic basis. Nonsteroidal anti-inflammatory drugs, activity modification, and corticosteroid injections all can provide pain relief. If conservative measures fail, various surgical interventions can be considered for definitive care. Urgent orthopedic consultation is unnecessary if the diagnosis of osteoarthritis is made because these patients can be followed as an outpatient.

## Rheumatoid Arthritis

- Anatomy

Histologically, RA is characterized by infiltrative and erosive joint destruction. Untreated, this autoimmune disease destroys joints and ligaments and can lead to gross deformity. The smooth surfaces that tendons glide over around the wrist become roughened, sometimes leading to tendon attrition and eventual rupture.

- History

RA is an atraumatic autoimmune disease that often affects the wrist. It is more common in women than in men and usually has an onset between 40 and 50 years of age. Although RA is classically thought of as a symmetric polyarthritis, isolated wrist disease is often one of the first manifestations. RA is more common in individuals with a family history of the disease and in patients who have Sjögren syndrome.

Patients with RA generally have a characteristic pattern of pain, in which they experience morning stiffness for more than 30 minutes, with the stiffness often recurring after prolonged inactivity or very rigorous activity. RA can cause many different diseases in the wrist, leading to more specific patterns of pain.

One of the earliest changes to the wrist is dorsal swelling within extensor tendon sheaths; the tendons of the extensor carpi ulnaris and extensor digitorum communis are most often affected. As the inflammatory process penetrates these tendons, they can eventually rupture causing the patient to experience acute onset of painless lack of function in the specific distribution of these muscles. A dorsal wrist finding that develops later in patients with RA is dorsal prominence of the ulnar head, termed *caput ulnae syndrome*. This finding is due to the inflammatory synovium stretching and eventually tearing the ligamentous restraints of the ulnar head. Similarly, the synovium can also infiltrate and compromise the function of the DRUJ, causing dysfunction during forearm supination and pronation.

RA also causes significant damage volarly. Cysts of synovial fluid, called synovial protrusion cysts, can develop and be palpated on the volar aspect of the wrist. The proliferative inflammatory synovium can cause the pressure within the carpal tunnel to increase significantly leading to compression of the median nerve and carpal tunnel syndrome. Similarly, the proliferative synovium can exert a large amount of pressure around the ulnar nerve at Guyon canal and cause ulnar nerve symptoms.

Eventually, if RA is allowed to progress, wrist function and structure are severely impaired. The carpus loses its normal height, there is a loss of joint space in the radiocarpal joints, and ankylosis occurs. These changes are accompanied by severe pain and dysfunction of the wrist.

In terms of prehospital care, there are no RA-specific issues. When there is a suspected tendon rupture, expedient follow-up care is warranted.

- Physical Examination
On inspection, the clinician should look for swelling and gross deformity in the joints commonly affected by RA (i.e., fingers, wrist, knees, and toes). In the fingers, the MCP joints are classically ulnarly deviated. Some patients may exhibit proximal interphalangeal joint hyperextension. In the wrist, the clinician should examine the head of the ulna for dorsal displacement and the carpus for volar subluxation. On palpation, the wrist is often tender. The dorsal aspect of the wrist is often swollen because of the presence of an infiltrative and expansive pannus. The tendons of the extensor carpi ulnaris and extensor digitorum communis should be examined as for tenosynovitis. On range of motion testing, the wrist commonly has a decreased arc of motion, which occurs secondary to inflammation. Range of motion testing is important because decreased wrist motion is often the first physical examination finding in patients with RA. The patient's ability to pronate and supinate should be thoroughly examined because the DRUJ may be compromised.

Finally, the patient's digital motion and nerve status should be examined. Extension deficits at the MCP joints could indicate extensor tendon rupture (in which the patient is unable to obtain or maintain extension) or extensor digitorum communis tendon subluxation secondary to sagittal band rupture (in which the patient cannot obtain but can maintain extension). It is also possible that the extensor lags are caused by posterior interosseous nerve compression from rheumatoid pannus at the elbow. Posterior interosseous nerve neuropathy can be differentiated from attritional tendon rupture by an intact tenodesis effect (in which passive wrist flexion produces digital extension). Patients should also be examined for carpal tunnel and ulnar tunnel syndromes. The clinician may suspect a carpal tunnel syndrome if a positive Tinel sign is elicited by tapping over the volar wrist or a positive Phalen sign is present (reproduction of volar numbness and tingling in the radial three and a half fingers with passive wrist flexion). Thenar muscle strength may be decreased in advanced cases. To test for ulnar nerve compression, the clinician should examine volar sensation in the ulnar one and a half fingers and the strength of the intrinsic hand muscles by testing abduction force of the index finger (first dorsal interosseous) and small finger (abductor digiti quinti). The clinician can differentiate between ulnar tunnel syndrome at the wrist and cubital tunnel syndrome at the elbow by understanding that the dorsal sensory branch of the ulnar nerve (which provides sensation to the dorsal and ulnar aspect of the hand) would not be compromised by ulnar nerve compression at Guyon canal. Cubital tunnel syndrome, which also could affect motor strength to the flexor digitorum profundus of the small and ring fingers, is far more common than ulnar tunnel syndrome.

- Diagnostic Testing
  - Imaging
  Radiographs of the hands and wrists should be obtained in a patient with a diagnosis of RA. In the early stages of RA, radiographic changes in the hands include swelling of the soft tissues and juxta-articular osteoporosis. As the disease progresses, an affected wrist develops joint space narrowing and subchondral cysts secondary to progressive cartilage loss. Typically, there is no osteophyte formation as in osteoarthritis. End-stage RA is characterized by bony ankylosis.
  - Serum studies
  Various laboratory markers are useful and can be obtained in patients with RA. Rheumatoid factor is a useful marker for prognosis, but it is not always positive in patients with RA. Not all patients with a positive test actually have RA. Anti–cyclic citrullinated peptide antibody is now regarded as a more specific test for diagnosing RA. Erythrocyte sedimentation rate and C-reactive protein are nonspecific markers of inflammation but can be followed to monitor the trends of disease activity.
- Treatment
The key in managing patients presenting to the emergency department with an acutely swollen wrist is to rule out any septic process. After a bacterial infection

in the wrist has been ruled out, other, more benign diagnoses such as RA can be considered. If RA is suspected, a referral to a primary care physician or rheumatologist is warranted.

## Systemic Lupus Erythematosus

■ Anatomy
The manifestations of systemic lupus erythematosus (SLE) in the hand and wrist resemble RA, but the pathogenesis of these two diseases is different. In SLE, deposition of autoantibody-containing immune complexes causes damage to periarticular tissue. This is in contrast to RA, in which an inflammatory synovium causes permanent damage to articular surfaces.

■ History
SLE is an atraumatic autoimmune disease that mainly affects women. SLE can cause significant musculoskeletal pathology, and the hands and wrists are often involved. Hand and wrist disease can be the first manifestation of SLE, so patients might not have any obvious disease when they initially present with musculoskeletal complaints. The pain experienced by patients with SLE and musculoskeletal problems is generally very similar to the pain experienced by patients with RA: morning stiffness, swelling, and pain after rigorous activity and prolonged inactivity. Raynaud phenomenon (in which vasospasm causes blanching discoloration of the fingers and toes) is often seen in patients with SLE but not in patients with RA.

At the wrist, SLE is known to weaken the function of the intrinsic ligaments that support and maintain the normal carpal architecture, leading to subluxation and dislocation of carpal bones. The most common sites of subluxation are the midcarpal joints and radiocarpal joint. The bone most commonly dislocated is the lunate. When subluxation occurs at either of the aforementioned joints or lunate dislocation occurs, the patient can experience resultant pain and dysfunction of the carpus.

In SLE, as in RA, several wrist problems can develop. In patients with SLE, the ulnar head often becomes dorsally displaced because of damage to the supporting ligaments. Dorsal displacement of the ulnar head compromises the DRUJ, leading to impaired supination and pronation. As in RA, dorsal displacement of the ulnar head can disrupt the extensor tendons that course through the dorsal forearm, leading to possible extensor tendon rupture. Similar to patients with RA and attritional tendon rupture, patients with SLE present acutely with painless loss of function of the specifically ruptured tendon. Similar to RA, the synovitis associated with SLE at the wrist can compress the median nerve and lead to carpal tunnel syndrome.

■ Physical Examination
The clinician should look for swelling and gross deformity, similar to in patients with RA. Palpation of the distal radius, distal ulna, and carpal bones and a thorough examination of range of motion and neurovascular status should be performed.

■ Diagnostic Testing
If a patient with SLE has significant wrist pain, the clinician can obtain radiographs to evaluate the problem further. Standard hand and wrist radiographs may show carpal subluxation and perilunate dislocations, if they are present. The distal ulna should be assessed for dorsal subluxation, and the structure of the DRUJ should be examined.

Serum studies can be performed in patients with SLE. Antinuclear antibody levels are often elevated in patients with SLE, but they can also be high in patients with other autoimmune conditions. Anti–double-stranded DNA antibodies can also be elevated in patients with SLE. Complement level is usually low in patients with SLE. Lupus anticoagulant, a type of antiphospholipid antibody, is elevated in many patients with SLE and is a risk factor for venous and arterial thrombosis.

■ Treatment
As with RA, the key in managing patients presenting to the emergency department with an acutely swollen wrist is to rule out any septic process. After a bacterial infection in the wrist has been ruled out, other, more benign diagnoses such as SLE can be considered. If SLE is suspected, a referral to a primary care physician or rheumatologist is warranted.

## Gout and Pseudogout (Calcium Pyrophosphate Dihydrate Crystal Deposition Disease)

■ Anatomy
Deposition of crystals into joints triggers an acute inflammatory response that causes localized inflammation. Tophi are collections of monosodium urate crystals that are seen in patients with chronic gout. They usually deposit along the extensor surfaces of joints and tendons.

■ History
Gout is an atraumatic disease in which patients either underexcrete or overproduce uric acid, leading to the formation of monosodium urate crystals that can deposit in the body. Risk factors for overproducing uric acid include obesity, alcoholism, and heavy consumption of red meat. Risk factors for underexcretion of uric acid include hypertension, thiazide and loop diuretics, and several antituberculosis medications. Classically, gout initially manifests by causing pain, redness, and swelling in the great toe owing to crystal deposition. Rarely, the initial gouty attack occurs in the wrist, causing the afflicted individual to experience acute onset of redness, swelling, and pain in the wrist owing to crystal deposition in this location.

In patients with chronic gout, attacks commonly occur at the wrist, causing the wrist to appear red and swollen. Patients with chronic gout can have tophi deposition on the flexor tendons and in other locations in the carpal tunnel, with the possible complication of carpal tunnel syndrome. If patients have chronic, recurring attacks of gout in the wrist, a debilitating arthritis can develop.

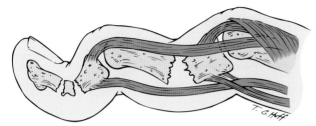

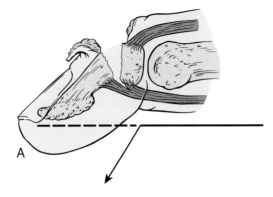

**FIGURE 12-22.** Transverse diaphyseal fractures of the phalanges displace as a result of intrinsic and extrinsic myotendinous forces. A transverse fracture of the middle phalanx distal to the insertion of the FDS will tend to angulate toward the volar apex. *(From Browner BD, Jupiter JB, Levine AM, et al, editors: Skeletal trauma: basic science, management, and reconstruction, ed 4, Philadelphia, 2008, Saunders.)*

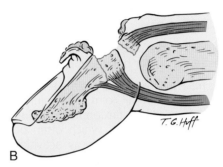

**FIGURE 12-23.** Two distinct physeal injuries of a pediatric distal phalanx include an open Salter-Harris type I or type II physeal separation in a preadolescent child **(A)** and a mallet-type fracture in an older adolescent **(B).** Either of these injuries can involve damage to the eponychial fold. *(From Browner BD, Jupiter JB, Levine AM, et al, editors: Skeletal trauma: basic science, management, and reconstruction, ed 4, Philadelphia, 2008, Saunders.)*

rotate dorsally. Closed reduction may be blocked by interposed soft tissues.

*Phalangeal condylar fractures of the proximal or middle phalanx:* Intracondylar fractures of the phalanges are divided into unicondylar and bicondylar subtypes. Unicondylar fractures are usually secondary to shearing forces, whereas bicondylar fractures are often the result of compressive loads to the head of the phalanx.

*Other intra-articular fractures of the PIP joint:* Fractures involving the articular base of the middle phalanx are the result of an axial load. The fracture pattern of displacement is determined by the nature of the deforming force. Avulsion fractures at the attachment of the volar plate are among the most common injuries. These fractures are the result of a direct axial load (or hyperextension force) and often involve only a small part of the volar aspect of the middle phalanx at the PIP joint. Stability is based on the amount of the articular surface avulsed by the volar plate, with fractures involving less than 30% of the joint surface thought to be stable and fractures involving greater than 50% almost always unstable. Higher energy axial loads can produce comminuted, pilon-type fractures of the PIP joint, which can be a devastating injury.

*Fractures at the dorsal aspect of the base of the middle phalanx:* Represent avulsion fractures of the central slip (insertion of the extensor digitorum communis tendon). These injuries are caused by hyperflexion forces at the PIP joint.

*Lateral plateau fractures of the phalanges:* Commonly are due to eccentric loading that results in the disruption of the base of the phalanx. This injury commonly causes impaction at the articular surface and may result in dorsal or rotational instability as the fragment rotates around the unaffected collateral ligament on the other side.

- Distal phalanx fractures

*Tuft and shaft fractures:* Tuft fractures are the most common subtype of distal phalanx fracture and are most often caused by a crushing mechanism. Shaft fractures also are usually secondary to a crushing-type mechanism. Both of these fracture types are associated with lacerations of the nail bed and frequently painful subungual hematomas.

*Base injuries:* Distal phalanx base fractures can be unstable injuries. The fragments of bone are subject to the deforming forces of the terminal extensor tendon and FDP tendon without the typical support of the nail plate. When these fractures are open, they are often associated with a significant amount of soft tissue injury including partial or complete amputation. In skeletally immature individuals, fractures at the base of the distal phalanx often involve the physis. Two types that are associated with age are commonly found in the pediatric age group (Fig. 12-23). The first is in the preadolescent child; the fracture is commonly open and is typically a Salter-Harris type I or type II. The extensor tendon pulls the proximal component dorsally, and the FDP tendon pulls the distal fragment volarly. The proximal aspect of the distal fragment may protrude through the wound and damage the eponychial fold. It is important to recognize this injury pattern to prevent deformity of the nail bed, growth plate arrest, and possible infection. The second group of pediatric distal phalanx base fractures is more common in the adolescent and more closely resembles a mallet-type fracture pattern.

*FDP avulsion injuries of the distal phalanx:* Relatively common injury caused by a hyperextension stress while the digit is in active flexion. Fractures can be associated with this injury pattern but are less common than an isolated FDP tendon rupture off of the bone. The ring finger is most commonly involved, and the classic patient is a rugby or football player grabbing an opponent's jersey when performing a tackle (thus the so-called jersey finger). Because there is a limited surgical window for treating certain types of FDP avulsion injuries (e.g., Leddy type 1 FDP ruptures, in which there is significant proximal retraction of the tendon into the palm), expedient follow-up with a hand surgeon is necessary when these injuries are suspected (Fig. 12-24).

*Mallet injuries of the distal phalanx:* Can be categorized as tendinous or bony and closed or open.

*Tendinous mallet injuries:* Injury to the terminal extensor tendon at the DIP joint. The injury is most commonly caused by a flexion force applied to the tip of an extended digit, which often occurs in sports but also in lower energy activities. Open mallet fingers can also be caused by a crushing mechanism or a laceration of the terminal tendon with a sharp object. Tendinous mallet injuries may be incomplete or complete (Fig. 12-25). An incomplete mallet injury is distinct from the other categories because of the patient can partially actively extend the distal phalanx. However, the digit is weaker compared with adjacent digits.

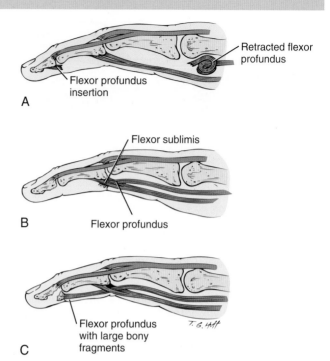

**FIGURE 12-24.** Classification system proposed by Leddy and Packer for FDP avulsion injuries. **A,** In type I, the FDP tendon ruptures off of the distal phalanx and retracts into the palm. This injury requires surgical repair within approximately 10 days. Expedient follow-up with a hand specialist is required after emergency department discharge. **B,** In type II, the FDP tendon ruptures and retracts only to the level of the PIP joint. A fleck of bone may or may not be present. **C,** In type III, a large bony fragment is avulsed along with the FDP tendon. *(From Browner BD, Jupiter JB, Levine AM, et al, editors: Skeletal trauma: basic science, management, and reconstruction, ed 4, Philadelphia, 2008, Saunders.)*

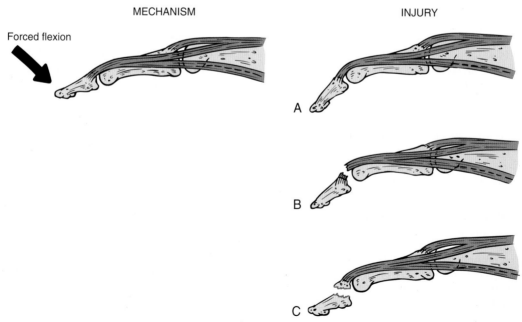

**FIGURE 12-25.** Closed tendinous mallet injuries are typically the result of a hyperflexion force to the distal phalanx. Three patterns are described: stretching of the terminal extensor tendon at its insertion **(A),** complete disruption of the terminal extensor tendon at its insertion **(B),** and complete disruption of the terminal extensor tendon with an associated avulsion of a fleck of bone pulled off of the distal phalanx at its insertion **(C).** *(From Browner BD, Jupiter JB, Levine AM, et al, editors: Skeletal Trauma: Basic Science, Management, and Reconstruction, ed 4, Philadelphia, 2008, Saunders.)*

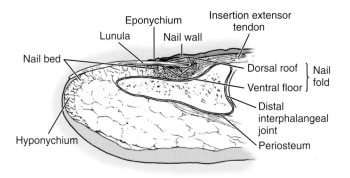

**FIGURE 12-35.** The anatomy of the nail bed illustrated in sagittal section. *(From Wolfe SW, Hotchkiss RN, Pederson WC, et al, editors: Green's operative hand surgery, ed 6, Philadelphia, 2011, Churchill Livingstone.)*

portion of the upper extremity and is often the place of interaction between an individual and his or her surroundings. Fingernails provide protection and significant function for the body. They provide tactile sensation and allow for scratching and picking up small objects.

■ Anatomy
  • Terminology
The perionychium consists of the paronychium and the nail bed (Fig. 12-35). The nail bed (matrix) consists of all the soft tissue immediately beneath the nail plate that participates in nail generation and migration. The nail bed comprises both germinal and sterile matrices. Growth of the nail plate occurs at a rate of approximately 0.1 mm/day. The proximal nail plate fits into a depression called the nail fold. The nail wall refers to the skin over the dorsum of the nail fold. The eponychium describes the thin membrane extending from the nail wall onto the dorsum of the nail. The lunula is the curved white opacity in the nail found just distal to the eponychium and resides approximately at the border between the sterile and germinal matrices. The hyponychium refers to the mass of keratin between the distal nail plate and the nail bed. This area is very resistant to infection.
  • Blood supply
The blood supply to the nail bed comes from the two terminal branches of the volar digital artery, which combine to form blood sinuses. The sinuses are surrounded by muscle fibers and participate in the regulation of blood pressure and blood supply to the distal extremities.
  Venous drainage occurs in the proximal nail bed and skin proximal to the nail fold. The veins course randomly along the dorsum of the finger.
Lymphatic vessels are abundant and are found most abundantly in the hyponychium.
  • Nerve supply
The nerve supply to the nail and nail bed is from the dorsal branch of the volar digital nerve.
■ Mechanism of Injury
Nail-bed injuries can be simply classified into one of the following four general categories:
  1. Simple lacerations (most common)
  2. Stellate lacerations

  3. Severe crush injury
  4. Avulsion
  Nail-bed injuries should be treated acutely and properly to prevent the development of future deformity. Late reconstruction of the nail bed is unpredictable, often with very little improvement. Nail deformity can be the result of anything causing deformation to the nail bed, including trauma, infection, and tumor. The focus here is on traumatic injury to the nail bed.
Sources of injury include the following:
  1. Doors (most common)
  2. Smashing between objects
  3. Lacerations from sharp objects
  4. Machinery such as knives, saws, lawnmowers in summer, and snow blowers in winter
  Nail-bed injuries occur most commonly in older children and young adults. The left hand and right hand are affected equally, with the frequency of injury occurring most commonly in the middle finger (most exposed) followed by the ring finger, index finger, and small finger. The thumb is the least frequently injured digit. Injuries to the nail bed alone are much less common than injuries that involve the surrounding paronychium and tip. The middle and distal thirds of the nail bed are the most frequent sites of injury. Simple lacerations are the most common types of injury followed by stellate, crush, and avulsion in order of decreasing frequency. Concomitant fracture of the distal phalanx is involved in 50% of nail-bed injuries.
  Injuries to the nail bed typically result from trauma to the nail, resulting in a compression between the broken or deformed nail and the bone; this typically results in a straight tearing laceration or stellate injury to the nail bed. When the nail is compressed by a much larger object and the bone, an exploding-type injury to the nail bed occurs resulting in a crush or avulsion type of pattern (Fig. 12-36).
■ History
History of the injury should elicit the mechanism and timing of the injury, any previous history of trauma to the hand, and hand dominance. The physician should also inquire about the most recent tetanus vaccine and significant medical history as it pertains to the injury and healing process. A full history can give indications of possible wound contamination and prognostic implications.
■ Diagnostic Testing
Anteroposterior, lateral, and oblique radiographs of the affected digit are necessary for diagnosis of concomitant distal phalanx fractures, DIP joint dislocations, or the presence of any foreign bodies.
■ Physical Examination
  • The patient should be supine and as comfortable as possible during the examination.
  • Observe the posture of the fingers near the nail bed, looking for deformities of nearby or underlying structures, lacerations, or crush wounds. The initial examination should be performed under sterile conditions to approximate the size of the wound, any skin loss, and the extent of the injury. Note the presence of any foreign objects and skin viability, including vascularity.

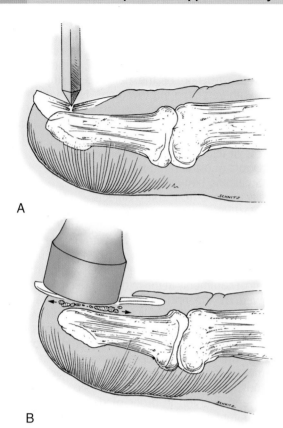

A

B

**FIGURE 12-36. A,** A relatively sharp object compressing the nail bed between the nail and bone causes a splitting laceration. **B,** A wider area of compression of the nail bed between the nail and the bone causes an exploding-type injury that results in fragmentation. *(From Wolfe SW, Hotchkiss RN, Pederson WC, et al, editors: Green's operative hand surgery, ed 6, Philadelphia, 2011, Churchill Livingstone.)*

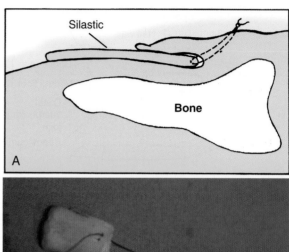

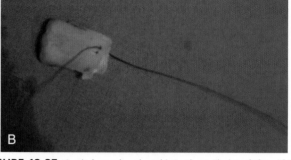

**FIGURE 12-37.** A stitch can be placed into the nail plate **(A)** or, if it is too badly damaged from the crush injury, into a silicone sheet or nonadherent gauze **(B)** and brought out dorsally through the nail wall to maintain the nail fold. *(A, From Wolfe SW, Hotchkiss RN, Pederson WC, et al, editors: Green's operative hand surgery, ed 6, Philadelphia, 2011, Churchill Livingstone.)*

- A digital block is sometimes needed to examine a nail-bed injury fully, to allow for a more comfortable assessment of motor function and vascularity. A complete sensory examination should be performed before the administration of the digital block.
- Successful repairs and outcomes are more likely when these injuries are treated acutely.
- Treatment
  - Subungual hematoma
  Small, painless subungual hematomas do not require treatment. If the hematoma is larger (>20% to 50% of the visible nail) and painful, nail trephination is recommended over removal of the nail. In this method, the heated tip of a paperclip or a microcautery device is passed through the nail to the hematoma. The physician should take care to make a hole large enough to allow sufficient drainage The hematoma is generally nonclotting blood, so it is rare for a clot to seal the hole. Care should be taken not to penetrate deep enough to injure the nail bed.
  - Simple nail-bed laceration
  Repair of a laceration of the nail bed occasionally may require removal of the nail plate. This might be considered if a subungual hematoma occupies greater than 50% of the visible nail or in the presence of a penetrating wound through the nail plate. Aggressive removal

of the nail plate for all fingertip injuries is not required because it has not been shown to improve outcomes.

A digital block and finger tourniquet are used to view the nail bed. The nail can be removed with either iris scissors slowly opening and closing under the nail bed or a periosteal elevator that is wedged underneath the distal end of the nail. The remaining soft tissue is cleaned from the removed nail, and the nail is allowed to soak in povidone-iodine (Betadine) during repair of the nail bed. If available, loupe magnification may be helpful to explore and repair the injury. Irregular edges should be trimmed cautiously because too much tissue loss results in tension on the wound.

Numerous suture options are available, but most commonly 5-0 or 6-0 chromic catgut is used (see Fig. 12-29), with a curved needle to allow for easy passage through the nail bed. Chromic catgut is absorbable, which avoids painful suture removal and disruption of healing in the future. The nail fold must be kept open to prevent scarring and allow for future nail growth. A hole can be drilled or burned in the nail approximately over the location of the injury to allow for serum or hematoma drainage of the repair site after the nail is replaced. It is best to keep the nail fold open by replacing the original nail, but a nail-shaped sheet of 0.02-inch reinforced silicone or nonadherent gauze may also be used if the nail is too badly damaged. If silicone is used, 5-0 or 6-0 suture is used to keep it in place; a horizontal mattress stitch is placed through the nail wall to hold the silicone sheet, nonadherent gauze, or nail plate in the nail fold (Fig. 12-37). The mattress stitch

A limited assessment of the wound can be done, and a thorough distal neurovascular examination looking for possible tendon or nerve injury should be performed. If any of these injuries are appreciated, telephone consultation in the emergency department with a hand surgeon should be obtained to facilitate surgical planning.

## INJECTION INJURIES

Despite benign-appearing superficial wounds and often painless presentations, injuries from high-pressure liquids are devastating injuries that often cause tissue loss and infection. The severity of the injury is often overlooked by the patient. Patients who do not seek treatment early may complain later of numbness, discoloration, or tenderness to palpation. If there is very little tenderness near the injection site within several hours, it is unlikely that significant injury has occurred. These injuries are becoming more common as hydrolic powered, pressure cleaning, and power painting tools are becoming less expensive to own and operate. The patient is most likely to be male laborer with an average age of 35 years. These tools produce fluid pressures greatly in excess of the minimum pressure needed to break human skin.

The fluid and resulting inflammatory reactions are thought to increase interstitial pressure in the finger, occluding the vascular supply and causing necrosis of the skin and subcutaneous tissue. Damage is related to the composition of the fluid injected and the volume, pressure, and location of injection. The most commonly affected digit is the nondominant index finger, with injury usually sustained while cleaning a high-pressure gun. The most common materials injected are grease, paint, paint thinner, hydraulic fluid, molding, plastic, and wax. Organic solvents, such as oil-based paints, are more damaging than water-based solvents.

Surgical decompression and débridement of all ischemic tissue within 6 hours of organic solvent injury reduces the risk of subsequent amputation. Delayed surgery increases both the risk of amputation and mortality. Paint injections are considered a surgical emergency; the use of solvents is not recommended because they can cause tissue damage. Water-based injuries also require immediate surgical exploration, treated with the same surgical urgency as any other compartment syndrome in the body.

Broad-spectrum antibiotics and a tetanus immunization if needed should be administered in the emergency department. The affected hand should be elevated to reduce pain and swelling. Steroid use has not been shown to decrease the amputation rate or incidence of infection. Digital block anesthesia should not be used as part of the primary treatment, but systemic pain medications should be used liberally to control pain. Urgent surgical treatment in the operating room under general anesthesia is indicated.

## HAND BURNS

Burns of the hand are common. Although most thermal injuries are minor, the most appropriate management of these injuries requires an aggressive and multidisciplinary approach best achieved at a specialized burn center. Detailed discussion of burn injuries in general and the comprehensive care given to a hand burn patient at a specialized center is beyond the scope of this chapter, but initial assessment and care are reviewed.

■ History

History should be obtained by the initial health care provider evaluating the patient, including occupation, hand dominance, preexisting extremity injury, mechanism of injury, and tetanus status. In pediatric patients, approximately 10% of burn injuries are suspicious for child abuse. Several typical types of abuse result in hand burns: (1) hot water immersion resulting in a glovelike burn distribution, (2) forced contact with a hot object, and (3) flame burn from a cigarette lighter.

■ Physical Examination

Examination of the injured hand must include perfusion, estimation of the depth and extent of injury, presence of circumferential components, and associated injuries. Warning signs of vascular compromise include skin that is cool to palpation or diminished capillary refill. Doppler may be used to assess the blood flow of the palmar arch and individual digits. A high suspicion of compromised flow should be maintained in patients with significant edema and deep dermal, circumferential, or near circumferential burns, and escharotomies should be performed in a timely manner to prevent ischemic necrosis of the hand.

■ Treatment

If a burn wound is supple, there is no need for an escharotomy. However, if a deep circumferential burn has produced an unyielding band of tissue that is restricting capillary perfusion and risking limb death, an escharotomy should be performed. Although experienced burn surgeons are the ideal physicians to perform any needed escharotomies, if urgently necessary to save a limb, the operation may be performed in the emergency department at the patient's bedside to release any restrictive burned tissue (Fig. 12-41). Forearm escharotomies are performed by making incisions longitudinally along the midaxial line of the radial or ulnar aspect of the forearm and can be extended past the MCP joints of the first and fifth digits. Intrinsic muscle and digital hand escharotomies can also be performed. The utility of digital escharotomies is debated in the literature with some authors believing that the risk of harm to underlying neurovascular structures outweighs the potential benefits.

The goals of initial emergency department management in a patient with a hand burn are to provide analgesia, prevent infection, minimize heat and water loss, and promote epithelialization. Any foreign material and loose or thin blisters should be débrided. There is debate regarding whether intact blisters should be left intact or débrided. For significant burns, application of silver sulfadiazine and dry gauze is appropriate. For burns of less depth, applying nonadherent greasy gauze and antibacterial ointment is adequate for bandaging.

Chemical burns of the hand warrant special note because they require specific care. All chemical burns should be treated with the following general principles:

**Digital, intrinsic, radial, ulnar escharotomies**

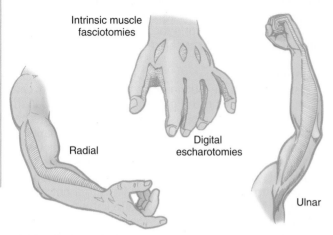

Intrinsic muscle fasciotomies

Radial

Digital escharotomies

Ulnar

**FIGURE 12-41.** Digital, intrinsic, radial, and ulnar escharotomies. Escharotomy is considered when circumferential burns are present and the burn wound is believed to be restricting capillary perfusion. *(From Hotchkiss RN, Pederson WC, Kozin SH, et al, editors. Green's operative hand surgery, ed 4, Philadelphia, Churchill Livingstone, 1999.)*

(1) removal of the chemical agent (i.e., brushing off the dry chemical); (2) copious irrigation of the affected area; (3) consideration of contacting a toxicology center because some agents have metabolic effects; (4) examination of the burn with the knowledge that most chemical burns are deeper than they initially appear; (5) special consideration for specific agents if appropriate (as in hydrofluoric acid burns); and (6) local care of the burn.

With respect to specific agents, hydrofluoric acid is highly dangerous and widely available in multiple household and industrial agents. The specific treatment of hydrofluoric acid burns warrants special attention. Treatment should be performed in a stepwise fashion, proceeding to the next step if pain persists after completion of the preceding one. Fluoride ions can cause extensive damage because they are absorbed into the tissue of the hand. Binding to calcium can neutralize them. Initial treatment is irrigation for 20 to 30 minutes with water. If pain persists, topical calcium gel is useful. If needed, mixing an ampule of calcium gluconate with two or three packages of Surgilube lubricating jelly can make an adequate gel. For larger burn areas, local injection of calcium gluconate or intra-arterial infusion may be necessary. Local infiltration is performed with 10% calcium gluconate; 0.5 mL/cm$^2$ of burned tissue is infiltrated with a 30-gauge needle. Traditionally, intra-arterial infusion is the next step if pain still persists.

## HAND AND DIGIT LACERATIONS

Lacerations of the hand are commonly occurring injuries that vary in severity from superficial breaches of skin to complete amputations. They are broadly categorized based on location (proximal or distal, dorsal or volar), amount of contamination, and mechanism of injury (simple cut or crush).

■ Anatomy and Classification
  • *Dorsal lacerations:* Are categorized based on zone of potential extensor tendon injury. Kleinert and Verdan described the most commonly used classification system that divided the hand and forearm into eight zones, beginning distally at the fingertips (zone I) and ending in the forearm (zone VIII). The odd-numbered zones overlie joints. Zone I covers from the tip of the finger to the DIP joints and contains the terminal tendon. Zone II extends across the middle phalanx and includes the extensor apparatus and the lateral bands, which travel from volar to dorsal in this zone. Zone III represents the PIP joint, and zone IV represents the proximal phalanx. Zone V covers the MCP joint and contains the extensor digitorum communis tendon and the sagittal bands. Zone VI extends over the metacarpals to the CMC joints. Zone VII represents the carpal bones. Zone VIII comprises the distal forearm. A ninth zone has been described to include the muscular portion of the extensors in the mid and proximal forearm (Fig. 12-42).
  • *Volar lacerations:* Similar to dorsal lacerations, are classified by zone as defined by Kleinert and Verdan. There are five flexor zones that apply to the index finger, middle finger, ring finger, and small finger; the thumb is classified separately (Fig. 12-43). Zone I flexor tendon injuries of the digits involve the FDP tendon only and extend from the tip of the finger to the insertion of the FDS tendon. Zone II, commonly referred to as "no man's land," is bounded distally by the insertion of the FDS tendon and extends proximally to the A-1 pulley just proximal to the MCP joint. Within this zone, the FDS tendon splits into two slips that surround the FDP tendon before reuniting at Camper chiasma (Fig. 12-44). Adhesions after injury are very common in this location. Zone III extends distally from the A-1 pulley to the proximal edge of the carpal tunnel. Zone IV represents the carpal tunnel, and zone V extends from the proximal edge of the carpal tunnel to the origins of the flexor tendons at their muscle bellies in the forearm.
  • *Amputations:* Are classified by mechanism of injury, the level and obliquity through which the amputation occurred, which digit or digits are involved, and the presence of exposed bone or nail-bed injuries.
■ Mechanism of Injury
  The mechanism of injury is a critical determinant of treatment and potential outcome. The mechanism of injury helps to define not only the energy of the injury but also the potential for contamination. High-energy mechanisms may have a much larger zone of injury than is initially apparent and may not manifest to the full extent immediately. Crushing, avulsion, and high-pressure mechanisms often result in a large zone of injury with damage to bone, neurovascular tissue, and surrounding soft tissue. Penetrating trauma mechanisms may have a more limited and specific zone of injury.
■ History
  The medical history, or the how, when, and where of what happened, is extremely helpful to guide treatment and offers prognostic information. How an injury

Peckler B, Hsu CK: Tourniquet syndrome: a review of constricting band removal. J Emerg Med 20:253–262, 2001.

Pinto MR, Turkula-Pinto LD, Cooney WP, et al: High-pressure injection injuries of the hand: review of 25 patients managed by open wound technique. J Hand Surg Am 18:125–130, 1993.

Satonik RC: Burns and cold injuries. In Hart RG, Uehara DT, Wagner MJ, editors: Emergency and primary care of the hand, Dallas, 2001, American College of Emergency Physicians, pp 247–255.

Schoo MJ, Scott FA, Boswick JA, Jr: High-pressure injection injuries of the hand. J Trauma 20:229–238, 1980.

Sheridan RL, Baryza MJ, Pessina MA, et al: Acute hand burns in children: management and long-term outcome based on a 10-year experience with 698 injured hands. Ann Surg 229:558–564, 1999.

Sheridan RL, Hurley J, Smith MA, et al: The acutely burned hand: management and outcome based on a ten-year experience with 1047 acute hand burns. J Trauma 38:406–411, 1995.

Simon RR, Sherman SC, Koenigsknecht SJ: Rheumatology. In Simon RR, et al, editors: Emergency orthopedics: the extremities, ed 5, New York, 2007, McGraw-Hill, pp 40–75.

Simon RR, Sherman SC, Koenigsknecht SJ: Hand. In Simon RR, et al, editors: Emergency orthopedics: the extremities, ed 5, New York, 2007, McGraw-Hill.

Smith MA, Munster AM, Spence RJ: Burns of the hand and upper limb: a review. Burns 24:493–505, 1998.

Stark HH, Ashworth CR, Boyes JH: Paint-gun injuries of the hand. J Bone Joint Surg Am 49:637–647, 1967.

Sterling J, Gibran NS, Klein MB: Acute management of hand burns. Hand Clin 25:453–459, 2009.

Sykes PJ: Severe burns of the hand: a practical guide to their management. J Hand Surg Br 16:6–12, 1991.

Thilagarajah M: An improved method of ring removal. J Hand Surg Br 24:118–119, 1999.

Tosti R, Ilyas AM: Empiric antibiotics for acute infections of the hand: evidence-based medicine. J Hand Surg Am 35:125–128, 2010.

Towheed TE, Maxwell L, Judd MG, et al: Acetaminophen for osteoarthritis. Cochrane Database Syst Rev (1):CD004257, 2009.

Tsai E, Failla J: Hand infections in the trauma patient. Hand Clin 15:373–386, 1999.

Turner TW: Do mammalian bites require antibiotic prophylaxis? Ann Emerg Med 44:274–276, 2004.

Urbaniak JR, Seaber AV, Chen LE: Assessment of ischemia and reperfusion injury. Clin Orthop Relat Res 334:30–36, 1997.

Verhoeven N, Hierner R: High-pressure injection injury of the hand: an often underestimated trauma: case report and study of the literature. Strategies in Trauma and Limb Reconstruction, 27-33, 2008.

Wee JT, Chandra D: A rapid method of removal of rings impacted in fingers. J Hand Surg Br 14:126–127, 1989.

Weiland AJ, Rohde RS: Acute management of hand injuries, Thorofare, NJ, 2009, Slack.

Wolanyk DE: Infections. In Hart RG, Uehara DT, Wagner MJ, editors: Emergency and primary care of the hand, Dallas, 2001, American College of Emergency Physicians, pp 219–246.

Zook EG: Discussion of "The etiologies and mechanisms of nail bed injury." Hand Clin 6:21, 1990.

Zook EG, Guy RJ, Russell RC: A study of nail bed injuries: causes, treatment, and prognosis. J Hand Surg Am 9:247–252, 1984.

# PART II
# Specific Anatomic Regions

## SECTION TWO
## Lower Extremity

*Hip and Thigh*
*Distal Femur, Knee, and Patella*
*Ankle*
*Foot*

# Chapter 13  *Hip and Thigh*

Fernando Checo, Mark Shekhman,
Alex Goldstein, and Andrew S. Erwteman

## ANATOMY

A good understanding of the femoroacetabular joint is necessary to appreciate hip pathology fully and help guide the physical examination. The hip is a diarthrodial joint consisting of bony and soft tissue constraints making it an inherently stable articulation.

- Bony Anatomy
  - Acetabulum, femoral head and neck, greater and lesser trochanter, and femoral shaft
  - Deep socket of the acetabulum allows for the large femoral head to be well seated and covered (Fig. 13-1)
  - This relationship along with a narrow femoral neck affords stability, while permitting a large arc of motion in the sagittal, coronal, and axial planes
- Soft Tissue
  - Labrum

    Ring of fibrocartilage that deepens the acetabular socket

    Increases the femoral head coverage and improves the overall stability of the hip joint

  - Ligamentum teres (round ligament of the femur)

    Triangular structure consisting of two fibrous bands that attach to the fovea capitis of the femoral head

    Traveling within the substance of the bands is the acetabular branch of the obturator artery

  - Capsule

    Formed by the coalescence of the iliofemoral, pubo-femoral, and ischiofemoral ligaments

    Fibrocapsular structure significantly increases stability of the hip joint

    Adheres anteriorly near the distal femoral neck and intertrochanteric region and posteriorly near the distal half of the femoral neck

    Knowledge of neurovascular anatomy of the proximal femur is important when evaluating fractures and dislocations

- Medial Femoral Circumflex Artery
  The medial femoral circumflex artery is the main blood supply of the femoral head and most of the neck via the terminal branches. It is a branch of the profunda femoris artery and gives rise to a deep branch. The deep branch initially is extracapsular running deep to the quadratus femoris. As it ascends along the greater trochanter, it pierces the capsule giving rise to multiple terminal branches that supply the femoral head. In adults, there is insignificant contribution from the lateral femoral circumflex artery, medial epiphyseal artery, obturator artery, and superior and inferior gluteal arteries.
- Femoral Nerve
  - Derived from the ventral rami of L2-4
  - Courses between the iliacus and the psoas muscles and then anteriorly over the iliacus before passing deep to the inguinal ligament
  - Innervates the quadriceps muscles, gives sensation to the anteromedial thigh, and terminates as the saphenous nerve
- Sciatic Nerve
  The sciatic nerve arises from the lumbosacral plexus (L4-S3). In the most common variation, the nerve exits the pelvis through the greater sciatic foramen and courses anterior to the piriformis muscle. The tibial

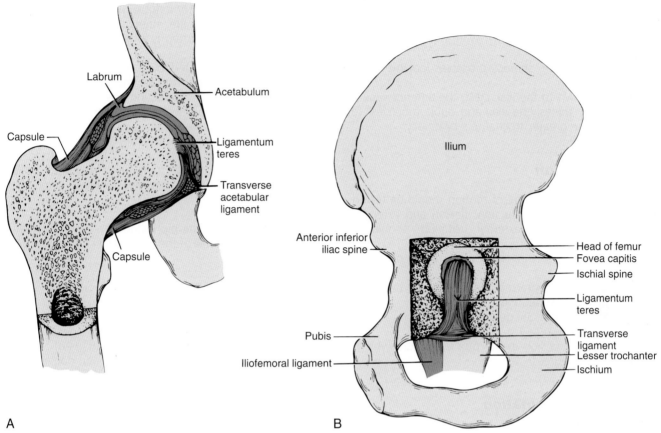

A                                                                                    B

**FIGURE 13-1.** Deep socket of the acetabulum allows for the large femoral head to be well seated and covered. *(From Browner BD, Jupiter JB, Levine AM, et al, editors: Skeletal trauma: basic science, management, and reconstruction, ed 3, Philadelphia, 2003, Saunders.)*

division arises from the anterior branch and innervates the long head of the biceps femoris, semitendinosus, and posterior compartment muscles. The peroneal division gives rise to the deep and superficial peroneal nerves. They innervate the anterior and lateral compartment muscles of the lower leg and provide sensation for the anterior and lateral aspect of the lower leg and the dorsum of the foot.

## HISTORY

- A comprehensive history regarding the mechanism of injury, trauma, or any antecedent pain or dysfunction should be obtained.
- Chronicity of symptoms should be determined.
- Location of pain or discomfort, quality, modifying factors, and radiation of the pain help narrow the differential diagnosis.
- The mechanism of injury can be from direct trauma or indirect trauma.
- A fall from a standing height leading to a fracture is typical of a fragility fracture.
- In young patients, significant energy is often required to fracture the femur or to cause a dislocation.
- Axial loading injuries can affect not only the lower limb but also the spine, so back and neck complaints should be sought.

## PHYSICAL EXAMINATION

- When evaluating a patient with hip complaints, it is imperative to be systematic in the musculoskeletal examination.
- Following general principles assists in honing in on the etiology of the symptoms.
- The physical examination comprises inspection, palpation, range of motion, neurologic examination, and vascular examination.

### Inspection

- Inspect the patient in a comfortable position either supine or standing.
- Evaluate gait when possible.
- Certain pathologic gaits such as antalgic, spastic, cerebellar ataxic, or Trendelenburg gait can aid in making the correct diagnosis.
- Initially the patient should be disrobed to expose the hip region.
- A thorough evaluation of the spine, pelvis, and hips should be performed.
- Look for any abrasions, lacerations, discolorations, hematomas, or soft tissue swelling.
- Assess for leg-length discrepancies, muscle atrophy, and the position of the extremity.

### Palpation

- Palpate to assess for any warmth, fluctuance, or tenderness.
- Start palpating the spinous processes looking for any stepoffs or pain.
- Continue down to the iliac crest, the anterior superior inferior iliac spines, the iliac and pubic tubercles, followed by the greater trochanters bilaterally.

### Range of Motion

- Active and passive range of motion should be tested.
- Hip abduction and adduction, flexion and extension, and internal and external rotation should be measured.
- With the patient supine, normal range of motion includes:
  - Abduction 45 degrees and adduction 20 degrees
  - Hip flexion 120 degrees
  - Internal rotation 35 degrees and external rotation 45 degrees
- Test for hip extension in the prone position, which is normally 30 degrees.

### Neurologic Examination

- Motor Examination
  - Muscle strength is graded with reference to the contralateral side and ranges from 0 to 5 (Table 13-1).
  - Hip flexors (iliopsoas, rectus femoris) are innervated by the femoral nerve.
  - Test hip flexors with the patient either supine or sitting and having the patient flex the hip against resistance.
  - Hip extensors (gluteus maximus and hamstrings) are innervated by the inferior gluteal nerve and the sciatic nerve.
  - Test hip extensors with the patient in prone position by having the patient elevate the thigh off the table against resistance while keeping the knee flexed to relax the hamstrings.
  - Abductors (gluteus minimus and medius) are innervated by the superior gluteal nerve.
  - To test abductors, the patient is placed in the lateral position and instructed to abduct the leg against resistance.

**TABLE 13-1** Medical Research Council Grading

| Grade | |
|---|---|
| 0 | No movement |
| 1 | Flicker of movement |
| 2 | Movement only with gravity eliminated |
| 3 | Full range of movement against gravity |
| 4 | Full range of movement against some resistance |
| 5 | Full power against resistance |

- Adductors (adductor longus, brevis, magnus, pectineus, and gracilis) are innervated by the obturator nerve (pectineus often is innervated by the femoral nerve).
- Adductors are tested by having the patient lay in the lateral position, making the leg being tested the bottom leg. After abducting the upper leg for the patient and supporting it, the patient is instructed to adduct the leg against resistance.
- Both abductors and adductors can be tested in the supine position by having both legs abducted and instructing the patient to abduct and adduct against resistance. This method allows for direct comparison of both sides.
- Sensation
  - Dermatomes of the hip include L1-4, with L1 being the most proximal at the hip and L4 coursing through the knee.

### Vascular Examination

- A thorough vascular evaluation is vital, especially when treating patients with fracture-dislocations of the hip.
- Palpate the popliteal, posterior tibial, and dorsalis pedis pulses.
- If pulses are not palpable, Doppler examination is warranted.

## DIAGNOSTIC TESTING

- Radiography
  - Radiographs should be the initial imaging studies.
  - Full-length images including the joint above and below are standard.
  - Anteroposterior pelvis and anteroposterior and lateral (cross-table) images of the hip should be obtained.
  - Anteroposterior and lateral knee radiographs should be obtained.
- Computed Tomography (CT) Scan
  - CT scans are reserved for pathologic fractures and for evaluating the congruency of the joint after a hip dislocation.
  - Patients who have sustained multiple trauma injuries should have a fine-cut CT scan (2-mm cuts) to evaluate for a nondisplaced femoral neck fracture.
- Magnetic Resonance Imaging (MRI)
  - MRI has some indication in the right clinical setting.
  - MRI is the preferred diagnostic study to evaluate for an occult femoral neck fracture in an elderly patient who is unable to bear weight after a fall and has negative hip radiographs.
  - MRI is useful in evaluating soft tissue injuries around the hip.
- Hip Joint Aspiration
  - Hip joint aspiration is rarely indicated in the emergency department.
  - In patients in whom there is concern for septic joint, joint fluid aspiration with ultrasound guidance could be attempted.

- Standard joint fluid studies include cell count, Gram stain, culture, glucose, protein, and crystals.
- In the setting of septic joint, C-reactive protein (CRP), erythrocyte sedimentation rate (ESR), and white blood cell (WBC) count assist in the diagnosis and evaluation of treatment response.

# PROXIMAL FEMUR FRACTURES

## *Femoral Head Fractures*

- Although these fractures are uncommon, timely diagnosis is important because delayed treatment can lead to significant morbidity.
- Femoral head fracture should be suspected in polytrauma patients, especially patients with hip dislocations.
- This fracture is estimated to be associated with 5% to 15% of all posterior hip dislocations.[1,2]
- Diagnosis
  - A thorough physical examination should be performed with emphasis on sciatic nerve function especially for posterior hip dislocations.
  - Femoral head fractures can be diagnosed with plain films when associated with a hip dislocation or with a CT scan after the hip has been relocated.
  - Clinically patients may have a shortened, adducted, and internally rotated extremity with a posterior hip dislocation and a shortened, abducted, and externally rotated extremity with an anterior hip dislocation.
- Classification
  - Femoral head fracture is classified by the Brumback or the Pipkin classification scheme.[3,4]
  - The Pipkin classification is the most widely used and reproducible.
  - Pipkin classification is based on the location of the femoral head fracture in reference to the fovea capitis femoris and the presence of an associated acetabular or femoral neck fracture (Fig. 13-2).
- Management
  - Treatment of these high-energy injuries should be prompt; immediate orthopedic consultation is recommended.

- Rapid restoration of blood perfusion is critical owing to the tenuous vascular supply of the femoral head and concomitant injuries.
- For femoral head fractures associated with a hip dislocation, reduction of the hip within 6 hours from injury has been associated with diminished risk of avascular necrosis (AVN) and osteoarthritis.[5]
- A fine-cut CT scan is recommended after reduction to evaluate for joint congruency and the quality of the fracture reduction.
- Patients with Pipkin I and II fractures can be treated conservatively when the fracture is less than 2 mm displaced, the joint is congruent, and the hip is stable to range of motion examination.
  - If these parameters are met, the patient can be made partial weight bearing with crutches.
- Patients with displaced Pipkin I and II fractures, Pipkin III and IV fractures, an incongruent joint, or an unstable hip joint are usually managed surgically.
- Objectives of treatment are anatomic reduction of the femoral head, neck, and acetabular fragments; congruency of the joint; and removal of intra-articular fragments.
- Common Pitfalls
  - Delayed closed reduction of the dislocated hip can lead to complications.
  - There is evidence that reduction within 6 to 12 hours reduces the risk of developing AVN.[5]
  - Overall incidence of AVN is 20%, including both surgical and nonsurgical treatment.[6,7]
  - Every patient with a femoral head fracture should be informed of the risk of developing AVN even with early reduction.
  - Risk of developing AVN is higher for Pipkin III and IV fractures.
  - There is a 10% to 23% incidence of sciatic nerve injury usually involving the peroneal division; 60% of patients regain partial motor and sensory function.[8]
  - Post-traumatic arthrosis is exceedingly common with a reported incidence ranging from 8% to 75%.[6,7]
  - Heterotopic ossification has been documented, especially in fracture-dislocations and in surgically treated injuries.
  - Overall incidence of heterotopic ossification is reported to be up to 75%.[6,7,9]

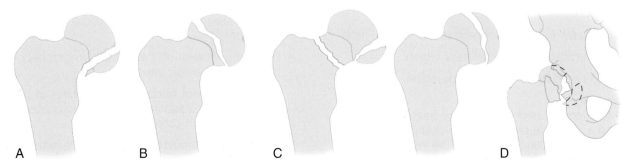

A          B          C          D

**FIGURE 13-2.** Pipkin classification. Notice the location of the femoral head fracture in reference to the fovea centralis and the presence of an associated acetabular or femoral neck fracture.

# HIP FRACTURES

- The mechanism of injury in elderly patients usually involves a low-energy fall.
- Hip fracture is a fragility fracture by definition.
- Attention should be paid to the ipsilateral upper extremity because concomitant proximal humerus and distal radius fractures can occur as the patient stretches out the hand trying to break the fall.[10,11]
- Younger patients sustain hip fractures secondary to high-energy trauma.
- Hip fracture in a young patient is usually a result of a motor vehicle or motorcycle accident or a fall from a height.
- There may be life-threatening injuries that take precedence over the limb injuries.
- A hip fracture is managed in an urgent fashion after the patient has been stabilized.[10,12,13]

## *Femoral Neck Fractures*

- These are mostly intracapsular fractures that occur below the femoral head and above the trochanters.
- Diagnosis
  - Any patient with suspected femoral neck fracture should have anteroposterior and lateral hip radiographs and anteroposterior and lateral knee radiographs.
  - In situations in which it is unclear whether the patient has a low femoral neck or intertrochanteric hip fracture, internal rotation traction hip radiographs including anteroposterior and lateral views can be helpful.
  - Distinguishing between the two fracture patterns is important because it may alter the definitive management.[12–14]
  - MRI is recommended for patients with acute trauma to the hip who are unable to bear weight and have negative radiographs.[15]
  - MRI is used to evaluate for occult femoral neck fracture.
  - A fine-cut (<2 mm) CT scan can be performed in patients with an absolute contraindication for MRI (i.e., metal implants in the eye, brain, or heart) or when MRI is unavailable.
- Classification
  - The Garden classification is used (Fig. 13-3).
  - Another method is to describe the fracture by its location:

    *Subcapital:* Below or adjacent to the femoral head

    *Transcervical:* Mid–femoral neck region

    *Basicervical:* Distal femoral neck region

- Management
  - Most femoral neck fractures are treated operatively, and a complete preoperative evaluation is required.
  - The decision concerning operative versus nonoperative treatment is based on the patient's age, medical comorbidities, fracture pattern, and concomitant injuries.

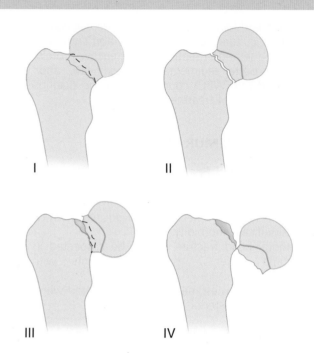

**FIGURE 13-3.** Garden classification.

  - At our institution, all patients have complete blood count, electrolytes, blood urea nitrogen and creatinine, prothrombin time/international normalized ratio, and partial thromboplastin time tests.
  - Patients older than 40 years also have a chest radiograph and electrocardiogram, and a type and crossmatch for 2 units of packed red blood cells is performed.[10,12]
  - Femoral neck fracture in a physiologically young patient (≤55 years old), whether displaced or not, is an orthopedic emergency.
  - Because of the retrograde femoral neck vascularity, timely reduction should be performed to preserve the native anatomy, and urgent orthopedic consultation is recommended.
- Emergency Department Management
  - Adequate pain control should be prescribed.
  - Buck's skin traction of 10 lb maximum can provide pain relief by limiting motion at the fracture site.[16]
- Common Pitfalls
  - Failure to recognize an occult femoral neck fracture

    All patients with acute hip pain after a fall who are unable to bear weight should undergo MRI (or CT as discussed) to rule out an occult femoral neck fracture.[15]

  - Delayed treatment of a displaced femoral neck fracture in a physiologic young patient

    Early reduction of femoral neck fractures in physiologic young patients has been associated with reduced risk of osteonecrosis.[17,18]

    Young patients should be informed of the increased risk of osteoarthritis, osteonecrosis, and nonunion when treated with open reduction and internal fixation; this is true for early and delayed treatment.[17,18]

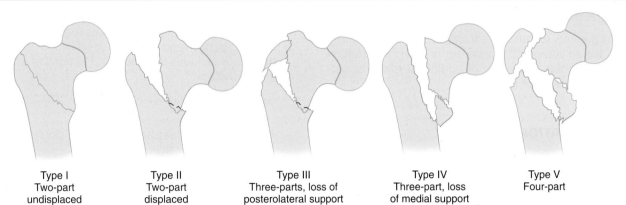

| Type I | Type II | Type III | Type IV | Type V |
| --- | --- | --- | --- | --- |
| Two-part undisplaced | Two-part displaced | Three-parts, loss of posterolateral support | Three-part, loss of medial support | Four-part |

**FIGURE 13-4.** Jensen classification.

- Inadequate radiographs

  Some femoral neck fractures are basicervical or low neck fractures, which can change the treatment plan.

  Internal rotation and traction views can help visualize the fracture pattern better and aid in the diagnosis.

  Radiographs of the joint above and below the fracture should always be obtained.

- Osteoporosis evaluation

  All patients sustaining a fragility fracture should be advised to be evaluated for osteoporosis.

  More recent literature shows the reduced incidence of fragility fractures with current pharmacologic treatment for osteoporosis.[19,20]

## Intertrochanteric Femur Fractures

- Intertrochanteric femur fractures are fractures located between the greater and lesser trochanter.
- These are among the most common hip fractures in elderly patients and are rare in young patients.[21]
- Diagnosis
  - Patients with intertrochanteric femur fractures typically complain of acute onset of hip pain after a fall.
  - Inability to bear weight and restricted range of motion are common findings.
  - Full-length anteroposterior and lateral radiographs including the knee should be obtained.
  - In a situation in which it is difficult to delineate between a low femoral neck fracture (basicervical) and an intertrochanteric femur fracture, traction internal rotation radiographs are helpful.
  - Occasionally a patient with negative radiographs who is unable to bear weight after an acute fall is encountered.
  - MRI is warranted to rule out an occult hip fracture.
  - A fine-cut CT scan with 2-mm cuts can be obtained in patients who are unable to undergo MRI.
- Classification
  - There have been many proposed classifications for intertrochanteric femur fractures, but no particular classification scheme has been universally accepted.

- Assess the number of fracture fragments, the direction of the main fracture, and the integrity of the posterior medial buttress.
- We prefer the Jensen classification because of its reproducibility, while offering guidance for surgical treatment (Fig. 13-4).[22]
- Management
  - All patients should have a baseline preinjury functional evaluation
  - Pain should be controlled with narcotics as appropriate.
  - Skin traction with Buck's inline traction can be used to reduce motion at the fracture site and theoretically to improve pain.
  - Because of the morbidity and mortality associated with untreated or neglected hip fractures, unless medically contraindicated, surgical treatment is nearly universal.[23]
  - Medical clearance is usually required because these patients are typically older and are likely to have multiple comorbidities.
  - The goal is to have the patient medically optimized as soon as possible before undergoing surgical management.
  - Patients with a significant cardiac history should have a cardiology consultation as soon as possible to have adequate time to obtain any necessary studies.
- Common Pitfalls
  - Inadequate radiographs

    Full-length films are required to evaluate for any pathologic lesions distal to the fracture and to assist in measuring the proper length of an intramedullary implant if one is used.

  - Missed occult fracture

    Any elderly patient with an acute history of trauma with inability to bear weight should undergo MRI if radiographs are negative.[15]

  - Incomplete work-up

    Hip fractures are usually surgically managed.

    Obtaining preoperative laboratory and imaging studies and consultations to optimize the patient medically before surgery is ideal.[23]

- Osteoporosis evaluation

  All patients with fragility fractures should be referred for an osteoporosis work-up or given information about the future risk of additional fractures secondary to osteoporosis.[20,24]

## HIP DISLOCATIONS

- Because of the bony and soft tissue anatomy, the femoroacetabular articulation is intrinsically stable.
- A hip dislocation requires significant force to disrupt the bony and soft tissue restraints.
- The most common etiology of hip dislocation is high-energy trauma usually from a motor vehicle accident or a fall.[25–28]
- Native hip dislocation when the anatomic femoral head dislodges from the anatomic acetabulum is a true orthopedic emergency.
- Reduction within a timely fashion, usually less than 6 to 8 hours after injury, is crucial for the survival of the femoral head, and prompt orthopedic consultation is recommended.[27,28]
- The goal of treatment is to obtain a stable concentric reduction as soon as possible.[29,30]
- A thorough initial evaluation should be performed because 80% of patients have other associated systemic injuries.

### Posterior Hip Dislocations

- Posterior hip dislocation is the most common type of dislocation; it occurs in up to 90% of all hip dislocations.[28-30]
- The classic mechanism includes an axial force to a flexed hip. This is commonly seen during a motor vehicle accident when the flexed knee strikes the dashboard.
- Diagnosis
  - Initial evaluation should follow the advanced trauma life support (ATLS) protocols.
  - For posterior dislocation, patients present with the lower extremity in a flexed, adducted, and internally rotated position.
  - A complete neurovascular examination should be performed with focus on the sciatic nerve distribution.
  - Standard radiographs include an anteroposterior pelvis view and a cross-table lateral view of the hip.
  - On the anteroposterior radiograph, there is an incongruous femoroacetabular joint with a smaller appearing femoral head relative to the contralateral femoral head.
  - Typically prereduction radiographs are sufficient.
  - If there is any concern for a no-displaced femoral neck fracture, a prereduction CT scan may be obtained.
  - CT scans can be performed relatively fast and should minimally delay time to reduction.
- Classification
  - Hip dislocation is classified by the direction of the femoral head relative to the acetabulum.

- The most commonly used and simplest classification is posterior and anterior hip dislocation.
- The Thompson and Epstein classification is useful because it includes any additional femoral or acetabular pathology:[31]

  *Type I:* Posterior dislocation with or without a minor fracture

  *Type II:* Posterior dislocation with large single fracture of the posterior acetabular rim

  *Type III:* Posterior dislocation with comminution of acetabular rim with or without a major fracture fragment

  *Type IV:* Posterior dislocation with a fracture of the acetabular floor

  *Type V:* Posterior dislocation with a fracture of the femoral head

- Management
  - Isolated posterior hip dislocations are treated with prompt closed reduction.
  - An uneventful closed reduction requires good muscle relaxation, analgesia, and conscious sedation.
  - If good muscle relaxation, analgesia, and conscious sedation are not possible in the emergency department, the closed reduction should be performed in the operating room.
- Reduction Technique
  - At our institution, the most commonly used method of reducing a posterior hip dislocation is the Allis technique.[29]
  - After sedation, analgesia, and muscle relaxation, the patient is positioned supine.
  - The operator applies inline traction to move the femoral head from under the acetabulum, while the assistant applies counterpressure to the pelvis.
  - This is followed by slow flexion of the hip with controlled internal and external rotation until the femoral head sinks into the acetabulum (Fig. 13-5).
  - Many other techniques have been described, including the Bigelow and East Baltimore lift.[29,30]
  - After obtaining a successful reduction, the hip should be put through a range of motion in all three planes to evaluate stability: flexion and extension, adduction and abduction, and internal and external rotation.
  - If the hip is stable, a knee immobilizer should be placed to prevent flexion.
- Postreduction Management
  - A postreduction examination should be performed, and radiographs should be obtained.
  - When evaluating the postreduction radiographs, the hip should be concentric.
  - It has become a standard practice at our institution to obtain a fine-cut (2-mm) CT scan after reduction to evaluate for osteochondral intra-articular fragments, femoral or acetabular fractures, and the overall congruency of the reduction.
  - This is especially important when there is an acetabular wall fracture because there is evidence that CT scan can augment the clinical examination when determining hip joint stability after reduction.[32,33]

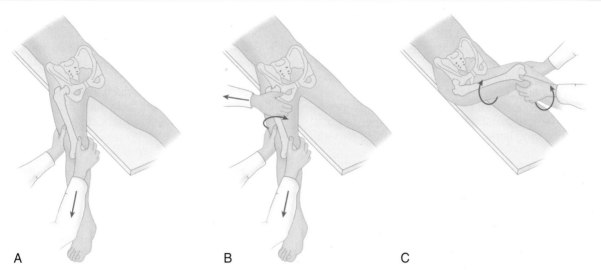

A            B            C

**FIGURE 13-5.** Slow flexion of the hip with controlled internal and external rotation until the femoral head sinks into the acetabulum.

- Keith et al.[32] determined the size of a posterior wall fragment that resulted in an unstable hip by studying cadavers.
- When less than 20% of the posterior wall was fractured, the hip was stable.
- When greater than 40% of the posterior wall was disrupted, the hip was unstable.
- Patients with successful closed reduction can be made foot flat touchdown weight bearing with crutches.
- Before discharge, the patient should be instructed to avoid any situations that require hip internal rotation and knee flexion.
- Indications for open reduction include incongruent reduction, unstable hip, incarcerated intra-articular fragment, and irreducible dislocation.

■ Common Pitfalls
  - Failure to obtain orthogonal radiographs

    All patients with hip dislocations require anteroposterior and cross-table lateral radiographs before reduction attempt.

  - Inadequate sedation and muscle relaxation

    For a successful reduction, it is crucial to obtain adequate muscle relaxation.

    Failure to obtain adequate muscle relaxation may lead to an iatrogenic acetabular or femoral neck fracture.

  - Neglecting associated injuries

    Strict ATLS protocol should be followed because 80% of patients have associated injuries.[29,30]

  - Accepting an incongruous reduction

    A postreduction CT scan is very helpful in evaluating for intra-articular fragments.

    An incongruous reduction is an indication for an open arthrotomy.[33–35]

- Osteonecrosis

  All patients should be informed of the risk of AVN regardless of timely reduction.

  AVN may develop in 30% of patients.[27,28,36]

- Osteoarthritis

  The rate of arthritis after dislocation ranges from 20% to 80%.

  Patients with associated posterior wall acetabular fractures have a higher incidence of osteoarthritis.[27,28]

- Delayed reduction

  Reduction within 12 hours has been associated with reduced incidence of osteonecrosis.[27]

- Nerve injury

  Sciatic nerve palsy, usually the peroneal division, can occur with 15% of posterior hip dislocations.[35]

## Anterior Hip Dislocations

■ Anterior hip dislocations are uncommon (10% to 15% of hip dislocations).[27,29]
■ The mechanism of injury usually involves axial force with an abducted leg, a posterior blow to the hip in a flexed position, or a fall from a height.
■ Biomechanically, the greater trochanter or the femoral neck impinges on the posterior rim of the acetabulum causing the femoral head to lever out, rupturing the anterior capsule in the process.
■ Diagnosis
  - Patients typically present with an extended, shortened, abducted, and externally rotated lower extremity.
  - The femoral head may be palpable near the anterior superior iliac spine or the obturator foramen.

- A complete motor and neurovascular examination should be performed with the focus on the femoral artery and nerve because the femoral head may impinge on these structures.
- Standard radiographs include an anteroposterior pelvis view and a cross-table lateral view.
- On the anteroposterior radiograph, there is an incongruous femoroacetabular joint with the femoral head appearing larger than the contralateral femoral head.
- Typically prereduction radiographs are sufficient.
- If there is concern for a nondisplaced femoral neck fracture, a prereduction CT scan may be obtained.

■ Classification
- Anterior hip dislocations can be subcategorized into superior, inferior, and obturator dislocations.
- Superior and inferior dislocations are described relative to the pubic ramus.
- Obturator dislocation is defined by the femoral head overlying the obturator foramen on the anteroposterior pelvic radiograph.[31]

■ Management
- Anterior hip dislocations are managed with prompt closed reduction.
- An uneventful closed reduction requires good muscle relaxation, analgesia, and conscious sedation.
- If good muscle relaxation, analgesia, and conscious sedation are not possible in the emergency department, the closed reduction should be performed in the operating room.

■ Reduction Technique
- After sedation, analgesia, and muscle relaxation, the patient is positioned supine.
- The operator applies inline traction with the leg in extension to move the femoral head from the anterior aspect the acetabulum, while the assistant applies counterpressure to the pelvis or pushes the femoral head inferiorly if it is palpable.
- Once the femoral head is overlying the acetabulum, the hip is gradually internally rotated to reduce the femoral head into the acetabulum.
- The hip can also be reduced using the previously described Allis technique.[29]
- After obtaining a successful reduction, the hip should be put through a range of motion in all three planes to evaluate stability: flexion and extension, adduction and abduction, and internal and external rotation
- If the hip is stable, a knee immobilizer with a foot extension should be placed to prevent flexion and external rotation.

■ Postreduction Management
- A postreduction examination should be performed, and radiographs should be obtained.
- When evaluating the postreduction radiographs, the hip should be concentric.
- It has become a standard practice at our institution to obtain a postreduction fine-cut (2-mm) CT scan to evaluate for osteochondral intra-articular fragments, femoral or acetabular fractures, and congruency of the joint.[32,33]

- The patient can be made foot flat touchdown weight bearing with crutches.
- Before discharge, the patient should be instructed to avoid any situations that require hip external rotation.
- Indications for open reduction include incongruent closed reduction, unstable hip, incarcerated intra-articular fragment, and irreducible dislocation.

■ Common Pitfalls
- Similar to posterior hip dislocation

    Orthogonal radiographs, congruent reduction, adequate sedation, analgesia, and muscle relaxation are mandatory.

    The risk of osteonecrosis and osteoarthritis should be discussed with the patient as previously described for posterior hip dislocation.[27,28,36]

- Delayed reduction

    Reduction within 12 hours has been associated with reduced incidence of osteonecrosis.[27]

- Femoral nerve and artery injury

    These injuries can occur secondary to femoral head compression injury.[29,31]

- Femoral head fracture

    CT scan may be considered to evaluate the femoral head for fractures.

    In some series, three fourths of anterior dislocations have an associated femoral head fracture.[37]

## SUBTROCHANTERIC FRACTURES

■ Subtrochanteric femoral fractures are fractures of the proximal femur that extend distally below the lesser trochanter down to the femoral isthmus and proximally to involve the piriformis fossa.
■ These fractures account for 10% to 30% of all proximal femur fractures.[38,39]
■ Fractures occur at any age but are most frequent in adults 20 to 30 years old and older than 65 years.[38,39]
■ Typically, fracture is due to a high-energy injury in younger patients, such as a fall from a height, motor vehicle accident, or a gunshot wound.
■ Typically, fracture is due to a lower energy injury in elderly patients.
■ In elderly patients, fracture is secondary to a fall leading to lateral hip trauma or a pathologic process such as metastatic disease.
■ Diagnosis
- Younger patients often have multiple associated injuries secondary to high-energy trauma.
- Standard ATLS protocol should be followed.
- Clinically patients present with a shortened and externally rotated leg.
- The thigh is usually very swollen owing to the fracture hematoma.
- Palpable crepitus is heard over the fracture site.

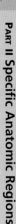

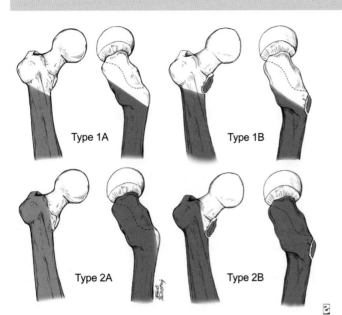

**FIGURE 13-6.** Russell-Taylor classification. *(From Lee MA, Ertle JP: Subtrochanteric hip fractures. Medscape Reference. Available at:* http://emedicine.medscape.com/article/1247329-overview. *Accessed November 11, 2011.)*

- Standard radiographs obtained include an anteroposterior pelvis view and full-length anteroposterior and lateral femur views.
- The proximal fragment is classically flexed and externally rotated by the pull of the iliopsoas and abducted by the gluteus medius and minimus muscles.
- The distal fragment is adducted and shortened by the pull of the adductors.

■ Classification
- The most frequently used classification is the Russell-Taylor classification (Fig. 13-6).
- This classification is based on involvement of the piriformis fossa and the lesser trochanter.
- This classification has implications for use of piriformis fossa entry intramedullary devices.
- It is possibly less useful currently because of increased use of trochanteric entry intramedullary nails.

■ Management
- Management occurs in the emergency department.
- The goals of treatment are stabilization and adequate resuscitation of the patient.
- Young patients often have associated injuries, which may include cranial, thoracic, and abdominal trauma (Waddell's triad).[40]
- Because the thigh compartment may accommodate significant volume, blood loss can be substantial.
- When this fracture has been diagnosed, immediate orthopedic consultation is recommended.
- Initial management involves the application of traction.
- Traction minimizes the thigh intracompartmental space, which decreases fracture-related blood loss.
- Pulling the fracture out to length reduces fracture-associated pain by minimizing motion at the fracture site.

- In elderly patients, 5 to 10 lb of Buck's traction should suffice.[16]
- In younger patients with good musculature, the pull of the surrounding muscles requires a more robust traction force.
- Skeletal traction is an option.
- A traction pin can be placed either in the distal femur or at the proximal tibia.
- It is imperative to obtain adequate radiographs before performing skeletal traction to ensure there are no fractures distally.
- In patients who are unstable and may not be able to undergo definitive fixation for a prolonged period, balanced skeletal traction is recommended.

■ Common Pitfalls
- Inadequate resuscitation

  This may occur especially in younger patients with high-energy trauma.

  The large potential space of the thigh along with associated injuries can lead to significant blood loss and hypovolemic shock.

- Missed associated injuries

  ATLS protocol should be followed to rule out cranial, cervical, thoracic, and abdominal injuries.[40]

- Inadequate radiographs

  An anteroposterior pelvis view and orthogonal full-length femur radiographs should be obtained.

## FEMORAL SHAFT FRACTURES

■ Femoral shaft fractures are common with an incidence of 1 in 10,000 people.[41,42]
■ Fractures have a bimodal age distribution: younger than 25 years and older than 65 years.[40,41]
■ In younger patients, this is a high-energy fracture usually associated with motor vehicle or motorcycle accident injuries, injuries sustained by a pedestrian struck by an automobile, or gunshot injuries.
■ In older patients, fracture is associated with a low-energy injury, such as a fall.
■ Diagnosis
- Patients usually present with polytrauma.
- The affected side may be shortened and internally or externally rotated depending on how the patient is positioned on the stretcher.
- Standard trauma radiographs should be obtained: anteroposterior pelvis view and full-length anteroposterior femur view including the knee.
- A fine-cut CT scan (<2 mm) is recommended for patients with high-energy trauma because there is a 1% to 8% incidence of associated femoral neck fracture, which can be misdiagnosed 30% of the time.[43]
- When the mechanism of injury is a significant axial load, patients should be examined carefully for calcaneus, tibial plateau, and spinal compression injuries, and appropriate radiographs should be obtained.

- Classification
  - The most widely used classification is the Winquist-Hansen classification, which is based on the amount of comminution and cortical contact:[44]

    0—no comminution, simple transverse or oblique fracture pattern

    I—small butterfly fracture fragment with no to minimal comminution

    II—butterfly fracture fragment with greater than 50% of the circumference of the cortices of the two major fragments intact

    III—butterfly fracture fragment with greater than 50% of the circumference of the two major fragments comminuted

    IV—segmental comminution, all cortical contact lost

- Management
  - ATLS protocol should be followed for patients with high-energy trauma, taking care to evaluate for concomitant head, chest, and visceral injuries.
  - The skin should be checked for evidence of lacerations, abrasions, or puncture wounds.
  - Although associated vascular injury is uncommon, distal pulses should be inspected; if pulses are not palpable, Doppler evaluation should be considered.
  - A thorough neurologic examination should be performed in awake patients with special focus on the sciatic nerve distribution.
  - The hip and knee are put through range of motion and tested for stability.
  - The incidence of ipsilateral knee ligamentous injuries can be 40%.[45]
  - Temporary fracture stabilization can be achieved with skeletal traction.
  - Skeletal traction is recommended if definitive operative treatment is expected to be delayed.
  - Skeletal traction stabilizes the fracture, reduces pain, and may diminish thigh intracompartmental bleeding
  - Traction can be applied at the distal femur or proximal tibia if there are no fractures or ligamentous injuries.
- Common Pitfalls
  - Missed open fractures

    All skin abrasions and lacerations should be explored.

    If the fracture is open, proper antibiotic and tetanus prophylaxis should be instituted.

  - Vascular injury

    The incidence of vascular injury is less than 1%, but it is important to examine for pulses before and after traction.[46]

  - Missed femoral neck fracture

    In 8% of midshaft fractures, an ipsilateral femoral neck fracture that may be nondisplaced may be present, and a fine-cut CT scan is recommended.[43]

  - Fat emboli syndrome

    These fractures tend to displace a significant amount of intramedullary fat into the circulation.

## SOFT TISSUE INJURIES OF THE HIP

- With the large muscle mass surrounding the hip joint, which includes the extensors, flexors, adductors, abductors, and rotators, hip soft tissue injuries are common.
- The most commonly hip soft tissue pathologies encountered in the emergency department are described.

### Proximal Hamstring Strains

- Proximal hamstring strains are due to direct or most commonly indirect trauma.
- The mechanism of injury involves either forceful hamstring concentric contraction or excessive eccentric contraction.
- Activities associated with proximal hamstring injury include sprinting, water-skiing, hurdling, and dancing.
- Strains can occur at the muscle origin, at the muscle insertion, at the muscle belly, or most commonly at the myotendinous junction.[47,48]
- Diagnosis
  - Patients may report hearing or feeling a pop in the back of their hip.
  - Patients may limit weight bearing on the affected side.
  - Tenderness to palpation and ecchymosis over the posterior hip region may be found.
  - Check for a palpable mass defect with the patient in the prone position.
  - There is pain with resisted active knee flexion and passive knee extension with the hip flexed at 90 degrees.
  - Radiographs include anteroposterior pelvis and lateral hip views.
  - Radiographs are usually normal, but avulsion of the ischial tuberosity can be seen.
  - Ultrasound can be performed to visualize the hamstrings; however, ultrasound scans are technician dependent.
  - MRI is the most sensitive and specific diagnostic study, but it is costly, not readily available, and often unnecessary in the emergency department.
  - MRI can be used when the diagnosis is equivocal or for grading the injury.[49]
- Classification
  - The American Medical Association classification system is commonly used.[47,48]
  - There are three degrees of injury:

    First-degree strain: Partial tear secondary to a stretching injury

    Second-degree strain: More severe injury at the myotendinous junction without complete tear

    Third-degree strain: Complete tear at the myotendinous junction

■ Management
- Swelling can be reduced with RICE (rest, ice, compression, and elevation).
- Pain should be controlled with nonsteroidal anti-inflammatory drugs (NSAIDs) or acetaminophen (Tylenol).
- Crutches can be used to unload the affected side until pain has subsided.[47,48]
- The hallmark treatment is physical therapy with the focus on obtaining full range of motion.
- Patients should be scheduled to be evaluated by an orthopedic surgeon preferably with specialization in treating sports-related injuries.[46,47]

## Adductor Strain

■ Injury to the hip adductors commonly occurs during extreme eccentric contraction during side-to-side motion.

■ The most commonly involved muscles are the adductor longus and gracilis with most strains occurring at the myotendinous junction.[50]

■ Diagnosis
- Patients typically have pain, swelling, and ecchymosis at the superior medial thigh.
- A palpable defect is occasionally present.
- Pain can be elicited with resisted active adduction and passive abduction.[50,51]
- Radiographs include an anteroposterior pelvis view; they are usually normal.
- An ultrasound scan can be performed; however, this scan is operator dependent.
- MRI is highly sensitive and specific but is not generally required to make the diagnosis.[50,52]

■ Management
- Swelling can be reduced with RICE (rest, ice, compression, and elevation).
- The affected side should be protected with limited weight bearing and the use of crutches.
- NSAIDs or acetaminophen (Tylenol) should be prescribed.
- The role of muscle relaxers is not clearly defined, but they may help with pain control.[50,51]
- Corticosteroid injection is controversial and generally not recommended.[52,53]
- The hallmark of treatment is rehabilitation; however, outpatient orthopedic evaluation is recommended, especially in patients with a palpable defect.

## Quadriceps Contusion

■ Direct trauma to the quadriceps can lead to muscle and connective tissue tears with subsequent hematoma and soft tissue swelling.

■ Quadriceps contusion is common in individuals participating in contact sports, most notably football.[54]

■ Diagnosis
- Anterior thigh pain associated with swelling and a tense anterior thigh compartment.

- Gait may range from normal to a severely antalgic gait.
- There is limited active and passive knee flexion; in complete tears, there is an extensor lag, which is the inability to maintain full knee extension during attempted straight leg raise.[54]
- Plain radiographs obtained immediately after injury may be negative, but radiographs obtained several weeks after contusion may show evidence of myositis ossificans.
- MRI is highly sensitive and specific for diagnosis but generally unnecessary in the emergency department.[55]
- Compartment syndrome is exceedingly rare in the absence of an associated fracture; however, if this is suspected, measuring the compartment pressure is indicated.[56]

■ Classification
- Contusions are graded depending on the limitation of knee flexion.
- A mild contusion has greater than 90 degrees of knee flexion.
- A moderate contusion has 45 to 90 degrees of knee flexion.
- A severe contusion has less than 45 degrees of knee flexion.[54,55]

■ Management
- Initial treatment involves immobilization of the knee in hyperflexion (120 degrees) with a hinged knee brace.
- Hyperflexion of the knee prevents the quadriceps from healing in a shortened position.
- Hyperflexion minimizes hematoma formation lowering the risk of developing myositis ossificans.
- Hyperflexion should be discontinued at 24 hours, and passive stretching should be initiated with icing between sessions.[53,54]
- Pain should be controlled with NSAIDs, and crutches should be used during ambulation.
- Follow-up evaluation with an orthopedist should be scheduled.

## Trochanteric Bursitis

■ Classified as an overuse syndrome, trochanteric bursitis results from friction of the iliotibial band over the trochanter.

■ This friction leads to painful inflammation of the trochanteric bursa, which is superficial to the greater trochanter of the femur

■ This condition is seen frequently in runners and other active individuals with a reported incidence of 1.8 in 1000.[57,58]

■ It is also seen in patients who recently underwent total hip arthroplasty.[59]

■ Prevalence is higher in women compared with men (up to 8× higher reported frequency).[57,58]

■ Diagnosis
- Lateral hip pain overlying the greater trochanter of the femur is present.

- Pain is usually elicited with direct pressure over the trochanteric bursa.
- This is best tested with the patient lying on the unaffected side.
- Onset of pain may be acute or chronic, and pain may radiate down to the knee because the iliotibial band attaches to Gerdy tubercle on the tibia.
- The pain may awaken the patient at night, especially when the patient lies on the affected side.
- Symptoms are worsened with most hip motion and with any increase in activity or exercise.
- Patients with acute trauma may have ecchymosis over the trochanteric region.
- Radiographs and advanced imaging are usually not required unless there is a history of trauma.
- When imaging is indicated, standard hip anteroposterior and lateral radiographs are sufficient.
- Management
  - The hallmark of treatment involves stretching the iliotibial band and a course of NSAIDs.
  - Corticosteroid injection seems to work best for severe trochanteric bursitis.
  - The point of maximal palpable pain is injected with a mixture of lidocaine/bupivacaine and methylprednisolone acetate or triamcinolone acetonide.[60-62]
  - Offending activities should be limited until resolution of the inflammation and pain.

## SEPTIC ARTHRITIS OF THE HIP

- Septic arthritis is caused by direct inoculation or more commonly by hematogenous seeding of the hip joint by bacteria, fungi, or viruses
- The most common bacterium is *Neisseria gonorrhoeae* in young, sexually active individuals, but *Staphylococcus aureus* is the most common pathogen overall.[63-65]
- Other organisms include *Streptococcus pneumoniae*, group B streptococci, viridans streptococci, *Pseudomonas aeruginosa*, and *Borrelia burgdorferi*.
- The main sequelae of bacterial invasion are direct articular cartilage damage and rapidly progressive arthritis.[64,65]
- Diagnosis
  - Early diagnosis is important to minimize injury to the native articular cartilage.
  - A thorough history detailing any risk factors should be obtained.
  - Subtle findings can aid your diagnosis.
  - Can the patient bear weight? What is the position of the hip?
  - Patients typically cannot fully bear weight and protect the involved extremity owing to pain with active and passive motion of the hip.
  - The hip is held in a position of flexion and external rotation to increase the joint space to accommodate the effusion.
  - In immunocompromised individuals, signs and symptoms may be blunted because of the diminished immune response to the pathogen.
  - Evaluate the skin integrity for any lacerations, abrasions, erythema, or tracking.
  - Palpate for any fluctuance or evidence of fluid collection.
  - Assess range of motion to check for any arc of motion that is pain-free.
  - In septic arthritis, all directions are usually very painful.
  - Baseline complete blood count, ESR, CRP, and uric acid levels should be obtained.
  - Elevated ESR and CRP in patients without inflammatory arthritis are highly specific and sensitive.
  - Hip joint aspiration can be done with ultrasound guidance or with the assistance of an interventional radiologist.
  - Joint fluid should be sent for cell count, Gram stain, culture, glucose, protein, and crystals.
  - WBC counts greater than 50,000/μL for native hips are worrisome for infection.
  - WBC counts greater than 1700 to 2500/μL for prosthetic hips with a neutrophil percentage greater than 65% are worrisome for septic hip.[66-68]
  - Anteroposterior and lateral radiographs should be obtained to ensure there are no fractures.
  - MRI is useful when there is concern for an abscess or significant effusion.
  - In patients with a contraindication to MRI, a CT scan is a reasonable option.[69]
- Management
  - Empiric antibiotic coverage is recommended.
  - In a nonseptic patient, antibiotics should be held until the aspiration has been obtained.
  - Adequate pain control should be initiated.
  - Orthopedic consultation should be obtained as soon as possible.
  - The choice of antibiotic should include coverage for both gram-negative and gram-positive bacteria.
  - An infectious disease consultant may be helpful in management of septic arthritis.
- Common Pitfalls
  - Giving antibiotics before obtaining hip aspirate

    This has the potential to lower the sensitivity of the hip aspirate.

  - Failure to diagnose *N. gonorrhoeae* or *B. burgdorferi* septic arthritis

    These pathogens can be successfully treated with antibiotics, whereas most other pathogens require surgical intervention.[63,70]

  - Incomplete work-up

    All patients with suspected septic joint should have a baseline CRP, ESR, and WBC count.

  - Failure to use strict sterile technique for joint aspiration

## AVASCULAR NECROSIS OF THE HIP (OSTEONECROSIS)

- In AVN, death of the cellular components of bone and bone marrow occurs.
- In the United States. the yearly incidence is approximately 15,000.[70,71]

- pain on superior, medial, lateral, or inferior aspect of patella
- Assess patella tracking in trochlea of femur as the knee goes from extension into flexion
- Palpate quadriceps tendon and patellar tendon for pain or defect
- Check knee for ligamentous stability in supine position
- Varus stress tests lateral ligaments: With one hand on femur and one hand on tibia, exert force to push knee laterally at both 0 degrees and 30 degrees of knee flexion
- Valgus stress tests medial ligaments: With one hand on femur and one hand on tibia, exert force to push knee medially at both 0 degrees and 30 degrees of knee flexion
- Lachman test assesses anterior cruciate ligament (ACL) integrity: With one hand on distal femur and one hand on proximal tibia at 30 degrees of knee flexion, exert force to bring tibia anterior to femur (Fig. 14-1)
- Posterior drawer test assesses posterior cruciate ligament (PCL) integrity: Flex knee to 90 degrees with foot on stretcher; with two hands on proximal tibia, exert force to push tibia posterior to femur (see Fig. 14-1)
- Test for meniscal injury: Medial or lateral joint line tenderness to palpation
- Flex knee and bring to extension with lower leg in internal and then external rotation; a palpable or audible click with pain is associated with a tear

- Apley test is performed with the patient in a prone position with the knee flexed to 90 degrees; an axial load is applied to the externally rotated tibia; pain is associated with tear
- Examine motor and sensory nerve function for nerves at risk—femoral, sciatic, tibial, superficial peroneal, deep peroneal
- Knee extension against resistance tests quadriceps and femoral nerve
- Knee flexion against resistance tests hamstrings and sciatic nerve
- Ankle dorsiflexion against resistance tests tibialis anterior and deep peroneal nerve
- Ankle eversion against resistance tests peroneus longus and brevis and superficial peroneal nerve
- Ankle plantar flexion against resistance tests gastrocnemius/soleus complex and tibial nerve
- Sensation on dorsum of foot tests superficial peroneal nerve
- Sensation on dorsum of first web space (between great and second toes) tests deep peroneal nerve
- Sensation on plantar aspect of foot tests tibial nerve
- Check distal pulses for strength and symmetry—dorsalis pedis and posterior tibial artery
- Assess ankle-brachial index if suspicion for vascular compromise
- Check for development of compartment syndrome (anterior and posterior thigh, anterior leg, lateral leg, posterior leg): Palpate compartments for significant tension and look for pain with passive stretch of muscles

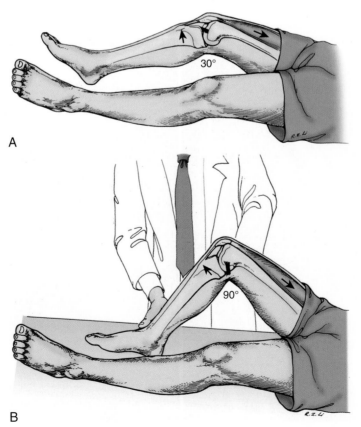

A

B

**FIGURE 14-1.** ACL and PCL testing. *(From Scott WN, editor: The knee, St Louis, 1994, Mosby.)*

■ Diagnostic Testing
  • X-ray
  Standard radiography for an acutely injured knee includes anteroposterior, lateral, and oblique views. Axial views should also be obtained if the patient is able to flex the knee appropriately.
  • Joint aspiration and injection (violated joint space)
  See under Physical Examination: Standard Focus Examination for description of joint aspiration.
■ Differential Diagnosis
  • True diagnosis typically determined via imaging
  • Distal femur fracture includes supracondylar, intracondylar, and condylar fractures (differentiated via imaging)
  • Traumatic versus pathologic fracture
  • Femoral shaft fracture
  • Knee dislocation
  • Tibial plateau or proximal tibia fracture

## Treatment of Specific Injuries

■ Develop Plan
  Patients with open fractures require immediate irrigation in the trauma bay and proceed to surgery urgently.
    The injury should be immobilized with a well-padded posterior long leg splint or knee immobilizer.
    Polytrauma affects surgical timing; confer with other surgical consultants.
    Elderly patients or patients with significant comorbidities require preoperative medical optimization and may benefit from admission to the hospital.

■ Discuss Alternative and Final Care Plan With Patient
  • Nonoperative treatment if fracture is nondisplaced and in severely ill or nonambulatory patients
  • Most distal femur fractures require hospital admission and surgery
  • Surgery includes open reduction and internal fixation (ORIF) or external fixation depending on the severity of other injuries and degree of comminution
  • Definitive treatment in balanced skeletal traction rarely performed
■ When to Consult a Specialist
  • Always obtain a telephone consultation with an orthopedic surgeon for any distal femur fracture
■ How and What to Communicate With Specialist
  • Open or closed

    Should be included in initial communication because open fractures require urgent operative attention

    Results of diagnostic injection if performed

    Gross contamination

    Patient received appropriate antibiotics and tetanus prophylaxis

  • X-ray description

    Goal is to be able to visualize fracture based on description (Fig. 14-2)

    Skeletal maturity (open versus closed physes)

    Fracture location—can measure distance from joint line

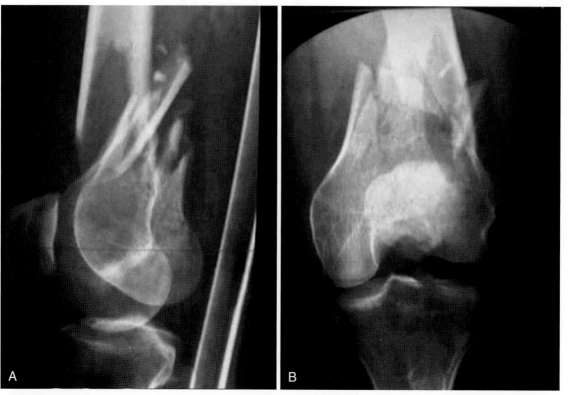

**FIGURE 14-2. A,** Lateral view of supracondylar femur fracture. **B,** Anteroposterior view of supracondylar femur fracture.

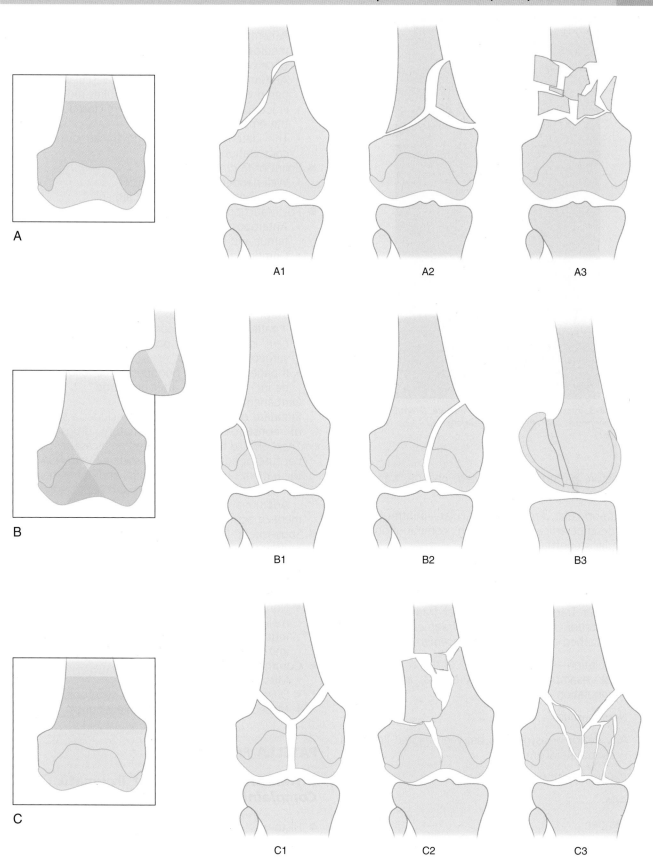

**FIGURE 14-2, cont'd  A,** Lateral view of supracondylar femur fracture. **B,** Anteroposterior view of supracondylar femur fracture. **C,** Distal femur fracture types.

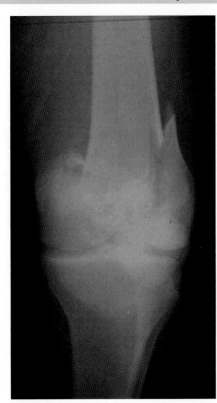

**FIGURE 14-3.** Intra-articular distal femur fracture. *(From Doherty GM: Current diagnosis and treatment: surgery, ed 13, New York, McGraw-Hill.)*

Fracture pattern—comminuted, oblique, transverse, spiral

Intra-articular versus extra-articular—if intra-articular, describe articular surface (e.g., comminution, articular stepoff) (Fig. 14-3)

Displacement in millimeters—convention dictates that fracture displacement is described based on position of *distal* fragment; for example, distal femur fracture with the distal fragment located posterior to the proximal fragment would be described as "posterior displacement"

Angulation—describe the apex of the angle formed; for example, "the fracture has apex-anterior angulation"

- Neurovascular

Any deficit or asymmetry between injured limb and contralateral limb

- Patient identifying information

Age

Gender

Medical comorbidities

Baseline ambulatory status

Mental status if abnormal

Mechanism of injury

- Analgesia, Anesthesia Block, and Sedation
  - Patients are likely to require intravenous pain medications.
- Reduce or Accept Alignment
  - Any limb with alteration in neurovascular status compared with unaffected limb requires reduction.
  - Fractures typically do not require closed reduction in the emergency department.
  - This determination is made by an orthopedist in consultation.
- Splint or Immobilize
  - Well-padded knee immobilizer
  - Well-padded posterior long leg splint
- Postreduction Imaging
  - Anteroposterior and lateral radiographs of distal femur and knee
  - Computed tomography (CT) scan through distal femur and knee helpful for intracondylar and condylar fractures; order thin-cut images for optimal visualization of articular surface injury
- Plan for Follow-up Care
  - If patient is admitted for operative fixation, follow-up care is determined postoperatively by orthopedic surgeon
  - If patient is treated nonoperatively, follow-up should be in 1 to 2 weeks after discharge
- Outpatient Pain Relief Options
  Standard outpatient pain relief includes a short course of nonsteroidal anti-inflammatory drugs (NSAIDs). These should be recommended on a case-by-case basis because of adverse effects associated with NSAIDs and the patient's renal function, age, and home medication list. Options include ibuprofen and naproxen.
  Additionally, opiates may be needed for management of acute injury pain over the first 1 to 3 days.
- Subsequent Management (Specialist Care Treatment Strategy, Anticipated Definitive Treatment)
  - ORIF likely required as definitive care
  - External fixation is a treatment option for definitive care of patients with polytrauma
  - Nonoperative management of nondisplaced or minimally displaced fractures in appropriate patients requires long-term non–weight bearing and immobilization
- Common Pitfalls
  - Missed neurovascular deficit
  - Development of compartment syndrome
  - Missed open fractures (pinhole wounds)

## PATELLA FRACTURES

### Differential Diagnosis of Traumatic Complaints

- History
  - Mechanism of injury
  - Numbness or tingling down leg
  - Age
  - Bone quality (history of osteoporosis)
  - Ascertain comorbidities (may influence treatment selection)

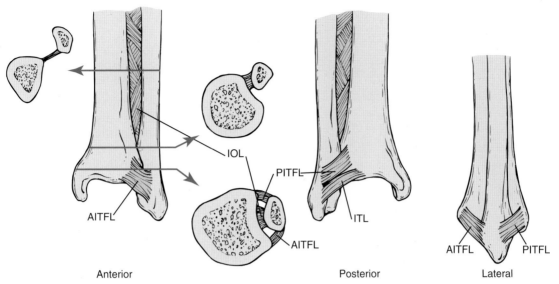

**FIGURE 15-10.** Syndesmotic ligament complex. *(From Browner BD, Jupiter JB, Levine AM, et al, editors: Skeletal trauma: basic science, management, and reconstruction, ed 4, Philadelphia, 2008, Saunders.)*

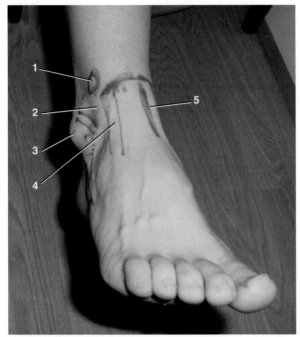

**FIGURE 15-11.** Important anterior surface landmarks: *1,* syndesmotic ligament; *2,* ankle joint; *3,* lateral malleolus; *4,* peroneus tertius; *5,* tibialis anterior tendon.

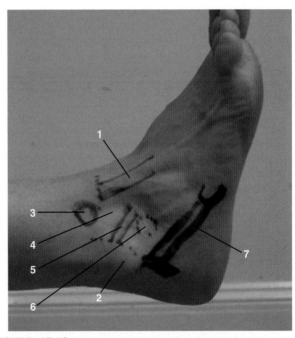

**FIGURE 15-12.** Important lateral surface landmarks: *1,* peroneus tertius; *2,* lateral malleolus; *3,* syndesmotic ligament; *4,* ankle joint; *5,* anterior talofibular ligament; *6,* sinus tarsi; *7,* peroneus brevis.

- Mechanism of Injury
  - An acute traumatic injury may lead to the onset of ankle pathology.
  - Generally, it is important to determine the mechanism of injury and use your knowledge of the commonly associated disorders to help guide the history taken, physical examination performed, and tests ordered.
  - High-energy direct trauma to the ankle secondary to high-speed motor vehicle accidents, falls from large heights, and direct blows such as crush injury may cause significant bone, cartilage, and soft tissue injury. These are more commonly associated with open injuries given the high energy of force exerted on the lower extremity.
  - Low-energy direct trauma may cause a range of injuries including minor contusions, sprain or rupture to ligaments or tendons, mild nondisplaced fractures, significant fractures in osteoporotic patients, and significant nerve disorders such as complex regional pain syndrome.
  - Repetitive activities or overuse may result in disorders such as tendinitis and stress fractures.

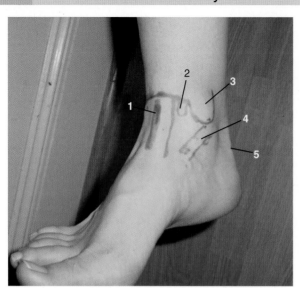

**FIGURE 15-13.** Important medial surface landmarks: *1,* tibialis anterior tendon; *2,* ankle joint; *3,* medial malleolus; *4,* tibialis posterior tendon; *5,* Achilles tendon.

- Indirect rotational injuries can lead to tendon and ligament injuries, fracture, and joint dislocation.
- Although uncommon, infection of the ankle joint can occur and accounts for approximately 7% of the total number of cases of septic arthritis.[4]

■ Timing
- There may be a history of symptoms developing acutely or being exacerbated after a specific ankle injury. Sometimes the symptoms may not occur or increase to the point that they become concerning until later in the day or on waking or ambulating the following day.
- With some ankle disorders, the patient may not have a specific inciting event, or the pathology may have increased slowly and progressively in severity.
- In overuse injuries such as tendinitis, there may be recent development of symptoms, whereas in degenerative disorders such as arthritis and tendinopathy, the symptoms may develop more slowly or be more intermittent.

■ Preexisting Illness
- Previous injuries to and disorders of the ankle, particularly previous conditions of a similar nature, and their response to treatment should be elicited.
- Any preexisting ankle symptoms and limitations should be sought.
- Preexisting medical conditions that may cause or exacerbate foot disorders or affect the treatment response to new injury, such as diabetes mellitus, rheumatoid arthritis, and obesity, should be noted.
- A history of previous lower leg surgery should be obtained.
- A history of generalized ligamentous laxity should be ascertained in patients with repetitive ankle sprains.

■ Pain
- The degree of pain is multifactorial, which must be taken into account when assessing the severity of injury and treatment options.

It depends on the extent, acuteness, and type of pathology.

Individual pain tolerance may vary in part owing to genetics, previous experience, age, and occasionally social or cultural factors.

- Previous treatment may reduce pain including recent reduction of fractures and dislocations, suturing of lacerations, and administration of narcotics and other medications.
- The character, location, timing, duration, progression, and exacerbating or relieving factors of pain are important to obtain from the patient because they aid in reaching the correct diagnosis.

Is the pain sharp, dull, burning, or pressure-like?

Is the pain global, or does it involve a specific tendon, bone, joint, or nerve distribution?

Is the pain present when the individual first gets up out of bed, as is commonly noted with ankle arthritis and rheumatologic conditions, or does it occur near the end of the day, at night, or all the time?

Is the pain acute and progressively getting worse, which may be seen in a compartment syndrome or infection, or is it chronic and stable?

Is the pain made worse by walking on uneven ground or concrete, wearing certain types of shoes versus going barefoot, or with motion of specific joints?

Is the pain made better by anti-inflammatory medication, bracing or orthoses, or elevation?

■ Dysfunction
- The important functional things that a patient cannot do, can do only to a limited fashion, or will not do secondary to discomfort or fear must be sorted out.
- After injury, was the patient able to bear weight, either unassisted or with support?
- Was the patient able to walk or run without a limp?
- Are there activities that the patient can no longer do or do well secondary to ankle pathology, and, if so, is it due to pain, weakness, instability, loss of balance, loss of endurance, or other factors?

■ Prehospital Care
- The nature, severity, and treatment urgency of the injury and the vascular status of the lower extremity and foot should be assessed.
- In patients with open fractures, gross contamination may be removed from the wounds.
- If the provider has the appropriate knowledge and experience, closed reduction of closed fractures and dislocations may be attempted, in particular if significant vascular compromise, tented skin at risk of becoming an open fracture, or significant patient discomfort is present.

The threshold for action depends in part on expected time to evaluation in the emergency department.

Contaminated open wounds ideally should undergo surgical débridement before reduction of fractures and joint dislocations.

- Patients should be splinted for comfort.
- In patients with intact vascular status, elevation, compression, and ice can improve swelling.
- Any amputated or extruded tissue should be preserved and transported with the patient to the emergency department.
- The patient should be kept from eating or drinking if there is a possibility that semiemergent surgery may be considered or required.

■ Physical examination
- A focused physical examination should be performed in all cases of suspected low-energy ankle fractures and in suspected high-energy ankle fractures after the patient is stabilized via the advanced trauma life support protocol.
- Inspection

    The lower leg, ankle, and foot should be inspected for deformity, ecchymosis, swelling, and perfusion.

    In closed injuries, evaluation of the skin for fracture blisters or significant swelling is an important aspect to relay to the orthopedic team.

    - Fracture blisters are thought to result from skin shearing at the dermal-epidermal junction during the initial injury.[5]
    - Two main subtypes exist; these differ in the amount of severity.
        - Serous blisters contain clear fluid and do not completely disrupt the epidermis.
        - Hemorrhagic blisters are more severe and represent increased injury to the dermal-epidermal junction; when viewed histologically, there is complete loss of epithelial cells.[6]

        Open injuries require immediate recognition to allow for appropriate antibiotics and tetanus prophylaxis.

        Any concern for communication with the ankle joint needs further investigation.

    - In the methylene blue dye test, fluid containing 1 to 2 drops of methylene blue dye added to normal saline is injected into the suspected joint.
    - If blue dye is seen coming from the open wound, the area communicates with the ankle joint.
    - If methylene blue dye is unavailable, the test may be performed with just normal saline.
    - Studies have shown 155 to 194 mL of saline is required to aid in diagnosis of an open knee joint with greater than 95% accuracy.[7,8] However, no studies have specifically looked at the amount of fluid needed to diagnose an open ankle joint, although given the smaller volume of the ankle joint, less than 150 mL seems reasonable.
- Palpation

    Palpation of both the medial and the lateral aspects of the ankle should be performed.

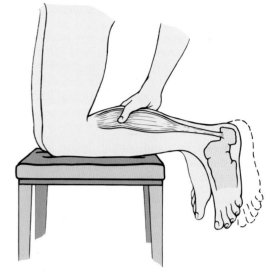

**FIGURE 15-14.** Thompson test for diagnosis of Achilles tendon rupture. If an intact tendon is present, squeezing the gastrocnemius and soleus muscular portion of the calf causes plantar flexion of the ankle. *(From Browner BD, Jupiter JB, Levine AM, et al, editors: Skeletal trauma: basic science, management, and reconstruction, ed 4, Philadelphia, 2008, Saunders.)*

- This includes the bony landmarks of the medial and lateral malleolus and adjacent soft tissue structures.
- On the medial side, the major soft tissue structure is the deltoid ligament complex.
- Tenderness along the medial malleolus does not mean fracture of the medial malleolus or disruption of the deltoid ligament complex.[9,10]

    The lateral ligament complex should be palpated, along with the syndesmosis and base of the fifth metatarsal.

    The peroneal tendons should be palpated to determine if there is any evidence of subluxation, partial tear, or complete tear.

    The Achilles tendon should also be palpated, and if any evidence of defect or concern about rupture is present, a Thompson test should be performed (Fig. 15-14).

    Always palpate and assess the joint above and the joint below the suspected fracture.

- In the ankle, this includes the knee, with specific attention paid to the proximal fibula. Distally, this includes the subtalar joint and foot.
- A spiral fracture of the proximal fibula can sometimes be missed without proper assessment of the surrounding structures, specifically palpation of the proximal fibula for pain. Although most isolated proximal fibula fractures require only supportive care, Maisonneuve fractures have associated injury to the interosseous membrane along with a deltoid ligament injury or medial malleolar fracture and may require surgical intervention.

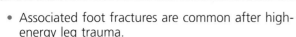
**PART II Specific Anatomic Regions**

- Associated foot fractures are common after high-energy leg trauma.
- In inversion-type injuries of the ankle, palpation of the foot is important to assess for fractures or ligamentous injury to the posterior and lateral processes of the talus, anterior process of the calcaneus, navicular tuberosity, cuboid, fifth metatarsal base, and tarsometatarsal joints.
- Range of motion

  Ankle dorsiflexion and plantar flexion and hindfoot inversion and eversion should be assessed for decreased or increased motion, instability, or pain.

- Neurovascular Examination (Table 15-1)
  - Neurologic status—specific nerves (Fig. 15-15)

    The saphenous nerve supplies sensation to the anterior and medial side of the lower leg and ankle region.

    The sural nerve provides sensation to the posterolateral aspect of the lower leg and lateral malleolus.

The superficial peroneal nerve provides sensation to the anterolateral aspect of the leg and ankle.

In patients with neuropathy, the proximal extent should be documented.

- Vascular status

  The dorsalis pedis pulse (Fig. 15-16) can be palpated between the extensor hallucis longus and extensor digitorum longus tendons just distal to the ankle. Active extension of the toes helps identify these tendons.

  The posterior tibial pulse can be palpated posterior to the medial malleolus.

  If the vascular examination reveals any abnormalities, a low threshold should exist for performing Doppler ultrasound, calculating an ankle-brachial index (ABI), and obtaining a vascular consultation.

- An ABI greater than 0.9 has been reliably proven to be not associated with vascular injury. Typically,

**TABLE 15-1** Tests for Assessment of Peripheral Nerves and Compartments of the Leg

| Nerve | Compartment | Motor Function | Sensory Function |
|---|---|---|---|
| Deep peroneal | Anterior | Ankle and toe dorsiflexion | First dorsal web space |
| Superficial peroneal | Lateral | Hindfoot eversion | Anterolateral leg and remaining dorsal foot including second dorsal web space |
| Tibial | Deep posterior | Ankle and toe plantar flexion; hindfoot inversion with ankle plantar-flexed | Plantar aspect of foot |
| Sural | None | None | Posterolateral leg and ankle; lateral border of foot |
| Saphenous | None | None | Medial leg and ankle |

Modified from Browner BD, Jupiter JB, Levine AM, et al, editors: Skeletal trauma: basic science, management, and reconstruction, ed 4, Philadelphia, 2008, Saunders.

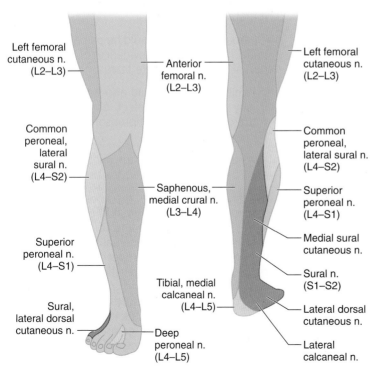

**FIGURE 15-15.** Cutaneous innervation of the lower leg. *(Redrawn from images in the Gray's Anatomy series, Oxford, Churchill Livingstone.)*

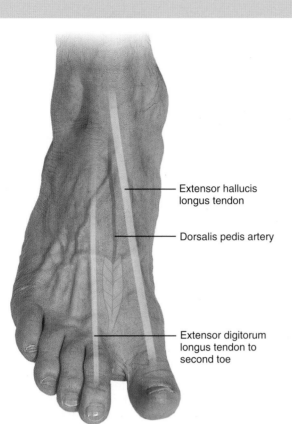

Extensor hallucis longus tendon

Dorsalis pedis artery

Extensor digitorum longus tendon to second toe

**FIGURE 15-16.** The dorsalis pedis pulse can be palpated between the tendons of the extensor hallucis longus and extensor digitorum longus. *(From Drake RL, Vogl WA, Mitchell AWM: Gray's anatomy for students, ed 2, Oxford, 2009, Churchill Livingstone.)*

an ABI less than 0.8 to 0.9 in a younger patient should be evaluated with angiography. In an older patient, clinical correlation is warranted because this patient population may have a lower baseline ABI.[11]

- Critical signs of ischemia such as cold or pallor with a pulse not detected by Doppler require urgent vascular consultation.

■ Assessment for Compartment Syndrome
  - With certain injuries, evaluation for signs and symptoms of compartment syndrome is extremely important both during the initial examination and subsequent reexamination in the emergency department.
  - Compartment syndrome occurs in approximately 4% of all tibial shaft fractures.[12]

    It is a common misconception that compartment syndrome cannot develop in an open fracture.

    Studies have shown a 9% incidence of compartment syndrome in association with open fractures, and this association was directly related to the severity of the injury.[13]

  - Parameters on physical examination that are suggestive of compartment syndrome include pain out of proportion to injury, paresthesias, pain with passive stretch of a tendon arising from the affected compartment, pallor of the extremity, and

sometimes paralysis and pulselessness in the later stages.[14]

Pulselessness is rarely seen with compartment syndrome because although the affected extremity compartment pressures are elevated, they usually are not above systolic pressure.

Palpation of the lower leg soft tissue for tenseness or firmness should be performed on initial evaluation to allow a baseline for further examinations.

Vascular occlusion, whether traumatic or nontraumatic, can cause compartment syndrome and should be in the differential diagnosis.

- Fasciotomy should be considered after prolonged acute ischemia to the muscles of a compartment.
- One study found that having one clinical sign of compartment syndrome increased the probability of compartment syndrome to 25%. This probability increased to 68% with two clinical findings, 93% with three clinical findings, and 98% with four clinical findings.[15]
- Compartment syndrome is a clinical diagnosis, confirmed by compartment pressure measurements. However, clinical evaluation is limited in various situations, and there may be a lower threshold for compartment pressure monitoring.

  Situations in which clinical evaluation is limited include unconscious or obtunded patients, patients with an unreliable examination or in whom examination is difficult such as young children, patients with equivocal signs and symptoms related to concomitant nerve injuries, and patients with multiple or distracting injuries.[16]

  If there is any clinical concern, it is better to err on the side of compartment pressure measurement because the subsequent clinical morbidity and medicolegal implications of missed compartment syndrome are significant.

- Intracompartment pressures can be obtained in various ways, including the use of commercially obtainable devices or arterial line monitors.

  If the difference between the patient's diastolic blood pressure and the measured intracompartment pressure is less than 30 mm Hg, this is considered diagnostic for compartment syndrome, and urgent fasciotomy is warranted.[16]

  An absolute measurement of 30 mm Hg in the presence of clinical symptoms also warrants emergent fasciotomy.

■ Description of Specific Tests
  - Thompson test (see Fig. 15-14)

    This test can be performed either with the patient prone on the examination table and the knee flexed to 90 degrees or with the patient placing the anterior lower leg on a chair with the knee flexed to 90 degrees.

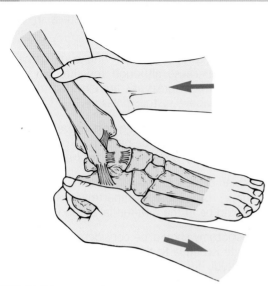

**FIGURE 15-17.** Anterior drawer test. Excessive anterior motion of the foot relative to the ankle mortise occurs if the anterior talofibular ligament and anterolateral capsule are compromised. *(From Browner BD, Jupiter JB, Levine AM, et al, editors: Skeletal trauma: basic science, management, and reconstruction, ed 4, Philadelphia, 2008, Saunders.)*

The gastrocnemius and soleus muscular portion of the calf is squeezed.[17]

If no plantar flexion of the ankle occurs, the test is considered positive, and a ruptured Achilles tendon is likely.

This test isolates the Achilles tendon and excludes the role of the secondary planter flexors of the ankle.

- Anterior drawer test (Fig. 15-17)

The anterior drawer test assesses the integrity of the anterior talofibular ligament and anterolateral capsule.

The knee is flexed and the foot is plantar-flexed to relax the gastrocnemius and soleus pull on the Achilles tendon.

The lower leg is stabilized just above the ankle joint with the thumb of that hand over the anterior talofibular ligament, while the other hand grasps the calcaneus and applies an anterior and internal rotation force.

If instability is present, there is excessive anterior motion of the foot relative to the ankle mortise with a palpable clunk sometimes felt or a vacuum effect felt by the thumb over the anterior talofibular ligament.[17]

To assess the deltoid ligament, the test is repeated with an anterior and external rotation force applied to the foot.

- Varus stress test (talar tilt test)

The varus stress test assesses the integrity of the lateral ligament complex.

The distal leg is stabilized by one hand, while the other hand grasps the calcaneus and applies a varus stress. The thumb of the hand supporting the leg palpates the lateral ligament complex; gapping of the lateral joint space indicates instability.[17]

This gapping may be difficult to distinguish clinically from normal subtalar inversion motion without radiographic assistance.

The calcaneofibular ligament is better assessed by performing this test with the ankle in dorsiflexion and the anterior talofibular ligament with the ankle in plantar flexion.

- Valgus stress test

The valgus stress test assesses the integrity of the deltoid ligament.

It is performed similarly to the varus stress test except a valgus and eversion stress is applied to the calcaneus with gapping of the medial joint space indicating instability.[17]

Similar to the varus stress test, gapping of the medial joint space may be difficult to assess clinically from normal subtalar motion without stress ankle mortise radiographs or fluoroscopy.

- Squeeze test

The squeeze test assesses for syndesmotic injury.

The proximal aspect of the lower leg is grasped, squeezing the fibula toward the tibia.

If a significant syndesmotic injury is present, this causes the distal tibiofibular joint to separate and cause pain.[18,19]

- Cotton abduction external rotation test

The Cotton test assesses for syndesmotic injury but may be difficult to perform in the acute setting secondary to patient discomfort.

With the knee in approximately 90 degrees of flexion, an abduction external rotation force is applied to the foot.

Pain over the syndesmosis indicates instability.[19]

There may be lateral shift of the talus in the ankle mortise relative to the medial malleolus.

This shift may be difficult to feel clinically but may be documented on stress radiographs.

■ Diagnostic Testing
- Plain radiographs

Anteroposterior and lateral views of the tibia and fibula are the standard views obtained to evaluate for suspected tibial or fibula shaft fractures.

Anteroposterior, lateral, and mortise views of the ankle are the standard views obtained to evaluate for a suspected ankle fracture.

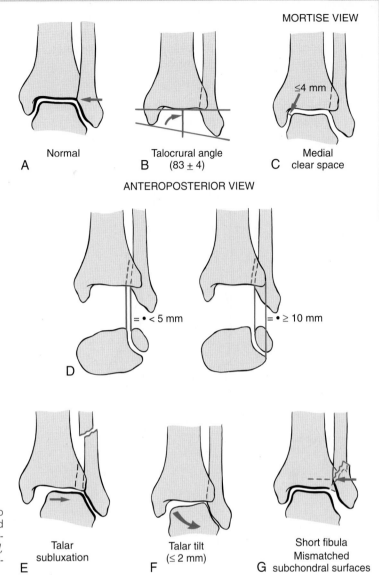

**FIGURE 15-18.** Important ankle radiographic parameters to measure. **A,** Medial clear space. **B,** Tibiofibular clear space and overlap measured 1 cm above the ankle joint line. **C,** Talar subluxation. **D,** Talar tilt. *(From Browner BD, Jupiter JB, Levine AM, et al, editors: Skeletal trauma: basic science, management, and reconstruction, ed 4, Philadelphia, 2008, Saunders.)*

The modified Ottawa ankle rules have been validated and are an excellent algorithm to determine the need for x-rays after a foot or ankle injury.[20]

Ankle x-rays should be obtained if there is evidence of bony tenderness along the distal 6 cm of the posterior edge of the tibia or fibula, bony tenderness at the tip of the medial or lateral malleolus, or an inability to bear weight for four steps both at the time of injury and in the emergency department.

- Ankle x-ray measurements may be used to assess for syndesmotic instability and acceptability of fracture displacement (Fig. 15-18).

Medial clear space

- This is the measurement of the space between the medial talar dome and subchondral bone of the articular surface of the medial malleolus. Typically, this should be 4 mm or less on anteroposterior or mortise views or equal to the superior clear space

between the talar dome and subchondral bone of the distal articular surface of the tibia.[21,22]

Tibiofibular clear space

- This measurement is the distance between the incisura fibularis of the tibia and the medial wall of the fibula.
- An increased tibiofibular clear space suggests significant enough syndesmotic ligament injury to lead to widening between the lateral tibia and the fibula.
- Typically, this measurement, which is made 1 cm above the ankle joint line, should be less than 5 to 6 mm on both anteroposterior and mortise views.[21,22]

Tibiofibular overlap

- This measurement is the overlap of the lateral malleolus of the fibula and the anterior tibial tubercle 1 cm above the ankle joint line.

- This value should be greater than 6 mm or greater than 42% of the fibular width on the anteroposterior view, whereas the overlap should be greater than 1 mm on the mortise view.[21-23]

Talocrural angle (Fig. 15-19)

- The talocrural angle assesses for adequate maintenance of fibular length after fracture.

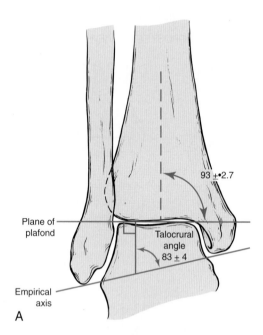

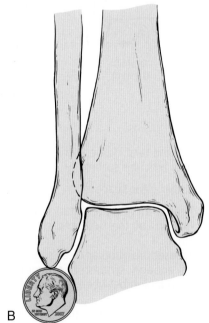

FIGURE 15-19. Measurements of fibular length. **A,** The talocrural angle represents the angle between a line perpendicular to the tibial plafond and a line connecting the distal tip of the lateral and medial malleoli. The normal angle range is 83 ± 4 degrees, or a deviation from the contralateral side. **B,** The dime sign is an unbroken arc connecting the recess in the distal tip of the fibula and the lateral process of the talus. A broken arc indicates shortening of the fibula. *(From Browner BD, Jupiter JB, Levine AM, et al, editors: Skeletal trauma: basic science, management, and reconstruction, ed 4, Philadelphia, 2008, Saunders.)*

- It is measured on the mortise view and represents the angle between a line perpendicular to the tibial plafond and a line connecting the distal tip of the lateral and medial malleolus.[21,22]
- The normal range is 83 ± 4 degrees or a deviation from the contralateral side.

"Dime" sign (see Fig. 15-19)

- The dime sign also assesses for adequate maintenance of fibular length after fracture.
- It is measured on the anteroposterior view, where normally there is an unbroken arc connecting the recess in the distal tip of the fibula and the lateral process of the talus.[21]
- If this arc is broken, it indicates shortening of the fibula.
- Additional radiographs

Based on clinical history and physical examination, additional extremity x-rays above and below the main level of injury should be considered.

- For significant ankle injuries, complete tibia and fibula and foot radiographs may be warranted.
- For injuries to the tibia or fibula shaft, knee and ankle radiographs should be obtained.

Radiographs should be assessed for the presence of air or swelling in the joints or soft tissues.

- The presence of air may be indicative of an open injury.
- Studies have shown that 5 mL of synovial fluid is required to be present in the ankle joint to diagnose a joint effusion on plain radiography.[24,25]

Stress radiographs are helpful when concern arises for ligamentous injury that may affect ankle fracture stability.

- A bimalleolar equivalent injury pattern consists of a fibula fracture with an associated deltoid ligament injury.
- To identify a possible deltoid ligament injury, a Cotton stress ankle mortise radiograph may be obtained with abduction and external rotation of the dorsiflexed foot.
  - In this situation, a medial clear space of 5 mm or greater has been shown to be the most reliable predictor of deep deltoid ligament status.[10]
- An alternative stress radiograph that is considered less painful is the gravity stress view.
  - An ankle mortise radiograph is taken with the patient placed in the lateral decubitus position on the injured side with the foot and ankle allowed to hang off the edge of the x-ray table, with the weight of the foot causing the ankle to be externally rotated.[26]
- Controversy exists regarding the treatment of bimalleolar equivalent fractures that exhibit a widened medial clear space on a stress view.
  - Some proponents believe that this test verifies an unstable ankle fracture that requires surgical fixation.

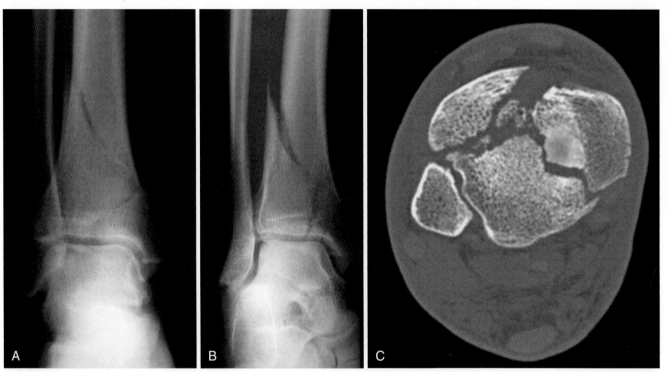

**FIGURE 15-20. A** and **B,** Plain radiographic images show a plafond/pilon fracture of the distal tibia with what appears to be a minimally displaced articular surface. **C,** Axial CT scan of the same patient shows extensive articular comminution that was not visualized on plain radiographs. *(From Browner BD, Jupiter JB, Levine AM, et al, editors: Skeletal trauma: basic science, management, and reconstruction, ed 4, Philadelphia, 2008, Saunders.)*

- ◆ Others believe that if an adequate reduction can be maintained with splint or cast application, nonoperative treatment would likely lead to long-term ligamentous stability secondary to appropriate deltoid ligament and fibular fracture healing.
- Computed tomography (CT) scan

  CT scan can help diagnose subtle fractures not seen clearly on plain x-rays or can help determine the extent of comminution or displacement of a known fracture (Fig. 15-20).

  CT may also play an important role in determining whether surgical treatment of a fracture is indicated and, if so, aid in surgical decision making with respect to incision location and type of fixation necessary.

- Magnetic resonance imaging (MRI)

  MRI may help diagnose soft tissue injuries including injuries involving tendons, ligaments, articular cartilage abnormalities, bone contusions, stress fractures, and subtle fractures (Fig. 15-21).

  MRI is typically not needed for the diagnosis and treatment of most acute ankle fractures, tibial and fibular shaft fractures, routine ankle sprains, and Achilles tendon ruptures.

  In cases of chronic ankle instability where surgical intervention is being considered, MRI may be ordered to rule out other associated pathology.

  In suspected cases of septic arthritis, MRI is typically performed only if there are clinical concerns regarding concomitant osteomyelitis or soft tissue abscess formation.[27]

- Ultrasound

  Ultrasound can be used diagnostically to assess for soft tissue pathology including Achilles tendon rupture or gastrocnemius and soleus muscle strain.

  Ultrasound may also be used therapeutically to guide injections or aspirations.

  Compared with MRI, ultrasound can be performed quickly, is relatively inexpensive, and allows for dynamic assessment of tendons. However, it is operator-dependent, and substantial experience is typically needed to perform and read the images.[28]

- Bone scan

  Bone scan may be helpful in assessing for increased bone activity secondary to pathology or injury. However, it is not specific and often cannot differentiate between stress fracture, traumatic fracture, osteomyelitis, arthritis, bone bruise, or other abnormalities.

- Joint aspiration

  Joint aspiration is performed to rule out the possibility of a septic joint or inflammatory process such as gout or pseudogout.

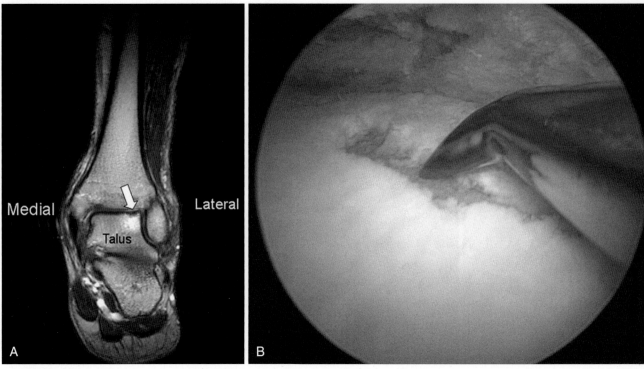

**FIGURE 15-21. A,** MRI shows a lucent region in the lateral aspect of the talus. **B,** Arthroscopic examination revealed an extensive osteochondral defect. *(From Browner BD, Jupiter JB, Levine AM, et al, editors: Skeletal trauma: basic science, management, and reconstruction, ed 4, Philadelphia, 2008, Saunders.)*

- Joint fluid should be sent for culture, cell count, Gram stain, glucose, protein, and crystal analysis.
- Aspiration can be done by knowledge of clinical anatomy or under fluoroscopy, CT, or ultrasound guidance.
- Clinicians should avoid placing the needle into an area with suspected overlying cellulitis whenever possible to decrease the risk of creating a septic joint.

  Joint injection with local anesthetic with or without corticosteroid can be performed for diagnostic and therapeutic purposes.

- Transient relief of symptoms after ankle anesthetic injection suggests that intra-articular pathology such as arthritis or mechanical impingement is the principal source of the patient's discomfort, whereas no relief suggests that the etiology is extra-articular.
- Incomplete transient symptom relief suggests the presence of both intra-articular and extra-articular pathology.
- Confirmation of intra-articular location of injection may be obtained by fluoroscopy or ultrasound.
- Disruption of adhesions or decreased inflammation with concurrent corticosteroid injection may also lead to longer term therapeutic benefit, although there is some evidence that both local anesthetic and corticosteroid may damage the chondrocytes responsible for maintaining the health of the articular cartilage.

- Typically 5 mL or less of local anesthetic and corticosteroid is injected.

  An anesthetic injection of local anesthetic into the ankle joint or fracture hematoma may be used to provide pain relief to allow for closed reduction of ankle fracture-dislocations.

- Adequate patient analgesia is imperative to avoid patient discomfort and allow for limb relaxation and manipulation.
- Intra-articular ankle blocks provide a similar amount of analgesia compared with conscious sedation in treatment of ankle fracture-dislocations and can be used effectively in significantly displaced ankle fractures that require reduction.[29]
- Blocks can be performed relatively quickly in the emergent setting and provide sufficient pain relief to allow for successful closed reduction.[30]
- After first confirming proper entry into the ankle joint by aspirating fracture hematoma, typically 10 to 12 mL of equal amounts of 1% lidocaine without epinephrine and 0.5% bupivacaine without epinephrine is injected into the ankle joint using a 20-gauge or 22-gauge needle.[21,31]

  Two approaches are commonly used for injection or aspiration of the ankle joint: the anterolateral approach and the more common anteromedial approach.[21,31]

- With either approach, the key is not to place the needle directly between the tibia and talus where

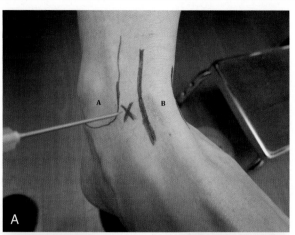

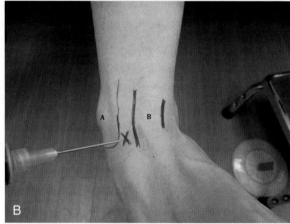

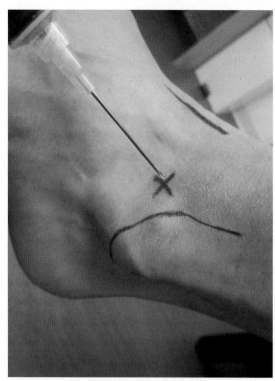

**FIGURE 15-23.** Anterolateral approach to ankle aspiration and injection. This approach uses the interval between the lateral malleolus and the peroneus tertius. The peroneus tertius muscle is absent in a percentage of the population, so typically a soft spot is palpated just medial to the lateral malleolus at the ankle joint line to find the correct mark.

**FIGURE 15-22.** Anteromedial approach to ankle aspiration and injection. This approach uses the interval between the lateral aspect of the medial malleolus and the tibialis anterior tendon. A soft spot is palpated just medial to the tibialis anterior tendon; this may be difficult to palpate in the emergency setting because of swelling of the soft tissue.

the articular cartilage may be damaged by the needle but rather in the joint space deep to the capsule that is directly anterior to the tibia and talus.

- Anteromedial approach (Fig. 15-22)
  - This approach allows entry into the joint between the medial malleolus and the tibialis anterior tendon.
  - A soft spot should be palpable just medial to the tibialis anterior tendon; this is where the needle should be inserted.
  - Dorsiflexion of the ankle allows better visualization and palpation of the soft spot medial to the anterior tibial tendon and places the anterior ankle capsule on less tension increasing the potential space between the capsule and articular surfaces in which to place the needle.
  - The needle should be advanced diagonally and laterally deep to the anterior tibial tendon; a "pop" can sometimes be felt when the needle penetrates the ankle joint capsule.
  - There is a risk of damage to the greater saphenous nerve and saphenous vein if initial needle placement is too medial.

- Anterolateral approach (Fig. 15-23)
  - This approach enters the joint through a palpable soft spot between the lateral malleolus and the peroneus tertius tendon or, if not present, extensor digitorum longus tendon.
  - Similar to the anteromedial approach, the landmarks are easier to palpate and the ankle joint space is easier to enter with the ankle dorsiflexed.
  - The needle should be advanced diagonally and medially deep to the peroneus tertius and extensor digitorum longus tendons; a "pop" can sometimes be felt when the needle penetrates the ankle joint capsule.
  - This approach can damage the dorsal intermediate cutaneous branch of the superficial peroneal nerve, which travels in the area of the injection site and sometimes can be palpated or visualized with the ankle held in plantar flexion and the hindfoot in inversion.
  - For this reason, the anteromedial approach is typically preferred unless there is anteromedial ankle cellulitis or principally anterolateral ankle joint pathology.
- ■ Differential Diagnosis
  - Acute traumatic injuries to the ankle include fractures, joint dislocations and subluxations, muscle and tendon tears, ligament sprains, nerve injuries, skin and soft tissue lacerations, soft tissue crush injuries, and lower leg compartment syndrome.

- Infectious processes include cellulitis, septic arthritis, and osteomyelitis.
- Patients with more chronic ankle or lower leg pathology, some of which is related to previous trauma, can also present in the emergency department secondary to acute or recent onset, an exacerbation of a chronic condition, or lack of access to health care providers secondary to insurance or other issues. These pathologies include:

  Degenerative or inflammatory processes including arthritis, Charcot arthropathy, and tendinopathy

  Chronic ligamentous instability in the ankle

## TREATMENT OF SPECIFIC INJURIES

- Develop Plan
  - Based on patient history and physical examination findings, obtain diagnostic testing to narrow the differential diagnosis and suggest treatment options.
  - Determine whether treatment needs to be emergent, semiurgent requiring partial or complete treatment during the emergency department visit or subsequent hospitalization, or nonemergent that could be completed at a follow-up outpatient visit.
  - Determine which of the following applies:

    Patient can definitively be treated at this emergency department visit.

    - If so, discuss treatment alternatives with the patient or family and carry out final treatment plan.

    Sufficient temporizing treatment can be provided to the patient to discharge home from the emergency department, but definitive follow-up treatment or diagnostic work-up is required by a primary care provider or a specialist.

    - If so, discuss treatment alternatives with the patient or family, carry out initial treatment plan, and arrange or stress the importance of scheduling an appropriate follow-up visit.

      A specialist is required to aid in determining the diagnosis or providing emergent or semiurgent treatment on an inpatient or outpatient basis.

    - If so, discuss treatment alternatives with the patient or family, carry out urgently required adjunctive treatment, and arrange specialist consultation.
  - In the emergent setting with injury owing to high-energy mechanisms, the initial management should follow advanced trauma life support guidelines. During the initial assessment, the physician should quickly check for signs of open injury or exsanguination and assess for peripheral pulses.

    Evidence of active bleeding from an injured extremity requires direct pressure while the primary survey is performed.

    A more detailed secondary survey is performed when the patient is stabilized and includes palpation of all extremities and passive range of motion of all joints to assess for deformity or pain. A more focused neurovascular examination is also performed at this time.

    Evidence of a pulseless or excessively bleeding lower extremity necessitates urgent assessment and potential vascular surgery consultation.

- Open Fractures
  - Initial management should consist of administration of prophylactic antibiotics and tetanus prophylaxis as soon as possible. An increased rate of wound infection has been seen if initiation of antibiotics occurs more than 3 hours after injury.
  - In the emergent setting, selection of appropriate antibiotics can be tentatively based on the Gustilo-Anderson classification.

    The Gustilo-Anderson classification is used to determine the extent of soft tissue injury in an open fracture. Typically, definitive classification of the wound occurs after initial surgical débridement in the operating room. However, initial use of this classification in the emergent setting can help aid the consulting orthopedic surgeon before his or her arrival in the emergency department.[21,32-36]

    - Type I injuries—a clean open wound less than 1 cm in length
    - Type II injuries—a clean open wound more than 1 cm in length but without extensive soft tissue injury
    - Type III injuries—associated with significant soft tissue injury and further divided into three subtypes[21,35,36]
    - Type IIIA injuries—adequate soft tissue coverage over the tibia
    - Type IIIB injuries—significant stripping of the periosteum overlying the tibia; these injuries typically have extensive contamination
    - Type IIIC injuries—most severe subtype and indicate arterial injury regardless of fracture pattern or soft tissue damage

      A first-generation cephalosporin is the antibiotic of choice for management of a Gustilo type I injury.[24,35,36]

      Clindamycin can be used if the patient has an allergy to penicillin.

      Addition of an aminoglycoside such as gentamicin or tobramycin is adequate in type II and type IIIA injuries.[21,35,36]

      In type IIIB fractures, penicillin G or ampicillin should be added to the regimen because of the potential risk of clostridial myonecrosis.[21,35,36]
  - Tetanus toxoid or immunoglobin should be administered based on the tetanus status of the patient.

    A patient with an unknown or no history of tetanus immunization should receive immunization with tetanus toxoid and prophylaxis with tetanus immune globulin.

studies have shown an incidence of ligamentous injury to the ipsilateral knee of 22%.[40]
- Mechanism

  Motor vehicle accident

  - Highest incidence of tibial shaft fractures
  - High rate of open injury with motorcycle crashes

  Pedestrian struck by motor vehicle (Fig. 15-27)

  Violence including direct blows, assault, and gunshot wounds (Fig. 15-28)

  - Less common but still can cause significant damage and comminution
- In open injuries, initial antibiotic and tetanus prophylaxis can be managed based on the Gustilo-Anderson classification as mentioned previously.

  Initial irrigation of exposed bone can be performed in the emergency department, but this does not substitute for a thorough irrigation and débridement in the operating room.

  Closed reduction of significantly displaced fractures should be attempted after assessment and débridement of the open wound.

  - This consists of longitudinal traction and application of a posterior and "U" splint. In some instances, a simple posterior splint may be adequate if the patient is being taken directly to the operating room.

- In patients who are severely unstable and require urgent CT imaging by the trauma surgery team, a long posterior plaster splint or prefabricated metal splint can be used to provide stability in emergent situations (Fig. 15-29).
- Adequate analgesia before reduction helps avoid excessive patient discomfort.
- An attempt should be made to reduce exposed fracture fragments with longitudinal traction, unless there is gross contamination of the fracture fragments.
- If difficulty arises in reduction, the fragments should not be forcibly thrust in the wound. Rather, a clean dressing should be applied before application of the splint in preparation for irrigation and débridement in the operating room.

■ Common Pitfalls
- In any high-energy fracture, it is imperative to perform a full secondary survey in the trauma bay to diagnose concurrent injuries.
- Prompt administration of appropriate antibiotics and tetanus prophylaxis based on presumed Gustilo and Anderson classification is imperative.

## Distal Tibia Pilon Fractures

■ General Considerations
- Fractures of the distal tibia are among the most challenging fractures to both the emergency physician and the orthopedic physician.

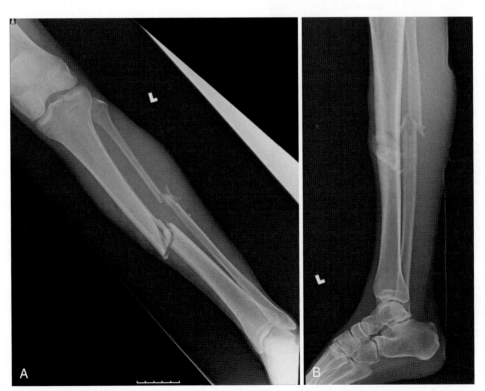

**FIGURE 15-27.** Anteroposterior and lateral radiographs of a 26-year-old man who sustained a grade I open midshaft tibia and fibula fracture after being struck by a car while riding his skateboard.

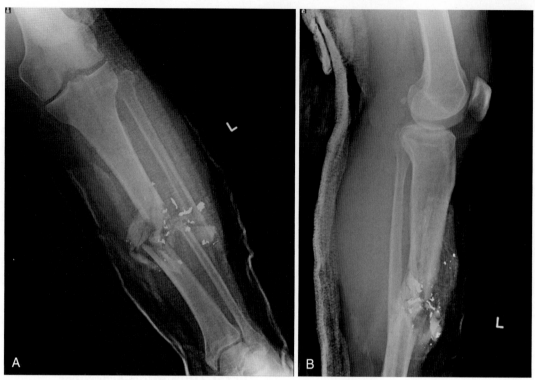

**FIGURE 15-28.** Anteroposterior and lateral radiographs of a 61-year-old man who sustained an accidental gunshot wound to the left tibia and fibula while hunting. He was taken to the operating room emergently for irrigation and débridement and placement of an external fixator.

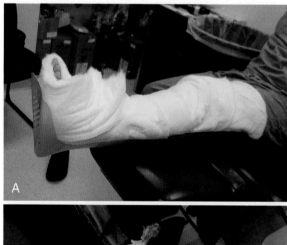

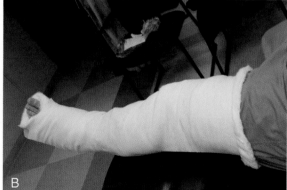

**FIGURE 15-29.** A prefabricated long metal posterior splint can be quickly applied in the trauma bay by the trauma team to provide temporary stability in unstable patients requiring immediate CT imaging. **A,** The leg should first be wrapped in either a Robert Jones dressing or cast padding before being placed in the metal splint. **B,** After the leg is placed in the metal splint, an Ace bandage is used as an overlying wrap.

- The French radiologist Destot first used the term *pilon fracture* in 1911, referring to the pestle-like shape of the talus that would apply a vertically directed crushing load onto the distal tibial articular surface during axial loading injuries.[41,42]
- A tibial pilon or plafond fracture by definition extends into the distal weight-bearing articular surface of the tibia where it articulates with the superior articular surface of the talar dome.[8,34]

  Fractures that involve just the medial or posterior malleolus typically are not considered to be pilon fractures.

  Depending on the amount of energy sustained, these fractures typically result in comminution and impaction of the tibial metaphysis with highly destructive forces onto the surrounding soft tissues.

  Pilon fractures constitute approximately 7% of all tibial fractures and 1% of all fractures of the lower extremity.

  These fractures have the second highest incidence of open fractures of the tibia and fibula after diaphyseal fractures.[42]

  Improvements in high-speed motor vehicle travel and lifesaving safety preventions have resulted in an increased incidence of distal tibial fractures.[41]

- Management of these fractures has changed over the past decades.

Although initially it was thought that early open reduction and internal fixation of pilon fractures provided the best outcomes, subsequent results in patients with high-energy pilon fractures have shown poorer soft tissue results and increased surgical complications.

Newer approaches, including early temporary spanning external fixation with or without open reduction and internal fixation of the fibula, are tailored toward protection of the fragile surrounding soft tissues.[43]

- Pilon fractures are often the result of high-energy axial loading injuries.

Most commonly, these fractures are the result of high-speed motor vehicle collisions, falls from heights, or workplace accidents (Fig. 15-30).

The foot is suddenly decelerated sending tremendous forces often greater than four times the body weight that overcome the surrounding ligamentous and osseous structures.[42]

There is a 25% to 50% chance of other associated injuries to the calcaneus, proximal tibial plateau, acetabulum, pelvis, and vertebral bodies.[44]

The distal fibula is usually fractured in higher energy injuries.

- Low-energy injuries typically occur with skiing or sports injuries and result from a spiral or rotational mechanism.

Although swelling commonly occurs, the soft tissue is generally intact and less compromised.

In contrast to high-energy fractures, the tibia is usually not comminuted, and the fibula is less often fractured.

- The location of the articular fracture lines is based on the position of the foot during impact (Fig. 15-31).

A foot in dorsiflexion results in fracture of the anterior distal tibia.

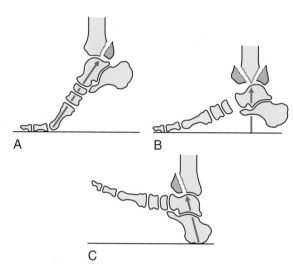

**FIGURE 15-31.** Pilon fracture patterns. *(From Browner BD, Jupiter JB, Levine AM, et al, editors: Skeletal trauma: basic science, management, and reconstruction, ed 4, Philadelphia, 2008, Saunders.)*

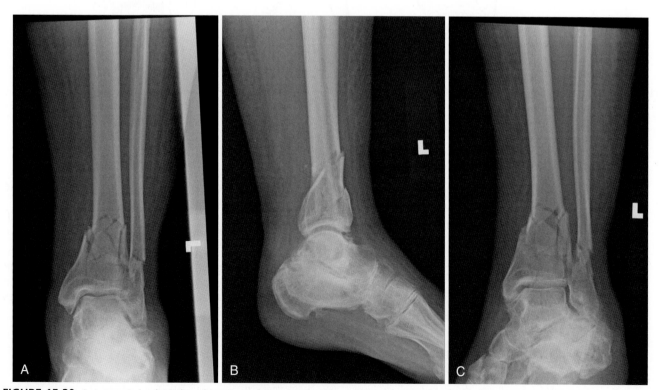

**FIGURE 15-30.** Anteroposterior, lateral, and mortise radiographs of a 50-year-old man with a history of alcohol abuse and cirrhosis who sustained a pilon fracture after falling down a flight of stairs while intoxicated.

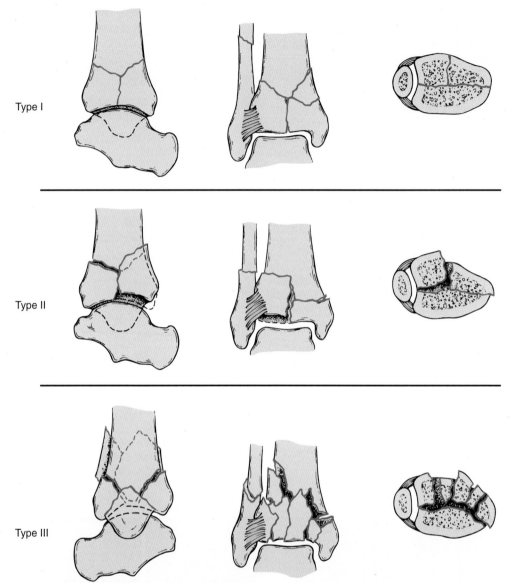

Type I

Type II

Type III

**FIGURE 15-32.** Ruedi and Allgower classification of distal tibia pilon fractures. *Type I* fractures include simple cleavage fractures with little to no articular displacement, *type II* fractures have articular displacement but no comminution, and *type III* fractures have articular displacement with comminution and metaphyseal impaction. *(From Browner BD, Jupiter JB, Levine AM, et al, editors: Skeletal trauma: basic science, management, and reconstruction, ed 4, Philadelphia, 2008, Saunders.)*

A foot in plantar flexion results in fracture of the posterior malleolus.

A foot in neutral dorsiflexion can result in fractures within any portion of the tibial plafond.

There may be multiple comminuted fracture fragments that often affect the surrounding soft tissues including a 25% chance of an open injury.

- Two main classification systems describe distal tibial fractures.

The Ruedi and Allgower classification separates fractures into three types (Fig. 15-32).[41,42]

- Type I—simple cleavage fracture, little or no articular displacement

- Type II—some articular displacement but no comminution
- Type III—intra-articular displacement with comminution and metaphyseal impaction

In 1996, the Arbeitsgemeinschaft fur Osteosynthesefragen/Orthopaedic Trauma Association (AO/OTA) developed a more intricate system to classify distal tibial fractures into nine categories (Fig. 15-33).[41,42]

- Type A—extra-articular fractures
- Type A1—simple
- Type A2—wedge
- Type A3—comminution
- Type B—partial articular surface
- Type B1—pure split

- Operative treatment

  The ruptured ends can be sutured together using open or percutaneous techniques.

  Compared with nonoperative treatment, surgical repair is associated with a significantly decreased Achilles tendon rerupture rate but an increased wound and nerve complication rate.[28,63]

  Some, but not all, studies comparing functional bracing with operative treatment showed comparable clinical results, including in young, active people more traditionally treated with surgery.[69,70]

  Ruptures that occur at the calcaneal insertion or that are associated with avulsion fractures of the calcaneus require operative treatment.

  Patients may take more than 1 year to reach full ankle plantar flexion strength, which may or may not be at the preinjury level.

## Gastrocnemius and Soleus Muscle Rupture

- General Considerations
  - Partial or complete tears of the calf musculature proximal to the Achilles tendon, which is sometimes referred to as "tennis leg," most commonly occur in the medial head of the gastrocnemius.
  - Historically, it was thought that these injuries were due to rupture or strain of the plantaris muscle. However, one study found that was rarely the case and that concomitant injury to the entire gastrocnemius-soleus complex occurred in 17% of individuals.[68]
- History
  - Similar to patients with Achilles tendon ruptures, patients often report a feeling of getting kicked in the back of the calf and report immediate pain and weakness after the injury.[71]
  - Similar to Achilles tendon injuries, injury often occurs in middle-aged, less conditioned individuals who overexert themselves while playing a recreational sport such as tennis.[71]
  - Preexisting gastrocnemius contractures may also be a predisposing factor; when the patient recovers from the rupture, the patient may note the same therapeutic benefit on foot disorders such as metatarsalgia and plantar fasciitis that surgical lengthening of the gastrocnemius contracture might provide.
- Physical Examination
  - There is typically tenderness, swelling, and occasionally a palpable defect over the proximal calf to midcalf, most commonly over the medial gastrocnemius.
  - Deep venous thrombosis is in the differential diagnosis and may need to be ruled out with a venous duplex examination.
  - In contrast to Achilles tendon ruptures, there is no palpable defect and usually minimal tenderness noted over the Achilles tendon, a Thompson test is negative, and passive ankle dorsiflexion with the knee flexed is usually not increased.

- The patient may or may not be able to do a single leg heel raise depending on pain tolerance.
- Treatment
  - Proximal gastrocnemius and soleus ruptures are treated nonoperatively.
  - The affected leg is wrapped with a compressive bandage and placed in a cam walker boot.
  - If significantly painful, a below-the-knee posterior and "U" plaster splint or bivalved cast may be applied for a short time.
  - Immobilization helps prevent further injury and limits increased bleeding from the torn muscle fibers.
  - Hemostasis may also be promoted during the first days after injury by icing the area and avoiding heat, massage, and nonsteroidal anti-inflammatory drugs.
  - The patient may be weight bearing as tolerated with crutches as needed.
  - When symptoms allow, a rehabilitation program stressing anti-inflammatory modalities, gentle stretching, and strengthening should be implemented.
  - Most patients can return to near-normal activity within 3 to 6 months.

## Septic Arthritis of the Ankle

- General Considerations
  - Accounts for approximately 7% of cases of septic arthritis
  - Common pathogens

    *Staphylococcus aureus* is the most common pathogen.[4]

    *Staphylococcus epidermidis* should be suspected if a patient has had previous ankle surgery.[72]

    Cases of *Mycobacterium tuberculosis* have been reported in patients living in areas endemic to the disease or in immunocompromised patients with previous history of exposure.[73]

  - Most common origin is via hematogenous spread of the offending organism

    Some patients may report a history of a "twisting" injury to the ankle in the recent past.

    In cases of *M. tuberculosis,* direct trauma introduction has been reported, but cases are typically associated with hematogenous spread.[73]

  - Patients typically present within first 24 to 48 hours of infection

    Only approximately one third to one half of patients report a history of fever before presentation.[4]

    Ankle pain is the most consistent finding on presentation followed by swelling around the ankle.[4]

    Patients may have difficulty bearing weight on the injured ankle.

    Erythema and warmth are less specific findings.[4]

    Patients typically report decreased ankle range of motion.

■ Preexisting Illness
  • Crystal arthropathy, gout, or chondrocalcinosis may mimic a septic presentation and a history of this should be sought in all patients.
  • A history of diabetes mellitus or neuropathy should also be sought because Charcot arthropathy can mimic a septic picture.
  • A recent or active history of a soft tissue infection in the foot, such as cellulitis, tenosynovitis, and abscesses, can increase the risk of developing septic arthritis.[27]
  • Patients with systemic diseases, such as rheumatoid arthritis, systemic lupus erythematosus, gout, and diabetes, have an increased risk of developing septic arthritis of the ankle.[4,74]
  • Concomitant osteomyelitis can occur and is most often seen in patients with significant comorbidities, such as diabetes mellitus or intravenous drug, alcohol, or corticosteroid use.[4]
■ Radiographic Studies
  • Weight-bearing anteroposterior, lateral, and mortise ankle radiographs should be obtained to assess for evidence of joint destruction or adjacent osteomyelitis; soft tissue swelling or fluid collections; and other potential causes of ankle pain including fracture, arthritis, and Charcot arthropathy.
■ Serum Studies
  • C-reactive protein and erythrocyte sedimentation rate are markers of inflammation.

    If elevated, the suspicion for infection increases.

    C-reactive protein and erythrocyte sedimentation rate are nonspecific and may be elevated in patients with inflammatory arthritis and other disorders.

  • Complete blood cell count with differential

    An elevated white blood cell count with an increased number of polymorphonuclear leukocytes is suggestive of infection.

    The white blood cell count may be elevated in less than 50% of patients with septic arthritis.[4]

  • Blood cultures are warranted in patients who have signs and symptoms of systemic infection such as fever or chills.

■ Joint Aspiration
  • If the differential diagnosis includes a septic ankle joint, joint aspiration and blood cultures should be performed before any antibiotics are given.
  • The aspirated joint fluid should be sent for:

    Synovial cell count and differential

    Synovial Gram stain

    Fungal and acid-fast staining if indicated based on history

    Crystal analysis

    Cultures

    • Aerobe
    • Anaerobe
    • Fungal and mycobacterial cultures may also be sent if indicated based on history
■ Joint Fluid Studies (Table 15-2)
  • Gold standard for diagnosis and treatment of possible septic arthritis
  • Synovial fluid typically appears clear and thick
■ Treatment
  • When the possibility of a septic ankle is considered, emergent treatment is indicated to decrease the risk of subsequent irreversible cartilage damage.
  • If the emergency physician feels comfortable with joint aspiration, an aspirate can be attempted before arrival of the orthopedic team to hasten laboratory diagnosis.
  • Antibiotics should not be started empirically until joint aspiration and blood draws have been performed and the surgeon has been consulted.
  • If imminent arthroscopic or open débridement of the joint is planned, empiric antibiotics ideally would be deferred until after intraoperative cultures have been taken.
  • Antibiotic treatment is begun empirically and subsequently adjusted based on culture results and often infectious disease consultation.

    Multiple acceptable empiric regimens are available, and the choice may be influenced by physician preference, cost, and prevalence of local organism and antibiotic resistance.

    One potential algorithm is as follows:

**TABLE 15-2** Characteristics of Different Synovial Fluid Pathology

| | Normal | Noninflammatory | Inflammatory | Septic |
|---|---|---|---|---|
| Viscosity | High | High | Low | Varies |
| Color | Clear | Straw-yellow | Yellow | Varies |
| WBC count | <200/mm$^3$ | 200-2000/mm$^3$ | 2000-75,000/mm$^3$ | >100,000/mm$^3$ |
| PMNs (%) | <25% | <25% | >50% | >75% |
| Glucose | ~ Blood | ~ Blood | ↓ | ↓↓ |
| Culture | Negative | Negative | Negative | Often positive |

*PMN*, Polymorphonuclear neutrophils; *WBC*, white blood cell.

- Intravenous oxacillin or nafcillin in combination with intravenous ceftriaxone[4]
  - Gram-positive cocci, staphylococci, and streptococci are the most common bacteria encountered.
  - Gram negative rods may also be present in lower extremity infections.
- If the patient has a penicillin allergy, intravenous clindamycin and an intravenous or well-absorbed parenteral quinolone such as ciprofloxacin may be given.

If methicillin-resistant *S. aureus* is suspected, intravenous vancomycin plus ceftazidime or a quinolone is an option.

Oxacillin-resistant *S. aureus* can occur in approximately 17% of cases of septic arthritis.[4]

- Emergent débridement of the ankle joint should be performed if the joint aspirate results are diagnostic or suspicious for a septic joint.
- Ankle arthroscopy allows better visualization and access for débridement of the posterior ankle joint than an open arthrotomy and has less surgical morbidity.

A small incision may be added for débridement of a concurrent extra-articular soft tissue abscess.

Serial joint aspirations do not allow any visualization of the joint, and they do not remove any infected or impinging synovial tissue.

- Depending on the intraoperative findings and the patient's clinical progress, repeat arthroscopic or open surgical débridement may be indicated.

■ Common Pitfalls
- Empiric antibiotics should not be initiated until after joint aspiration, blood cultures, and potentially intraoperative cultures have been obtained.
- It is helpful to verify that joint cultures have been received by the laboratory and do not need to be repeated before initiating empiric antibiotics.
- One should avoid placing the aspiration needle in an area of overlying suspected cellulitis whenever possible to avoid potentially seeding the joint.
- Unless there is a significant ankle effusion, the space between the tibial plafond and the talus seen on ankle radiographs does not represent joint space but radiolucent articular cartilage.
- Care should be taken not to plunge the aspiration needle into the articular cartilage but in the space deep to the ankle capsule and anterior to the distal tibial articular cartilage.

## References

1. Witvrouw E, Borre KV, Willems TM, et al: The significance of the peroneus tertius muscle in ankle injuries: a prospective study. Am J Sports Med 34:1159–1163, 2006.
2. Hastrup SG, Chen X, Bechtold JE, et al: Effect of nicotine and tobacco administration method on the mechanical properties of healing bone following closed fracture. J Orthop Res 28:1235–1239, 2010.
3. Hollinger JO, Schmitt JM, Hwang K, et al: Impact of nicotine on bone healing. J Biomed Mater Res 45:294–301, 1999.
4. Holtom PD, Borges L, Zalavras CG: Hematogenous septic ankle arthritis. Clin Orthop Relat Res 466:1388–1391, 2008.
5. Strauss EJ, Petrucelli G, Bong M, et al: Blisters associated with lower-extremity fracture: results of a prospective treatment protocol. J Orthop Trauma 20:618–622, 2006.
6. Giordano CP, Koval KJ, Zuckerman JD, et al: Fracture blisters. Clin Orthop Relat Res 307:214–221, 1994.
7. Keese GR, Boody AR, Wongworawat MD, et al: The accuracy of the saline load test in the diagnosis of traumatic knee arthrotomies. J Orthop Trauma 21:442–443, 2007.
8. Nord RM, Quach T, Walsh M, et al: Detection of traumatic arthrotomy of the knee using the saline solution load test. J Bone Joint Surg Am 91:66–70, 2009.
9. DeAngelis NA, Eskander MS, French BG: Does medial tenderness predict deep deltoid ligament incompetence in supination-external rotation type ankle fractures? J Orthop Trauma 21:244–247, 2007.
10. Park SS, Kubiak EN, Egol KA, et al: Stress radiographs after ankle fracture: the effect of ankle position and deltoid ligament status on medial clear space measurements. J Orthop Trauma 20:11–18, 2006.
11. Melvin JS, Dombroski DG, Torbert JT, et al: Open tibial shaft fractures: I. Evaluation and initial wound management. J Am Acad Orthop Surg 18:10–19, 2010.
12. Petrisor BA, Bhandari M, Schemitsch: Tibia and fibula fractures. In Bucholz RW, Heckman JD, Court-Brown C, et al, editors: Rockwood and Green's fractures in Adults, ed 7, Philadelphia, 2010, Lippincott Williams & Wilkins, pp 1867–1927.
13. Blick SS, Brumback RJ, Poka A, et al: Compartment syndrome in open tibial fractures. J Bone Joint Surg Am 68:1348–1353, 1986.
14. Schmidt AH, Anglen J, Nana AD, et al: Adult trauma: getting through the night. J Bone Joint Surg Am 92:490–505, 2010.
15. Ulmer T: The clinical diagnosis of compartment syndrome of the lower leg: are clinical findings predictive of the disorder? J Orthop Trauma 16:572–577, 2002.
16. McQueen MM, Christie J, Court-Brown CM: Acute compartment syndrome in tibial diaphyseal fractures. J Bone Joint Surg Br 78:95–98, 1996.
17. Hoppenfeld S: Physical examination of the spine and extremities, Upper Saddle River, NJ, 1976, Prentice Hall.
18. Teitz CC, Harrington RM: A biochemical analysis of the squeeze test for sprains of the syndesmotic ligaments of the ankle. Foot Ankle Int 19:489–492, 1998.
19. Zalavras CG, Thordarson D: Ankle syndesmotic injury. J Am Acad Orthop Surg 15:330–339, 2007.
20. Springer BA, Arciero RA, Tenuta JJ, et al: A prospective study of modified Ottawa ankle rules in a military population: interobserver agreement between physical therapists and orthopaedic surgeons. Am J Sports Med 28:864–868, 2000.
21. Davidovitch RI, Egol KA: Ankle fractures. In Bucholz RW, Heckman JD, Court-Brown C, et al, editors: Rockwood and Green's fractures in adults, ed 7, Philadelphia, 2010, Lippincott Williams & Wilkins, pp 1975–2021.
22. Vander Griend R, Michelson JD, Bone LB: Fractures of the ankle and the distal part of the tibia. Instr Course Lect 46:311–321, 1997.
23. Ostrum RF, De Meo P, Subramanian R: A critical analysis of the anterior-posterior radiographic anatomy of the ankle syndesmosis. Foot Ankle Int 16:128–131, 1995.
24. Jacobson JA, Andresen R, Jaovisidha S, et al: Detection of ankle effusions: comparison study in cadavers using radiography, sonography, and MR imaging. AJR Am J Roentgenol 170:1231–1238, 1998.
25. Schweitzer ME, van Leersum M, Ehrlich SS, et al: Fluid in normal and abnormal ankle joints: amount and distribution as seen on MR images. AJR Am J Roentgenol 162:111–114, 1994.
26. Schock HJ, Pinzur M, Manion L, et al: The use of gravity or manual-stress radiographs in the assessment of supination-external rotation fractures of the ankle. J Bone Joint Surg Br 89:1055–1059, 2007.
27. Yu KH, Luo SF, Liou LB, et al: Concomitant septic and gouty arthritis—an analysis of 30 cases. Rheumatology (Oxford) 42:1062–1066, 2003.
28. Saltzman CL, Tearse DS: Achilles tendon injuries. J Am Acad Orthop Surg 6:316–325, 1998.
29. White BJ, Walsh M, Egol KA, et al: Intra-articular block compared with conscious sedation for closed reduction of ankle

fracture-dislocations: a prospective randomized trial. J Bone Joint Surg Am 90:731–734, 2008.

30. Alioto RJ, Furia JP, Marquardt JD: Hematoma block for ankle fractures: a safe and efficacious technique for manipulations. J Orthop Trauma 9:113–116, 1995.

31. Saunders S, Longworth S, editors: Injection Techniques in Orthopaedics and Sports Medicine, ed 3, Oxford, UK, 2006, Blackwell, pp 122–134.

32. Garbuz DS, Masri BA, Esdaile J, et al: Classification systems in orthopaedics. J Am Acad Orthop Surg 10:290–297, 2002.

33. Horn BD, Rettig ME: Interobserver reliability in the Gustilo and Anderson classification of open fractures. J Orthop Trauma 7:357–360, 1993.

34. Olson SA, Schemitsch EH: Open fractures of the tibial shaft: an update. Instr Course Lect 52:623–631, 2003.

35. Zalavras CG, Patzakis MJ: Open fractures: evaluation and management. J Am Acad Orthop Surg 11:212–219, 2003.

36. Zalavras CG, Patzakis MJ, Holtom PD, et al: Management of open fractures. Infect Dis Clin North Am 19:915–929, 2005.

37. Quinn RH, Macias DJ: The management of open fractures. Wilderness Environ Med 17:41–48, 2006.

38. Tull F, Borrelli J, Jr: Soft-tissue injury associated with closed fractures: evaluation and management. J Am Acad Orthop Surg 11:431–438, 2003.

39. Gaston P, Will E, Elton RA, et al: Fractures of the tibia. Can their outcome be predicted? J Bone Joint Surg Br 81:71–76, 1999.

40. Brodell JD, Axon DL, Evarts CM: The Robert Jones bandage. J Bone Joint Surg Br 68:776–779, 1986.

41. Barei DP, Nork S: Fractures of the tibial plafond. Foot Ankle Clin N Am 13:571–591, 2008.

42. Chowdhry M, Porter K: The pilon fracture. Trauma 12:89–103, 2010.

43. Borrelli J, Ellis E: Pilon fractures: assessment and treatment. Orthop Clin North Am 33:231–245, 2002.

44. Germann CA, Perron AD, Sweeney TW, et al: Orthopedic pitfalls in the ED: tibial plafond fractures. Am J Emerg Med 23:357–362, 2005.

45. Barrett JA, Baron JA, Karagas MR, et al: Fracture risk in the U.S. Medicare population. J Clin Epidemiol 52:243–249, 1999.

46. Michelson JD: Ankle fractures resulting from rotational injuries. J Am Acad Orthop Surg 11:403–412, 2003.

47. Alexandropoulos C, Tsourvakas S, Papachristos J, et al: Ankle fracture classification: an evaluation of three classification systems: Lauge-Hansen, A.O. and Broos-Bisschop. Acta Orthop Belg 76:521–525, 2010.

48. Lauge-Hansen N: Fractures of the ankle. II. Combined experimental-surgical and experimental-roentgenologic investigations. Arch Surg 60:957–985, 1950.

49. Quigley TB: A simple aid to the reduction of abduction-external rotation fractures of the ankle. Am J Surg 97:488–493, 1959.

50. Anderson RB, Hunt KJ, McCormick JJ: Management of common sports-related injuries about the foot and ankle. J Am Acad Orthop Surg 18:546–556, 2010.

51. Maffulli N, Ferran NA: Management of acute and chronic ankle instability. J Am Acad Orthop Surg 16:608–615, 2008.

52. Hintermann B, Knupp M, Pagenstert GI: Deltoid ligament injuries: diagnosis and management. Foot Ankle Clin 11:625–637, 2006.

53. Philbin TM, Landis GS, Smith B: Peroneal tendon injuries. J Am Acad Orthop Surg 17:306–317, 2009.

54. Edwards M: The relations of the peroneal tendons to the fibula, calcaneus and cuboideum. Am J Anat 42:213–253, 1988.

55. Eckert WR, Davis EA Jr: Acute rupture of the peroneal retinaculum. J Bone Joint Surg Am 58:670–672, 1976.

56. Sammarco GJ: Peroneus longus tendon tears: acute and chronic. Foot Ankle Int 16:245–253, 1995.

57. Slater HK: Acute peroneal tendon tears. Foot Ankle Clin 12:659–674, 2007.

58. Arrowsmith SR, Fleming LL, Allman FL: Traumatic dislocations of the peroneal tendons. Am J Sports Med 11:142–146, 1983.

59. McGarvey WC, Clanton TO: Peroneal tendon dislocations. Foot Ankle Clin 1:325–342, 1996.

60. Ogawa BK, Thordarson DB: Current concepts review: peroneal tendon subluxation and dislocation. Foot Ankle Int 28:1034–1040, 2007.

61. Carr AJ, Norris SH: The blood supply of the calcaneal tendon. J Bone Joint Surg Br 71:100–101, 1989.

62. Maffulli N, Wong J: Rupture of the Achilles and patellar tendons. Clin Sports Med 22:761–776, 2003.

63. Schepsis AA, Jones H, Haas AL: Achilles tendon disorders in athletes. Am J Sports Med 30:287–305, 2002.

64. Haddow LJ, Chandra Sekhar M, Hajela V, et al: Spontaneous Achilles tendon rupture in patients treated with levofloxacin. J Antimicrob Chemother 51:747–748, 2003.

65. Haines JF: Bilateral rupture of the Achilles tendon in patients on steroid therapy. Ann Rheum Dis 42:652–654, 1983.

66. Ureten K, Oztürk MA, Ozbek M, et al: Spontaneous and simultaneous rupture of both Achilles tendons and pathological fracture of the femur neck in a patient receiving long-term hemodialysis. Int Urol Nephrol 40:1103–1106, 2008.

67. Chiodo CP, Glazebrook M, Bluman EM, et al; American Academy of Orthopaedic Surgeons: Diagnosis and treatment of acute Achilles tendon rupture. J Am Acad Orthop Surg 18:503–510, 2010.

68. Dixon JB: Gastrocnemius vs. soleus strain: how to differentiate and deal with calf muscle injuries. Curr Rev Musculoskelet Med 2:74–77, 2009.

69. Aronow MS: Commentary on an article by Kevin Willits, MA, MD, FRCSC, et al: Operative versus nonoperative treatment of acute Achilles tendon ruptures: a multicenter randomized trial using accelerated functional rehabilitation. J Bone Joint Surg Am 92:e321–e322, 2010.

70. Willits K, Amendola A, Bryant D, et al: Operative versus nonoperative treatment of acute Achilles tendon ruptures: a multicenter randomized trial using accelerated functional rehabilitation. J Bone Joint Surg Am 92:2767–2775, 2010.

71. Kwak HS, Lee KB, Han YM: Ruptures of the medial head of the gastrocnemius ("tennis leg"): clinical outcome and compression effect. Clin Imaging 30:48–53, 2006.

72. Thordarson DB, Ahlmann E, Shepherd LE, et al: Sepsis and osteomyelitis about the ankle joint. Foot Ankle Clin 5:913–928, 2000.

73. Shams F, Asnis D, Lombardi C, et al: A report of two cases of tuberculous arthritis of the ankle. J Foot Ankle Surg 48:452–456, 2009.

74. Waguri-Nagaya Y, Kobayashi M, Goto H, et al: Septic arthritis of the right ankle caused by *Staphylococcus aureus* infection in a rheumatoid arthritis patient treated with etanercept. Mod Rheumatol 17:338–340, 2007.

Krause JO, Brodsky JW: Peroneus brevis tendon tears: pathophysiology, surgical reconstruction, and clinical results. Foot Ankle Int 19:271–279, 1998.

Templeman DC, Marder RA: Injuries of the knee associated with fractures of the tibial shaft: detection by examination under anesthesia: a prospective study. J Bone Joint Surg Am 71:1392–1395, 1989.

# Chapter 16 *Foot*

Lauren Geaney, Michael Aronow, and Benjamin H. Evenchik

## ANATOMIC CONSIDERATIONS

A strong foundation in the anatomy of the foot is important for appropriate diagnosis and treatment of foot disorders in the emergency department. A complete pictorial atlas of the foot is beyond the scope of this chapter. Nevertheless, appropriate knowledge of the bone (Figs. 16-1 through 16-4), joint (Fig. 16-5), and surface anatomy of the foot (Figs. 16-6 through 16-11), including the sensory nerve innervation areas (Fig. 16-12), is extremely beneficial with respect to appropriate clinical diagnosis, accurate reading of radiographic studies, and performance of procedures involving the foot.

## Bones

- Talus
  - Of the surface area of the talus, 70% is articular cartilage, rendering many fractures intra-articular.

    The medial and superior talar dome articulates with the medial malleolus and tibial plafond of the ankle.

    The lateral talar dome articulates with the lateral malleolus.

    The talar head articulates with the navicular and the anterior facet of the calcaneus.

    The posterior, middle, and anterior facets articulate at the subtalar joint with the posterior, middle, and anterior facets of the calcaneus.

  - The lateral process of the talus includes articulations with the distal fibula and the posterior facet of the calcaneus.
  - There are no tendon insertions to the talus.
  - The vascular supply to the talar neck and head comes from three major sources.

    The largest contributor is the posterior tibial artery, which supplies the artery of the tarsal canal.

    The artery of the tarsal sinus is supplied by perforating vessels of the peroneal artery.

    The dorsal portion of the talar neck is supplied by branches of the dorsalis pedis.

  - The vascular supply to the talar body is principally intraosseous from the talar neck and is very susceptible to injury.
  - The vascular supply also receives contributions to the medial talar dome through the deltoid ligament and posterolaterally through distal branches of the peroneal artery.
- Calcaneus
  - The calcaneus is an end-bearing bone and absorbs most of the axial load on the hindfoot.
  - The calcaneus articulates with the talus at the subtalar joint through its posterior, middle, and anterior facets.
  - The posterior and middle facets are separated by the tarsal canal and thick talocalcaneal interosseous ligament, whereas the anterior and middle facets are often contiguous.
  - The anterior process contains the anterior facet and the articulation with the cuboid at the calcaneocuboid joint.
  - Although the calcaneus does not have a true cartilage articulation with the navicular, occasionally a fibrous or bony tarsal coalition is present.
  - The calcaneal tuberosity contains the Achilles tendon insertion on its posterior-superior origin, and the plantar fascia origin is on its anterior-inferior aspect.
  - The plantar fat pad is attached inferiorly, and there is a thin layer of skin and subcutaneous tissue medially, laterally, and posteriorly.
  - The sustentaculum tali emerges from the medial wall, contains the middle facet, and has the flexor hallucis longus traveling inferior to it.
- Navicular
  - The navicular articulates proximally with the talus to form the talonavicular joint and distally with the three cuneiforms to form the naviculocuneiform joint.

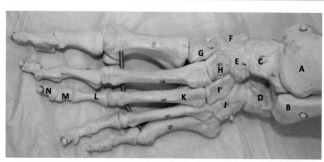

**FIGURE 16-1.** Anterior bone anatomy. Distal tibia *(A)*, lateral malleolus *(B)*, talar head *(C)*, anterior process of calcaneus *(D)*, navicular *(E)*, navicular tuberosity *(F)*, medial cuneiform *(G)*, intermediate cuneiform *(H)*, lateral cuneiform *(I)*, cuboid *(J)*, third metatarsal *(K)*, third proximal phalanx *(L)*, third middle phalanx *(M)*, and third distal phalanx *(N)*.

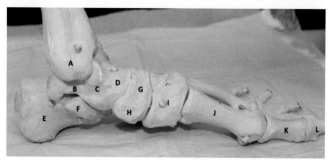

**FIGURE 16-2.** Medial bone anatomy. Medial malleolus *(A)*, talar body *(B)*, talar neck *(C)*, talar head *(D)*, calcaneal tuberosity *(E)*, sustentaculum tali *(F)*, navicular *(G)*, navicular tuberosity *(H)*, medial cuneiform *(I)*, first metatarsal *(J)*, hallux proximal phalanx *(K)*, and hallux distal phalanx *(L)*.

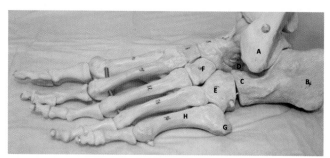

**FIGURE 16-3.** Lateral bone anatomy. Lateral malleolus *(A)*, calcaneal tuberosity *(B)*, anterior process of calcaneus *(C)*, sinus tarsi *(D)*, cuboid *(E)*, lateral cuneiform *(F)*, fifth metatarsal base *(G)*, and fifth metatarsal *(H)*.

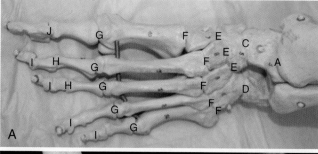

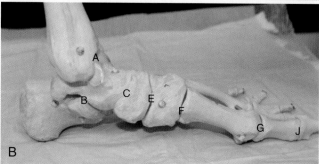

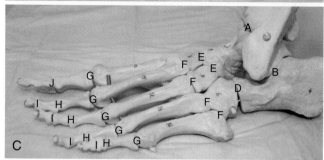

**FIGURE 16-5.** Anterior **(A)**, medial **(B)**, and lateral **(C)** joint anatomy. Ankle joint *(A)*, subtalar joint *(B)*, talonavicular joint *(C)*, calcaneocuboid joint *(D)*, naviculocuneiform joint *(E)*, tarsometatarsal joints *(F)*, metatarsophalangeal joints *(G)*, proximal interphalangeal joints *(H)*, distal interphalangeal joints *(I)*, and hallux interphalangeal joint *(J)*.

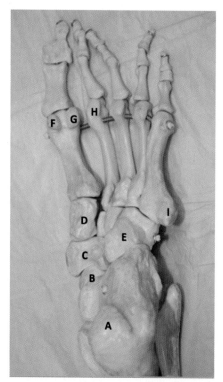

**FIGURE 16-4.** Plantar bone anatomy. Calcaneal tuberosity *(A)*, talar head *(B)*, navicular *(C)*, medial cuneiform *(D)*, cuboid *(E)*, medial (tibial) sesamoid *(F)*, lateral (fibular) sesamoid *(G)*, second metatarsal head *(H)*, and base of fifth metatarsal *(I)*.

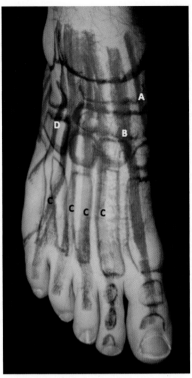

**FIGURE 16-6.** Anterior anatomy. Anterior tibial tendon *(A)*, extensor hallucis longus tendon *(B)*, extensor digitorum longus tendons *(C)*, and peroneus tertius tendon *(D)*.

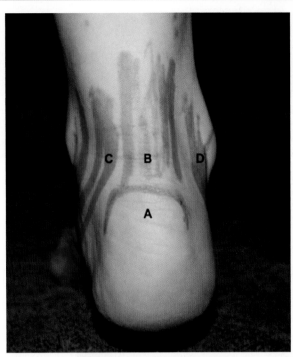

**FIGURE 16-9.** Posterior anatomy. Calcaneal tuberosity *(A)*, Achilles tendon *(B)*, flexor hallucis longus tendon *(C)*, and peroneus longus and peroneus brevis tendons *(D)*.

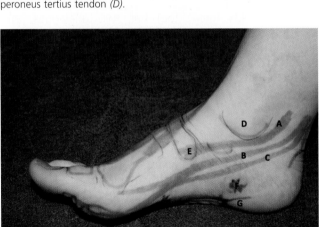

**FIGURE 16-7.** Medial anatomy. Posterior tibial tendon *(A)*, flexor digitorum longus tendon *(B)*, flexor hallucis longus tendon *(C)*, medial malleolus *(D)*, navicular tuberosity *(E)*, first branch of lateral plantar nerve *(F)*, and posteromedial origin of plantar fascia *(G)*.

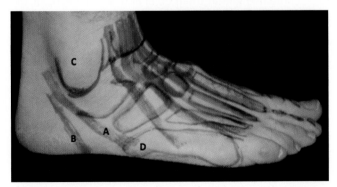

**FIGURE 16-8.** Lateral anatomy. Peroneus brevis *(A)*, peroneus longus *(B)*, lateral malleolus *(C)*, and fifth metatarsal base *(D)*.

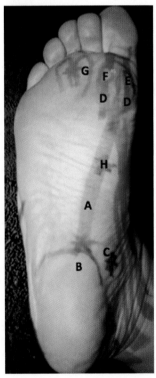

**FIGURE 16-10.** Plantar anatomy. Medial cord of plantar fascia *(A)*, posteromedial origin of plantar fascia from medial calcaneal tuberosity *(B)*, first branch of lateral plantar nerve *(C)*, flexor digitorum brevis (medial and lateral heads) *(D)*, medial (tibial) sesamoid *(E)*, lateral (fibular) sesamoid *(F)*, second metatarsal head *(G)*, and plantar medial cuneiform–second metatarsal base articulation (location of plantar ecchymosis sign in Lisfranc injury) *(H)*.

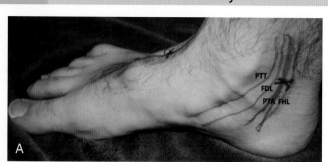

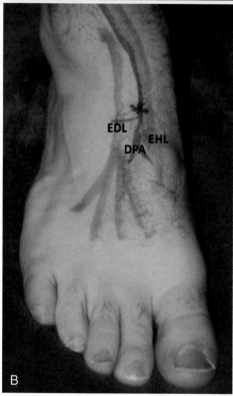

**FIGURE 16-11.** Vascular anatomy. **A,** The posterior tibial pulse is found behind the medial malleolus between the flexor digitorum longus (*FDL*) and flexor hallucis longus (*FHL*) tendons. **B,** The dorsalis pedis pulse is found between the extensor hallucis longus (*EHL*) and extensor digitorum longus (*EDL*) tendons at the level of the navicular. *DPA,* Dorsalis pedis artery; *PTA,* posterior tibial artery; *PTT,* posterior tibial tendon.

- The blood supply to the navicular is structured in a radial manner, rendering the central aspect susceptible to avascular necrosis and stress fracture.
- Shortening of the medial column of the foot through loss of navicular length may lead to a higher arched, cavus foot.
- ◼ Cuboid
  - The cuboid articulates proximally with the calcaneus to form the calcaneocuboid joint and distally with the fourth and fifth metatarsals to form the fourth and fifth tarsometatarsal (TMT) joints.
  - Shortening of the lateral column of the foot through loss of cuboid length may lead to a more planovalgus flatfoot deformity.
- ◼ Medial, Intermediate, and Lateral Cuneiforms
  - The cuneiforms articulate proximally with the navicular to form the naviculocuneiform joint and distally

with the first, second, and third metatarsals to form the first, second, and third TMT joints.
  - The cuneiforms also articulate with each other and the cuboid to form the relatively immobile intercuneiform joints.
- ◼ Metatarsals
  - The metatarsal bases articulate proximally with the cuneiforms and cuboid to form the TMT joints and the metatarsal heads distally with the proximal phalangeal bases to form the first through fifth metatarsophalangeal (MTP) joints.
  - The second through fifth metatarsals are connected by proximal and distal transverse metatarsal ligaments.
  - The interosseous Lisfranc ligament connects the second metatarsal to the medial cuneiform, and the deep transverse metatarsal ligament runs between the second metatarsal neck and the lateral sesamoid.
  - There are no ligamentous connections between the first and second metatarsals, which may lead to the development of hallux valgus bunion deformities.
  - The first metatarsal usually contributes most to weight bearing and balance.
  - There is a watershed area of vascular supply at the proximal metadiaphyseal-diaphyseal junction of the fifth metatarsal, making fractures more susceptible to nonunion.
- ◼ Phalanges
  - The hallux (great toe) has two phalanges, and the second through fifth toes usually have three phalanges.
  - The proximal phalangeal bases articulate with the metatarsal heads to form the MTP joints.
  - The hallux proximal phalangeal head articulates with the distal phalangeal base to form the interphalangeal joint.
  - The second through fifth proximal phalangeal heads articulate with the middle phalangeal bases to form the proximal interphalangeal joints.
  - The second through fifth middle phalangeal heads articulate with the distal phalangeal bases to form the distal interphalangeal joints.
  - Tendon imbalance and ligamentous laxity across the MTP and interphalangeal joints can lead to deformity, including hallux valgus, hammer toes, and mallet toes.
- ◼ Sesamoid Bones
  - The medial (tibial) and lateral (fibular) sesamoids are contained within the medial and lateral heads of the flexor hallucis brevis muscle, and the flexor hallucis longus tendon runs between the two sesamoids.
  - The sesamoids articulate with the first metatarsal head as part of the first MTP joint.
  - The sesamoids are weight-bearing bones and may develop pathology including fracture, avascular necrosis, and sesamoiditis from overuse.

### *Joints*

- ◼ Ankle Joint
  - The ankle joint provides approximately 70% of the dorsiflexion and plantar flexion motion of the foot relative to the leg.

- Previous treatment may reduce pain, including recent reduction of fractures and dislocations, suturing of lacerations, and administration of narcotics and other medications.
- The character, location, timing, duration, progression, and exacerbating or relieving factors of the pain are important to elicit and aid in diagnosis.

  Is the pain sharp, dull, burning, or pressure-like?

  Is the pain global or over a specific tendon, bone, joint, or nerve distribution?

  Is the pain present when the patient first gets out of bed as is commonly noted with plantar fasciitis, near the end of the day, at night, or all the time?

  Is the pain acute and progressively getting worse, which may be seen in a compartment syndrome or infection, or is it chronic and stable?

  Is the pain made worse by walking on uneven ground or concrete, wearing certain types of shoes versus going barefoot, or with motion of specific joints?

  Is the pain made better by anti-inflammatory medication, orthotics, or elevation?

- **Dysfunction**
  - The important functional things that a patient cannot do, can do only to a limited degree, or will not do secondary to discomfort or fear must be sorted out.

    After the injury, was the patient able to bear weight, either unassisted or with support?

    Is the patient able to walk or run without a limp?

    Are there activities that the patient can no longer do or do well secondary to foot pathology, and if so, is this due to pain, weakness, instability, loss of balance, loss of endurance, or other factors?

    Are there certain shoes that the patient can no longer wear because of pain or deformity?

- **Prehospital Care**
  - The nature, severity, and treatment urgency of the injury and the vascular status of the foot should be assessed.
  - In patients with open fractures, gross contamination may be removed from the wounds.
  - If the clinician has appropriate knowledge and experience, restoration of the normal anatomic position for nonopen fractures and dislocations may be attempted. In particular, restoration of anatomic position should be attempted if significant vascular compromise, tented skin at risk of becoming an open fracture, or significant patient discomfort exists.

    The threshold for action depends partly on expected time to evaluation in the emergency department.

    Contaminated open wounds ideally should undergo surgical débridement before reduction of fractures and joint dislocations.

- Patients should be splinted for comfort.
- In a patient with intact vascular status, elevation, compression, and ice can reduce swelling.
- Any amputated or extruded tissue should be transported with the patient to the emergency department. Ideally, amputated parts should be kept cool and be wrapped in moist gauze in a plastic bag.
- The patient should be kept from eating or drinking if there is a possibility that semiemergent surgery may be considered or required.

- **Physical Examination**
  - Inspection

    Assess both feet for obvious deformities.

    - Compare the symptomatic foot with the contralateral foot for asymmetry.
    - Assess the foot weight bearing if not contraindicated and the patient is able to stand on it.
    - Weight bearing accentuates deformities, including deformity secondary to bunions, hammer toes, Charcot arthropathy, posterior tibial tendon dysfunction, and Lisfranc ligament injuries.

      Any open traumatic wounds, chronic ulcers, or breaks in the skin should be noted and sterilely probed to assess whether they communicate with a fracture site, intact bone, joint, or tendon.

      Small wounds may be associated with open fractures including over the medial calcaneus.

      Look for any tenting of the skin, particularly posteriorly with tongue-type calcaneal fractures and talar fracture-dislocations.

      Edema and ecchymosis are usually present in the area of the injury.

      Fracture blisters may occur in high-energy injuries associated with significant swelling, although sometimes the manifestation of fracture blisters is delayed.

  - Palpation

    Assess for tenderness or defects over commonly injured fracture sites, tendons, joints, and ligaments, particularly in areas where the patient complains of pain.

  - Range of motion

    Assess for any limitation of active or passive joint range of motion or associated discomfort, particularly of the more mobile ankle, subtalar, talonavicular, calcaneocuboid, fourth and fifth TMT, MTP, and interphalangeal joints.

    Use stress testing to assess for abnormal increased joint range of motion secondary to ligament rupture.

    Assess for weakness secondary to muscle or tendon injury.

  - Vascular examination

    Assess the dorsalis pedis and posterior tibial pulses.

    A Doppler examination should be performed if pulses are nonpalpable.

Ankle-brachial index may be used to quantitate vascular status.

Cyanosis, loss of hair, and pallor may indicate vascular injury or chronic arterial insufficiency.

- Neurologic examination

Sensation to light touch, pinprick, or two-point discrimination should be assessed for all five sensory nerves to the foot and distal to any lacerations.

Sensation to a Semmes-Weinstein 5.07 monofilament or to vibration may be used to assess for neuropathy.

A Tinel sign may be present over nerves irritated secondary to compression, stretch, or direct injury.

Motor function should be assessed.

- Diagnostic Testing
  - Plain radiographs

Anteroposterior, lateral, and oblique views of the foot are the standard views obtained (Fig. 16-13).

These x-rays should be taken with the patient weight bearing with the knee straight and ankle dorsiflexed unless contraindicated secondary to obvious displaced foot fractures or dislocations, significant pain, or other concurrent extremity or body injuries.

Non–weight bearing x-rays often underestimate the extent of chronic foot deformity, the amount of joint space narrowing in ankle and subtalar arthritis, and the presence of latent ligamentous instability in Lisfranc ligament injuries and Charcot deformity.

Anteroposterior, lateral, and mortise ankle x-rays are helpful in diagnosing fractures of the talus including fractures of the lateral and medial processes; fractures of the body, neck, and head; and osteochondral fractures of the talar dome.

Avulsion fractures off the calcaneus and cuboid are sometimes also seen on the anteroposterior or mortise view.

A weight-bearing Cobey (Fig. 16-14) view is helpful in evaluating patients with varus or valgus deformities of the hindfoot because it shows the angle between the axis of the tibia and the axis of the calcaneus.

A Canale view (Fig. 16-15) is helpful in assessing the talar neck for fracture. This view is obtained with the foot in maximum plantar flexion and pronated 15 degrees and aiming the beam 75 degrees cephalad.

A Broden view (Fig. 16-16) shows alignment of the posterior facets of the subtalar joint and may be helpful in evaluating subtalar arthritis and intra-articular fractures of the calcaneus and lateral process of the talus. This view is obtained with the foot resting in neutral dorsiflexion on the

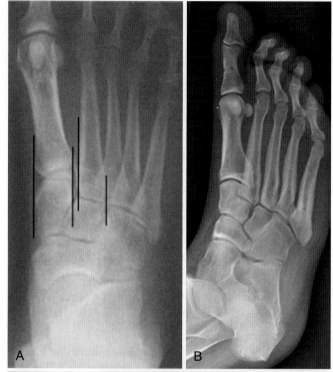

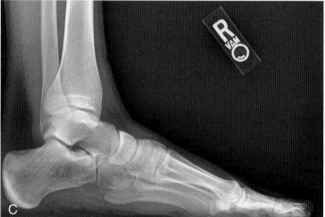

**FIGURE 16-13.** Anteroposterior **(A)**, 30-degree oblique **(B)**, and lateral **(C)** x-ray views of a normal foot. On the anteroposterior view, the lateral first metatarsal aligns with the lateral border of the medial cuneiform, and the medial second metatarsal aligns with medial border of the middle cuneiform. On the 30-degree oblique view, the medial border of the fourth metatarsal aligns with the medial border of the cuboid. The third metatarsal aligns with the lateral cuneiform. The TMT joints can be seen better on the anteroposterior and oblique films if the angle of the beam is modified such that it is parallel to the TMT joint surfaces.

cassette with the foot internally rotated 45 degrees. Films are obtained with 10 degrees, 20 degrees, 30 degrees, or 40 degrees of cephalic tilt.

A Harris axial view (Fig. 16-17) is helpful in evaluating calcaneal fractures for varus, lateral, and superior displacement of the tuberosity and posterior facet congruity. It also is helpful in diagnosing isolated tuberosity or sustentaculum tali fractures.

Sesamoid and metatarsal head views (Fig. 16-18) are taken parallel to the plantar aspect of the

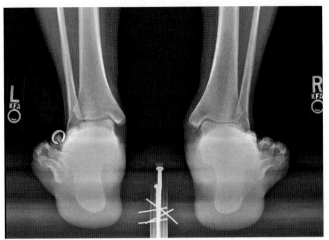

**FIGURE 16-14.** Cobey view. This weight-bearing view is also helpful in evaluating patients with varus or valgus deformities of the hindfoot because it shows the angle between the axis of the tibia and the axis of the calcaneus.

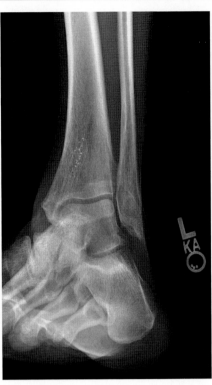

**FIGURE 16-16.** Broden view. This view is obtained with the foot resting in neutral dorsiflexion on the cassette with the foot internally rotated 45 degrees and the beam aimed with 10 degrees, 20 degrees, 30 degrees, or 40 degrees of cephalic tilt. This view shows the posterior facet of the subtalar joint and is useful to assess for subtalar arthritis or intra-articular displacement in calcaneal fractures.

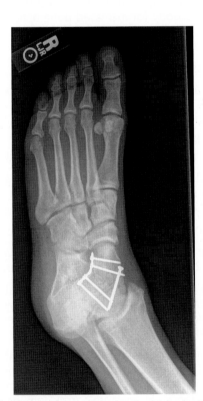

**FIGURE 16-15.** Canale view. This view is obtained with the foot in maximum plantar flexion and pronated 15 degrees and aiming the beam 75 degrees cephalad. This view allows assessment of the talar neck angulation after a fracture.

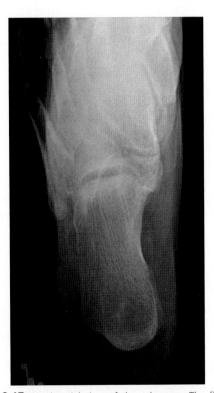

**FIGURE 16-17.** Harris axial view of the calcaneus. The film is taken with the plantar foot placed on the cassette and the beam angled 45 degrees toward the midline on the heel. This view is useful in assessing subtalar arthritis and tuberosity displacement in calcaneal fractures.

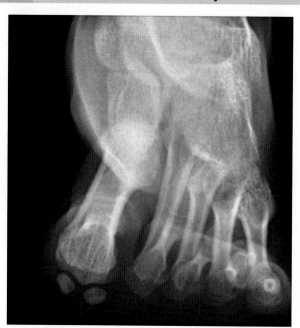

**FIGURE 16-18.** Metatarsal head view. This view is taken parallel to the plantar aspect of the metatarsal heads with the toes dorsiflexed. A sesamoid view is a similar radiograph centered on the first metatarsal sesamoid articulation.

metatarsal heads and sesamoids with the toes dorsiflexed.

These views are helpful in diagnosing sesamoid fractures or avascular necrosis, metatarsosesamoid arthritis, the extent of first MTP joint malalignment in hallux valgus, and dorsal and plantar position of the metatarsal heads in patients with metatarsalgia or metatarsal fractures.

- Computed tomography (CT)

  CT scans provide better three-dimensional bone and to a lesser extent soft tissue visualization than plain radiographs but with increased patient radiation exposure and cost.

  CT is helpful for diagnosing subtle fractures including stress fractures and intra-articular fragments not seen on plain x-rays and tarsal coalitions.

  CT scan, usually as part of outpatient clinic follow-up, is considered when there is a high clinical suspicion for fractures that may require treatment but have negative plain x-rays.

  CT scan may also aid in clinical decision making with respect to the need for surgery and intraoperative planning by showing size and displacement of intra-articular and extra-articular fracture fragments and the extent of preexisting arthritis.

  CT scans may show subtle static subluxation of joints including the TMT joints but if obtained in standard fashion may miss latent subluxation that occurs only with weight bearing or stress testing.

- Magnetic resonance imaging (MRI)

  MRI can also be helpful in diagnosing subtle fractures, including stress fractures, and static joint subluxation.

  Although less optimal than CT scan with respect to bone definition, MRI requires significantly less patient radiation exposure than CT scan and is preferable for assessing bone edema, cartilage abnormalities, tendon and ligament injury, soft tissue masses, infections, and tumors.

- Ultrasound

  Ultrasound is user-dependent but is helpful is assessing tendon and soft tissue pathology such as Morton neuromas.

  Ultrasound can be used dynamically to assess specific anatomic structures of the foot for direct tenderness or specific tendons for subluxation or triggering with provocative maneuvers.

- Bone scan

  Bone scan may be helpful in assessing a larger area of the body for increased bone activity but often cannot differentiate between fracture, osteomyelitis, arthritis, and other abnormalities.

- Joint aspiration

  Joint aspiration is performed to rule out a septic joint or inflammatory process such as gout or pseudogout.

  Joint fluid should be sent for culture, cell count, Gram stain, glucose, protein, and crystal analysis.

  Aspiration can be performed by knowledge of clinical anatomy or under fluoroscopy, CT, or ultrasound guidance.

- Joint injection

  Joint injections with local anesthetic have traditionally been performed for diagnostic purposes.

  Transient relief of symptoms suggests that arthritis or mechanical impingement in the joint injected is the source of the patient's discomfort, whereas lack of relief suggests a different etiology.

  Disruption of adhesions or decreased inflammation with concurrent corticosteroid injection may also be therapeutic, although there is some evidence that the local anesthetic may damage the chondrocytes responsible for maintaining the articular cartilage.

  Leakage of fluid or methylene blue dye from a traumatic wound after injection into the joint from a different site suggests that there is an open joint injury that might benefit from surgical irrigation.

- Compartment pressure

  Compartment pressure should be measured when clinical suspicion exists for a foot compartment syndrome.

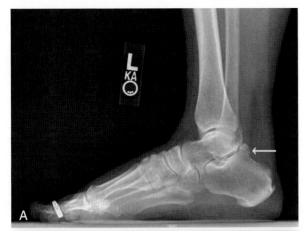

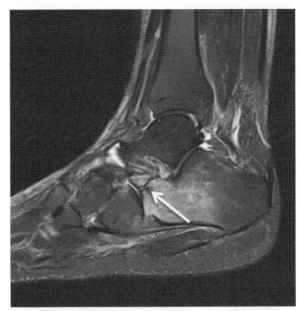

**FIGURE 16-22.** MRI showing fracture of the anterior process of the calcaneus.

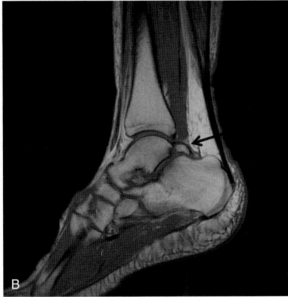

**FIGURE 16-21.** Os trigonum. **A,** Lateral x-ray view. **B,** MRI.

to the body of the talus by a stable fibrous synchondrosis instead of being one contiguous bone.
- A normal os trigonum usually has a nondisplaced smooth border at the talar body junction, as opposed to the more irregular border and often increased displacement seen with fractures.
- Pain is usually increased with full plantar flexion of the ankle, and tenderness is present over the posterolateral talus.

These fractures are treated with cast immobilization; surgical excision is reserved for chronically symptomatic fractures.

- If the patient is symptomatic and a fracture or disrupted os trigonum synchondrosis cannot be ruled out by available radiographic studies, it is preferable to immobilize the injury in a well-padded short leg splint with specialist follow-up within 1 week.
- Medial process of the talus fractures may need to be differentiated from medial malleolar avulsion fractures.

Unless large and displaced, these fractures are usually initially treated with a brace or splint, with surgical excision reserved for the rare chronically symptomatic ones.

- Common Pitfalls
  - Fractures of the lateral process and posterior tubercle are often missed on plain radiographs.
  - Fracture-dislocations must be adequately reduced in a timely fashion to minimize soft tissue necrosis.

## Calcaneus Fractures
- General Considerations
  - Fractures of the calcaneus commonly seen in the emergency department include fractures of the body (either extra-articular or with intra-articular involvement of the subtalar or calcaneocuboid joints), anterior process, sustentaculum tali, and calcaneal tuberosity.
  - Fractures of the anterior process of the calcaneus (Fig. 16-22) can occur after dorsiflexion and eversion of the foot causes compression between the cuboid and the talus or after inversion of the plantar-flexed ankle results in an avulsion injury from the bifurcate ligament.
  - Tuberosity fractures can occur on the plantar aspect as a result of direct trauma on the heel or at the posterosuperior aspect as a result of an avulsion fracture at the Achilles tendon insertion (Fig. 16-23).
  - The mechanism of injury for calcaneal body fractures is usually an axial load, often secondary to a fall from a height or a motor vehicle collision, where the lateral process of the talus is driven into the floor of the sinus tarsi.
    - There are usually four main fracture fragments, which may often have additional fracture fragments within them.

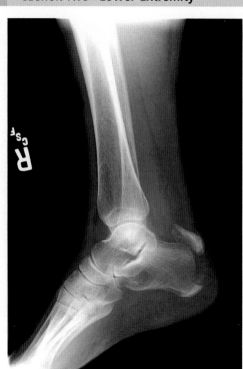

**FIGURE 16-23.** Avulsion fracture of the calcaneal tuberosity including the Achilles tendon insertion.

The primary fracture line runs from the anterolateral calcaneus at the level of the inferior aspect of the sinus tarsi and extends posteromedially through the medial calcaneal wall.

The posterior fragment is divided further into a posterolateral tongue or joint depression fragment, which involves the lateral aspect of the posterior facet of the subtalar joint and the tuberosity fragment.

- The tuberosity fragment usually is displaced superiorly, anteriorly, laterally, and into varus.

The anterior fragment is usually divided into a constant sustentaculum tali fragment and the anterior process fragment.

- The sustentaculum tali fragment usually contains the anteromedial portion of the posterior facet of the subtalar joint and the posterior portion of the middle facet and is usually nondisplaced owing to its attachment to the interosseous talocalcaneal ligament.
- The anterior process fragment may have additional fracture lines involving the calcaneocuboid joint.
- On examination, there is often extensive soft tissue swelling and ecchymosis.

With displaced intra-articular calcaneal body fractures, the calcaneus is often shortened and widened, similar to a crushed soda can.

- The posterior heel often appears wide when viewed in the prone position, and the lateral calcaneal wall may be prominent such that when the

examiner's thumb is placed against it instead of resting underneath the lateral malleolus, the thumb is lateral to the malleolus.
- This calcaneal widening may also be associated with peroneal tendon dislocation from the fibular groove and sural neurapraxia.

With anterior process fractures, tenderness is noted over the dorsal aspect of the anterior process at the anterior border of the sinus tarsi.

With sustentaculum tali fractures, tenderness is noted over the sustentaculum tali, which is a palpable prominence a couple centimeters inferior and slightly anterior to the tip of the medial malleolus.

- Standard radiographs obtained include anteroposterior, lateral, Harris axial, and Broden views of the foot.

The anteroposterior view may show intra-articular extension and displacement of the calcaneocuboid joint and widening of the lateral calcaneal wall in body fractures (Fig. 16-24A).

The Harris axial view shows the primary fracture line of a calcaneal body fracture exiting the medial calcaneal wall and the lateral and superior displacement of the tuberosity fragment (Fig. 16-24B). It would also show a displaced sustentaculum tali fracture.

The lateral view may show a fracture in the dorsal aspect of the anterior process involving the calcaneocuboid joint in an anterior process fracture.

- In a displaced intra-articular body fracture, there may be dorsal subluxation of the entire anterior process of the calcaneus relative to the cuboid, loss of Bohler angle, and visible displacement of the subchondral bone of the posterolateral fragment.
  - *Bohler angle* is the angle between a line extending from the dorsal aspect of the anterior calcaneus to the posterior facet and another line from the posterior facet to the dorsal aspect of the posterior calcaneal tuberosity (Fig. 16-24C). A normal angle is between 140 degrees and 160 degrees, and this angle becomes closer to a straight line as the posterior facet articular surface depresses and the calcaneal tuberosity displaces proximally.
  - The subchondral bone of the posterior facet of the calcaneus is normally parallel to the subchondral bone of the posterior facet of the talus. As the posterolateral fragment rotates anteriorly and inferiorly, the subchondral joint line also rotates anteriorly and inferiorly so that the anterior aspect is no longer parallel to the posterior facet of the talus (Fig. 16-25).

A Broden view shows stepoff of the posterior facet of the calcaneus.

- CT scan is helpful for diagnosing subtle fractures and for surgical decision making in intra-articular

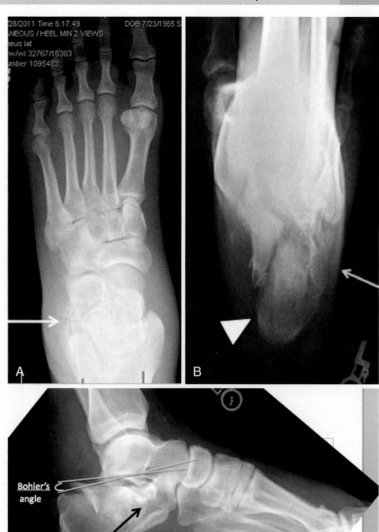

**FIGURE 16-24. A,** Anteroposterior view of joint depression fracture of the calcaneus with disruption of the calcaneocuboid joint and lateral calcaneal wall blow-out *(arrow).* **B,** Axial view of joint depression fracture. Note widening of the lateral calcaneal wall *(arrow)* with lateral and proximal displacement of the tuberosity fragment *(arrowhead)* relative to the sustentaculum tali fragment. **C,** Lateral view of a joint depression fracture of the calcaneus showing loss of Bohler angle and depression of the lateral joint posterior facet fragment *(arrow* is on articular surface of depressed posterior facet fragment).

fractures by showing the extent and displacement of the fracture fragments.

■ Fracture Classifications
  ● Essex-Lopresti classification

  In a tongue-type fracture, the posterolateral fragment exits through the posterior tuberosity (Fig. 16-26).

  In a joint depression–type fracture, the posterolateral fragment exits through the superior aspect of the calcaneal tuberosity (see Fig. 16-24).

  ● Sanders classification (Fig. 16-27):

  The fracture is classified based on coronal plane CT scan images and the number and location of the fracture fragments involving the posterior facet of the calcaneus that are at least 2 mm displaced.

  ● Type I—nondisplaced fracture
  ● Type II—two-part fracture with one fracture line
  ● Type III—three-part fracture with two fracture lines
  ● Type IV—four-part or more fracture

The fracture is subclassified further by whether the posterior facet fracture lines are medial (A), central (B), or lateral (C).

■ Treatment
  ● Minimally displaced fractures with less than 2 mm displacement are treated nonoperatively with cast or boot immobilization and limited weight bearing.
  ● Patients with anterior process fractures with intra-articular fragments that are displaced and involve greater than 1 cm of the joint may benefit from ORIF. Otherwise, patients are generally treated with cast immobilization for approximately 6 weeks with delayed ORIF or excision reserved for symptomatic nonunions.
  ● The treatment of displaced intra-articular body fractures is controversial.

  Barring significant surgical complications, patients who undergo ORIF by a surgeon capable of performing a near-anatomic reduction on average do better than patients treated nonoperatively.

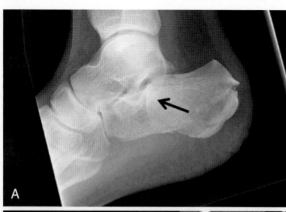

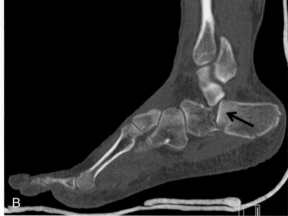

**FIGURE 16-25.** Tongue-type fracture of the calcaneus with depressed tongue fragment including lateral posterior facet *(arrow)*. **A,** Lateral x-ray view. **B,** CT sagittal reconstruction.

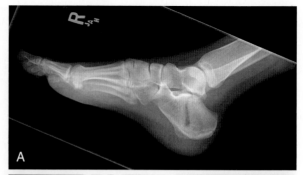

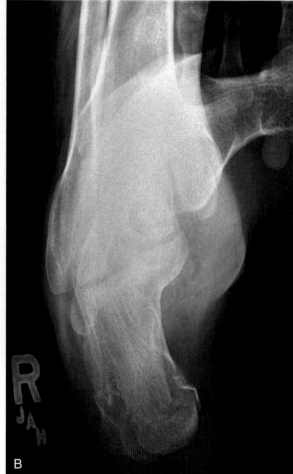

**FIGURE 16-26.** Tongue-type fracture of the calcaneus. **A,** Lateral x-ray view. **B,** Axial view. The varus deformity is better appreciated by looking at the tibiocalcaneal angle between the axes of the tibia and the calcaneal tuberosity.

Some patients develop significant wound problems and infections after surgery and may still develop malunion or post-traumatic subtalar or calcaneocuboid arthritis secondary to significant chondrocyte and cartilage damage from the initial injury despite the quality of the reduction obtained by the surgeon.

Some patients do well despite significant residual articular and extra-articular displacement after nonoperative treatment.

Patients with diabetes, peripheral vascular disease, or significant tobacco use may be candidates for nonoperative or limited percutaneous surgical treatment because of a significantly increased risk of surgical complications.

- If nonoperative treatment is chosen, the patient is kept non–weight bearing for 6 to 10 weeks and then begun on early hindfoot range of motion exercises to limit the expected subsequent subtalar joint stiffness.
- The timing of surgery depends on the amount of soft tissue swelling and the presence of fracture blisters. Although surgery ideally would be performed early before the fracture fragments begin to heal in their malreduced positions, the risk of wound problems and infections is significantly increased until swelling

reduces to the point that the skin is wrinkling and fracture blisters have healed.
- Semiurgent reduction is usually required if there is a large posteriorly displaced tongue fracture or tuberosity avulsion fracture impinging on the skin overlying the Achilles tendon insertion that may cause skin necrosis.
- The specialist should be notified while the patient is in the emergency department to confirm whether or not to obtain a CT scan for further clinical decision

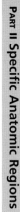

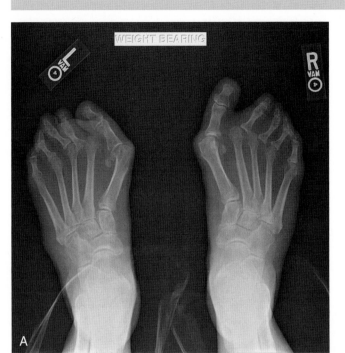

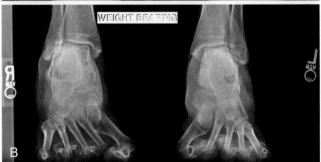

**FIGURE 16-44.** Chronic dislocations of the right second and third and left second MTP joints in a patient with rheumatoid arthritis. Bilateral hallux valgus (bunions) is also present. Anteroposterior **(A)** and metatarsal head **(B)** x-ray views.

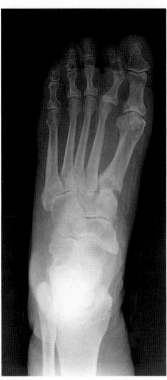

**FIGURE 16-45.** Anteroposterior view of an acute dislocation of the second MTP joint.

such as erosions or cystic changes of the proximal phalangeal base or metatarsal head.

There may also be signs of chronic lesser metatarsal overload such as a short first metatarsal, a long second and third metatarsal, or significant cortical diaphyseal thickening of the affected lesser metatarsals.

■ Treatment
  • Acute lesser MTP joint dislocations require semi-urgent reduction similar to first MTP joint dislocations.

    An initial attempt at closed reduction should be made with longitudinal traction manually or with the use of finger traps, exaggeration of the usual hyperdorsiflexion deformity, and then correction of the deformity usually with plantar flexion.

    If reduction is confirmed by repeat foot x-rays, and the MTP joint is stable on examination, the patient is placed into a hard-soled shoe with a stiff fore-foot rocker.

    Irreducible or unstable lesser MTP joint dislocations often have an interposed plantar plate and require open reduction and occasional Kirschner wire fixation.

  • Chronic lesser MTP joint dislocations are not reducible by closed means.

    Initial treatment consists of accommodative shoe wear and orthotic offloading of symptomatic metatarsalgia.

    Surgical treatment includes open capsular release with a stable reduction usually also requiring shortening of the corresponding metatarsal and often tendon balancing across the MTP joint.

## Metatarsophalangeal Synovitis, Instability, and Interdigital Neuritis

■ General Considerations
  • MTP synovitis is inflammation that occurs in the lesser MTP joints, most commonly the second followed by the third, fourth, and fifth MTP joints, usually secondary to biomechanical overload or inflammatory arthropathies.
  • MTP synovitis may be associated with or lead to MTP instability, in which tearing or attenuation of the plantar plate or collateral ligaments may cause pain, joint laxity, and deformity.
  • An acute traumatic hyperdorsiflexion injury can injure the plantar plate, and overuse such as a sudden

increase in running can lead to synovitis within the MTP joint.

- Biomechanical factors that increase weight-bearing stress on the metatarsal head that may lead to metatarsalgia, MTP synovitis, or MTP instability include a relatively long or plantar-flexed second or third metatarsal relative to the first metatarsal, hypermobility of the first TMT joint, triceps surae contractures (Achilles tendon or isolated gastrocnemius contractures), and significant hammer toe, which leads to distal migration of the plantar fat pad that cushions the metatarsal head.
- Pain is located in the area of the affected MTP joint.
- In MTP synovitis, there is usually tenderness underneath the plantar base of the proximal phalanx where the plantar plate inserts and underneath and over the MTP joint.
- By contrast, in isolated metatarsalgia, there is usually a tender callus underneath the affected metatarsal head without associated swelling or instability.
- There is usually swelling of the affected MTP joint, and deformity and instability may be present.
- Medial or lateral angulation of the affected toe may develop with asymmetric splaying between the affected toe and adjacent one, most commonly between the second and third toes.

    There can be progressive dorsiflexion, dorsal subluxation, medial or lateral angulation, and hammering of the affected toe that may progress to the point that the hammer toe may cross over the adjacent toe or dorsally dislocate.

    Most commonly, the second toe crosses over the hallux, which may have a hallux valgus bunion deformity.

- In MTP synovitis without MTP instability, an attempted Lachman test (Fig. 16-46) produces pain but not abnormal motion of the proximal phalanx relative to the metatarsal head.
- In the presence of MTP instability, dorsal stress to the proximal phalanx causes abnormal, usually painful dorsal subluxation of the proximal phalanx relative to the corresponding metatarsal head.
- Significant swelling of the MTP joint can compress or irritate the adjacent interdigital nerve and cause symptoms of interdigital neuritis similar to a Morton neuroma.

    In Morton neuroma, the plantar interdigital nerve is compressed underneath the deep transverse metatarsal ligament and may cause pain and paresthesias radiating into the adjacent web space and toes, most commonly the third and then second web space.

    Compared with patients with isolated MTP synovitis, who often note benefit with cushioned shoe wear, patients with Morton neuroma often complain of pain related to tight shoe wear that is relieved by shoe removal and sometimes by walking barefoot.

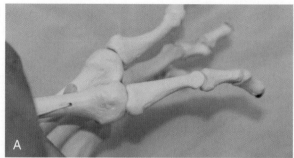
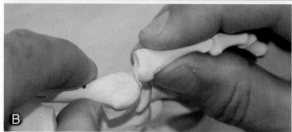

**FIGURE 16-46.** Lachman test of the second MTP joint. **A,** Normal relationship. **B,** With the thumb and index finger of one hand stabilizing the metatarsal head, the thumb and index finger of the other hand attempt to sublux the proximal phalangeal base dorsally to test for instability of the plantar plate.

Although patients with MTP synovitis tend to have maximum tenderness over the MTP joint that is aggravated by an attempted Lachman test, patients with Morton neuroma have maximum tenderness over the interdigital web space at the level of the metatarsal neck and head that is aggravated by squeezing the metatarsal heads together from medial to lateral and may demonstrate a Mulder click, in which a painful snapping sensation is noted when the adjacent metatarsal heads are moved dorsally and laterally relative to each other.

- Standard anteroposterior, lateral, oblique, and metatarsal head weight-bearing views of the foot should be obtained.

    Assess for MTP subluxation, angulation, or arthritis; relative metatarsal length on anteroposterior and oblique views; and plantar position of the lesser metatarsal heads and sesamoids relative to each other on lateral and metatarsal head views.

■ Treatment
- Initial treatment is nonoperative and involves stabilizing the affected MTP joint; unloading the affected metatarsal head; and decreasing inflammation to decrease pain, improve function, and limit further deformity.

    The affected MTP joint can be taped for stability (Fig. 16-47).

- Half-inch tape is placed along the plantar aspect of the metatarsal shaft, through the web space over the dorsal proximal phalanx and back through the adjacent web space, and then back proximal along the plantar metatarsal crossing over the

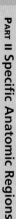

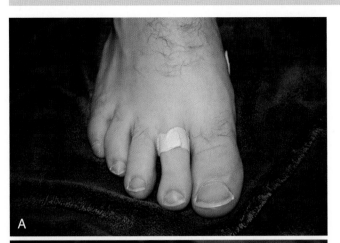

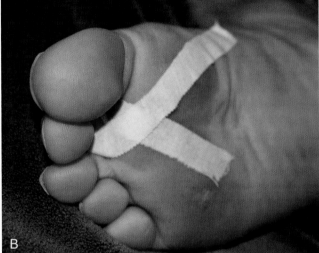

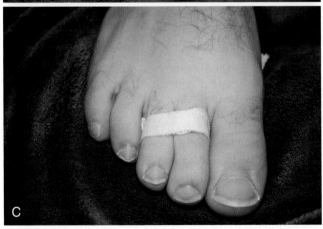

**FIGURE 16-47.** Taping technique for MTP subluxation. **A** and **B,** A piece of ½ -inch tape is placed over the unstable dorsal proximal phalanx **(A)** and crossed on the plantar surface to resist dorsal translation **(B)**. **C,** The toe is buddy taped to the neighboring toe for additional stability.

Although splints and taping can hold the toe in a more normal position, decrease pain, and limit the development of further deformity, the deformity cannot be corrected with nonoperative treatment.

A shoe with a stiff forefoot rocker is recommended to limit the dorsal translation force to the proximal phalanx that occurs during gait with push-off and a dorsiflexed MTP joint.

A cushioned insole with a metatarsal pad or bar proximal to the affected metatarsal head biomechanically offloads the metatarsal head and decreases inflammation in the affected MTP joint, as does gastrocnemius and Achilles tendon stretching exercises.

- Systemic anti-inflammatory medications can decrease inflammation in the MTP joint and periostitis underneath the metatarsal head.
- Although a corticosteroid injection into the affected MTP joint can decrease pain and inflammation, it can also increase attenuation of the plantar plate and increase the associated deformity.

If an injection is performed, the affected toe should be protected with taping and a shoe with a stiff forefoot rocker for at least 1 to 2 months afterward.

- In patients refractory to conservative treatment, surgical options include biomechanically offloading the affected metatarsal with a metatarsal osteotomy or gastrocnemius lengthening, stabilizing the MTP joint with a plantar plate repair or tendon transfer such as the FDL to the base of the proximal phalanx, and correcting toe deformity.
- Interdigital neuritis or Morton neuroma is initially treated with wide accommodative shoes, anti-inflammatory medications, and corticosteroid or alcohol injections.

Orthoses or metatarsal pads are sometimes helpful in decreasing the inflammation surrounding the interdigital nerve, but they may also irritate it further by crowding the foot within the shoe or putting pressure directly on the neuroma.

If conservative treatment is unsuccessful, surgical decompression of the nerve by releasing the deep transverse metatarsal ligament over it or excision of a Morton neuroma if present may be performed.

■ Common Pitfalls
- Failure to recognize early MTP synovitis may lead to progressive toe deformity that cannot be corrected without surgical intervention.

initially placed tape at the level of the metatarsal head.
- A second piece of tape is used to buddy tape the proximal phalanx to the proximal phalanx of the adjacent toe.

Over-the-counter splints such as a Budin splint also can stabilize the toe.

# Gout
■ General Considerations
- Gout is a systemic disorder in which there is overproduction, underexcretion, or both, of uric acid.

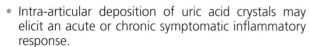

- Intra-articular deposition of uric acid crystals may elicit an acute or chronic symptomatic inflammatory response.
- Tophi, subcutaneous lumps that may drain chalky white material and may or may not be symptomatic, may also develop.
- Patients often present with severe pain, erythema, and swelling of the affected joints, which often feel warm to the touch.

   The MTP joint of the great toe is affected in 75% of patients.

- Acute gout attacks may be associated with many things, including stress, alcohol intake, medications such as diuretics and cyclosporine, and foods such as sardines and red meat.
- The differential diagnosis includes pseudogout caused by calcium pyrophosphate crystal deposition and septic arthritis.
- The diagnosis is made by fluid analysis after aspiration.

   Uric acid crystals are negatively birefringent on microscopic examination under polarizing light, whereas calcium pyrophosphate crystals have positive birefringence.

   Cell count, Gram stain, and culture are performed to assess for infection.

- There is often, but not always, an elevated serum uric acid.
- Plain radiographs may show soft tissue swelling, a lacy pattern of subcortical bone erosion, or periarticular bone erosions.

■ Treatment
- Treatment is primarily medical to decrease inflammation, decrease uric acid formation, and increase uric acid excretion.

   In the acute phase, nonsteroidal anti-inflammatory drugs such as indomethacin, ibuprofen, or colchicine are often effective.

   If these medications are ineffective, a specialist may prescribe other medications including corticosteroids, and in some patients with chronic symptoms, medications such as allopurinol or probenecid may be prescribed to reduce uric acid levels and decrease the likelihood of future attacks.

- In the absence of infection, corticosteroid injection may be beneficial in decreasing symptoms if oral medication is ineffective.
- Food, beverages, medications, and activities that increase uric acid levels should be avoided.
- The affected joint should be rested.
- In the case of the first MTP joint, an accommodative shoe with a stiff rocker sole may be sufficient.
- For significant symptoms involving the hindfoot and midfoot joints, a cam walker boot may be helpful.
- Surgical treatment is reserved for a concurrent septic joint or chronic symptoms secondary to gout-associated arthritis, deformity, or tophi.

## Puncture Wounds

■ General Considerations
- Patients may present to the emergency department acutely at the time of injury or at a delayed time secondary to subsequent related infection or discomfort related to a retained foreign body.

   A reaction to a retained foreign body may occur, which often manifests as a tender granuloma that may have associated drainage.

   Infection can range from local cellulitis to deep abscess or osteomyelitis.

   Staphylococcal infections are the most common pathogen, although *Pseudomonas* infection commonly develops in patients after a nail puncture through a sneaker sole.

- X-rays are often negative, particularly in cases of wood splinters or other radiolucent foreign bodies.

   MRI or ultrasound may be helpful in these cases

■ Treatment
- When patients present acutely, tetanus status should be addressed, the wound should be irrigated, and an attempt should be made to determine if a residual foreign body is present and, if so, remove it.

   If a foreign body is identified but is too deep to be safely removed in the emergency department, a specialist should be consulted to determine if and when it needs to be surgically removed.

- If infection is present, antibiotics that provide adequate *Staphylococcus* and *Pseudomonas* coverage should be given after appropriate cultures have been taken.
- Deep abscess or osteomyelitis is treated by semiurgent surgical débridement and intravenous antibiotics after deep cultures have been taken.
- Chronic granulomas can be removed by surgical excision if symptomatic.

## Compartment Syndrome of the Foot

■ General Considerations
- Acute compartment syndrome of the foot is underdiagnosed and should be suspected whenever there is significant foot trauma, especially crush injuries, calcaneal fractures, multiple forefoot fractures, and Lisfranc injuries, or when there is prolonged arterial ischemia.
- More chronic exercise-induced compartment syndromes can also occur with activity, most commonly in the medial compartment of the foot ("jogger's foot").
- As noted in the anatomy section earlier, there are nine compartments in the foot: medial, lateral, superficial, calcaneal (which communicates with the deep posterior compartment of the leg), adductor, and four interosseous compartments.

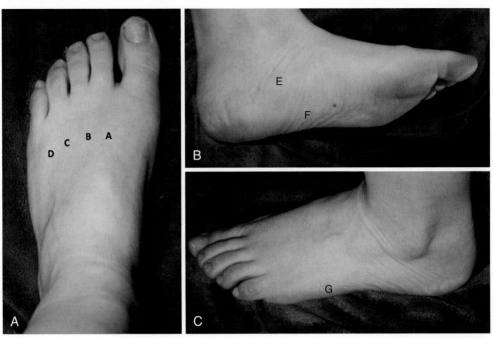

**FIGURE 16-48.** Location of foot compartment pressure measurement. *A-D,* The pressure in the four interosseous compartments is measured by inserting the measuring needle from a dorsal approach in each of the four intermetatarsal spaces. The adductor compartment (*A* and *B*) may be accessed by inserting the needle more plantarly through the first or second intermetatarsal space. *E,* The medial compartment is measured 4 cm inferior to the medial malleolus and 6 cm anterior to the posterior heel over the abductor hallucis, and the calcaneal compartment is measured by advancing the needle further laterally. *F,* The superficial compartment pressure is measured in the midplantar arch with the needle placed through the plantar fascia over the FDB. *G,* The lateral compartment is measured by placing the needle directly plantar to the fifth metatarsal over the abductor digiti minimi.

- Patients often present with significant swelling of the foot, pain out of proportion to the injury, loss of two-point discrimination, and, in particular, pain with passive dorsiflexion stretch of the toes at the MTP joints.
- Although all nine compartments may be involved, there are also situations in which only some of the compartments have elevated pressures.

  In some Lisfranc injuries, only the adductor and interosseous compartments may be elevated, whereas in some calcaneal fractures only the calcaneal or other hindfoot compartments may be elevated.

- Similar to compartment syndromes of the leg, compartment syndromes of the foot can occur in the presence of open fractures.
- Because of the significant potential morbidity of an untreated compartment syndrome of the foot, compartment pressures should be measured whenever clinical suspicion is present (Fig. 16-48).

  The pressure in the four interosseous compartments is measured by inserting the measuring needle from a dorsal approach in each of the four intermetatarsal spaces.

  The adductor compartment may be accessed by inserting the needle more plantarly through the first or second intermetatarsal space.

  The medial compartment is typically measured over the abductor hallucis 4 cm inferior to the medial malleolus and 6 cm anterior to the posterior heel,

and the calcaneal compartment is measured by advancing the needle further laterally.

The lateral compartment pressure is measured just plantar to the fifth metatarsal over the abductor digiti minimi.

The superficial compartment pressure is measured in the midplantar arch with the measuring needle placed through the plantar fascia over the FDB.

Compartment pressure measurements that are less than 30 mm Hg below diastolic blood pressure or greater than 30 mm Hg are considered diagnostic for acute compartment syndrome.

- Treatment
  - Patients with compartment syndrome of the foot are semiemergently taken to the operating room for fasciotomies.
  - The safest and the most reliable way to release all nine compartments is through a three-incision approach (Fig. 16-49).

    A medial hindfoot incision is used to release the medial, lateral, superficial, and calcaneal compartments.

  - The incision is along the abductor hallucis, and the superficial fascia is released.
  - Plantar retraction of the abductor hallucis muscle exposes the deep fascia over the calcaneal compartment, which also decompresses the medial plantar nerve, lateral plantar nerve, and first branch of the lateral plantar nerve.

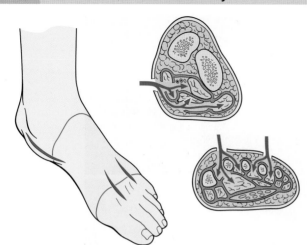

**FIGURE 16-49.** Location of the nine compartments of the foot and the two dorsal and one medial incision used to perform fasciotomies of them. The medial incision allows sequential release of the medial, calcaneal, superficial, and lateral compartments. The dorsal incisions allow release of the four interosseous compartments and the adductor compartment, which is deep to the first and second interosseous compartments. *(From Browner BD, Jupiter JB, Levine AM, et al, editors: Skeletal trauma: basic science, management, and reconstruction, ed 4, Philadelphia, 2008, Saunders, p. 2725.)*

- The abductor hallucis muscle is retracted dorsally exposing the medial fascia of the superficial compartment, which is released.
- The FDB muscle is also retracted plantarly, and staying well superficial to the quadratus plantae to avoid the medial and lateral plantar nerves and vessels, the medial fascia of the lateral compartment is identified and released.

Two dorsal incisions are made over the medial aspect of the second and lateral aspect of the fourth metatarsals.

- From the second metatarsal incision, the fascia over the first dorsal interosseous muscle in the first intermetatarsal space is released, and then the fascia over the second dorsal interosseous and first plantar interosseous muscle is released in the second intermetatarsal space.
- Dissection is carried more plantarly in the first or second intermetatarsal space, and the fascia over the adductor hallucis muscle is released.
- From the fourth metatarsal incision, the third intermetatarsal space is used to access the fascia overlying the third dorsal and second plantar interosseous muscles, and the fourth intermetatarsal space is used to access the fascia overlying the fourth dorsal and third plantar interosseous muscles.
- The dorsal incisions may also be used to perform ORIF of associated Lisfranc injuries and metatarsal fractures.
- Although all nine compartments can be released through one extended medial incision, the release of the adductor and interosseous compartments is done bluntly, and there is increased risk of damaging the neurovascular structures.

- Wounds are usually left open initially, and delayed closure occurs when swelling has improved, although immediate covering of the dorsal incisions with a split-thickness skin graft has been described.
- ■ Common Pitfalls
  - Lack of diagnosis and appropriate treatment of foot compartment syndromes can lead to painful, nonfunctional claw toe deformities, an increased cavus foot, and sensory abnormalities of the plantar aspect of the foot.

## *Soft Tissue Disorders*

### Plantar Fasciitis
- ■ General Considerations
  - Plantar fasciitis is the most common cause of plantar heel pain.
  - Inflammation and microtearing occurs in the plantar fascia, which can be secondary to an acute traumatic injury such as stepping on a pebble or repetitive trauma such as working on hard surfaces in poorly cushioned shoes.
  - More commonly, it is due to recurrent biomechanical strain on the plantar fascia, which may be secondary to a contracted plantar fascia in a cavus foot, gastrocnemius or Achilles tendon contracture, excess body weight, or overuse.
  - Patients complain of pain in the plantar heel that is often most pronounced with the first few steps after getting out of bed or after prolonged sitting and may be exacerbated with increased weight-bearing activity.
  - Tenderness is most commonly noted at the posteromedial origin of the plantar fascia at the medial tubercle of the calcaneus, but it may also occur at the central or lateral origin or along the medial aspect in the midfoot.

    Fully dorsiflexing the first MTP joint increases tension in the plantar fascia, which may be painful but also facilitates palpating the plantar fascia and locating the posteromedial origin.

  - Another common cause of heel pain that often occurs in conjunction with plantar fasciitis is compression of the first branch of the lateral plantar calcaneal nerve under the deep fascia of the abductor hallucis.

    Compared with plantar fasciitis, the pain may be more burning in nature and more noticeable at night while in bed.

    Tenderness over the nerve is typically approximately 2 cm anterior and 1 cm dorsal to the posteromedial origin of the plantar fascia.

  - In patients presenting with the typical history and physical examination of plantar fasciitis, plain radiographs are usually unnecessary.

    Exceptions would be patients with a history of acute trauma to the heel or tenderness over the

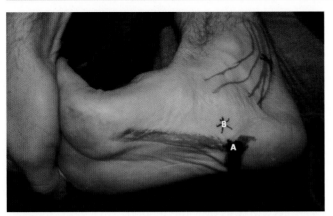

**FIGURE 16-50.** Plantar fasciitis stretch. The stretch is performed by simultaneously dorsiflexing the ankle and first MTP joint. The medial cord of plantar fascia *(green)* becomes taut during the stretch. *A,* The posteromedial origin of the plantar fascia is the most common location for point tenderness in plantar fasciitis. *B,* If there is compression of the first branch of the plantar nerve underneath the deep fascia of the abductor hallucis, point tenderness is usually 1 to 2 cm more anterior and dorsal.

calcaneal body as opposed to the plantar fascia origin where there is suspicion that a calcaneal fracture, stress fracture, or, less likely, tumor may be present. Another exception would be a patient with chronic symptoms that have been nonresponsive to initial treatment.

Although a heel spur may be noted anterior to the inferior aspect of the calcaneal tuberosity in many patients with plantar fasciitis, it is usually not the cause of the patient's pain except in the uncommon situations in which it is fractured or directed plantarly as opposed to anteriorly.

■ Treatment
- Initial treatment for plantar fasciitis is nonoperative consisting of gastrocnemius and plantar fascia stretching exercises (Fig. 16-50) that should be performed at least three times a day including before getting out of bed in the morning and after prolonged sitting, wearing shoes with a cushioned heel with possible addition of a gel heel cup or soft orthotic insert, and rest from high-impact activity.
- Icing of the heel and nonsteroidal anti-inflammatory drugs may also be considered.
- If the aforementioned treatments are ineffective, second-line conservative options include night splints, a corticosteroid injection into the posteromedial origin of the plantar fascia, and immobilization in a cast with a footplate that extends distal to the toes.

## Posterior Tibial Tendon Dysfunction
■ General Considerations
- Posterior tibial tendon dysfunction includes tenosynovitis, tendinopathy, and rupture of the posterior tibial tendon. Although it may lead to the development of asymmetric flatfoot deformity, more often than not there was a preexisting flatfoot deformity that may or may not be increased.

Tenosynovitis is typically secondary to an overuse phenomenon in athletes or may manifest in patients was systemic inflammatory disorders including rheumatoid arthritis.

Rupture may occur with significant eversion force on the hindfoot or with normal activity in a patient with preexisting tendinopathy.

- Patients with posterior tibial tendon dysfunction usually initially complain of medial ankle pain that is worse with activity and weight bearing.

If there is an associated flatfoot deformity these patients may later complain of lateral hindfoot pain secondary to inflammation or impingement in the sinus tarsi area.

- On examination, tenderness and swelling is usually present over all or part of the posterior tibial tendon, most commonly inferior to the medial malleolus.

There may be associated discomfort with and weakness of hindfoot inversion, which is tested with the ankle in plantar flexion to limit the contribution of the tibialis anterior.

With weight bearing, there may be loss of the longitudinal arch, increased hindfoot valgus, and abduction of the midfoot with a "too many toes" sign, in which an increased number of lateral toes can be seen when viewing the patient from behind (Fig. 16-51).

The patient may be unable to perform a single leg heel raise, or it may be painful or associated with lack of the normal recreation of the longitudinal arch and normal movement of the calcaneus into varus.

- Most of the time the diagnosis of posterior tibial tendon dysfunction can be made clinically, and radiographic studies can be deferred until the patient is evaluated by a specialist.
- In the presence of acute trauma or neuropathy, weight-bearing foot and ankle x-rays may show an avulsion fracture of the navicular, a displaced accessory navicular, a Charcot lateral subtalar dislocation, or a Lisfranc injury.
- MRI can show pathology of the posterior tibial tendon, injury to the spring ligament, or edema around the synchondrosis of a type II accessory navicular.

■ Treatment
- Initial treatment is conservative with biomechanical support, rest, and anti-inflammatory modalities including anti-inflammatory medication and ice.

Biomechanical support may range from an over-the-counter arch support or ankle brace in mild cases to immobilization in a splint or walking boot if there is acute significant discomfort, tenderness over an accessory navicular, or suspicion of an acute tendon tear or Charcot process.

- Additional treatment may be offered by a specialist including physical therapy, custom orthoses, injections, and surgery.

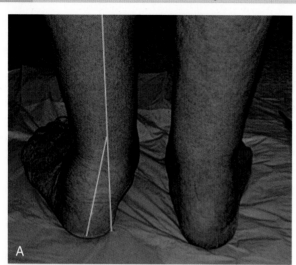

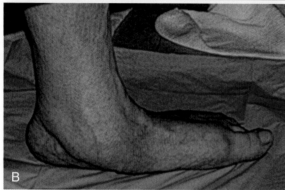

**FIGURE 16-51.** Clinical signs of posterior tibial tendon dysfunction. **A,** Posterior view showing too many toes sign of the left foot with increased valgus angulation of the calcaneus and abduction of the midfoot at the talonavicular joint. **B,** Medial view showing pes planovalgus with loss of the longitudinal arch.

## Flexor Hallucis Longus Tenosynovitis and Hallux Saltans ("Trigger Toe")

- General Considerations
  - FHL tenosynovitis most commonly occurs at the level of the medial calcaneus where the FHL's fibro-osseous sheath is located.
  - Less commonly, it occurs where the FDL tendon crosses superficial to the FHL at the master knot of Henry or where the FHL tendon runs between the medial and lateral sesamoids.
  - FHL tendinitis occurs commonly in ballet and other dancers and is sometimes referred to as "dancer's tendinitis."
  - There may be a partial tendon tear, tenosynovitis, or a nodule in the FHL tendon that causes pain as it passes through the tight fibro-osseous sheath.
  - Occasionally with plantar flexion of the first MTP joint and hallux interphalangeal joint, a nodule may get temporarily stuck at the proximal aspect of the fibro-osseous sheath resulting in a trigger toe.
  - Patients often complain of posteromedial ankle pain with activity and may give a history of triggering of the hallux.
  - On examination, the FHL tendon may have tenderness to palpation in the posteromedial ankle, which

may be increased with active resisted plantar flexion of the first MTP and interphalangeal joints or as the FHL tendon is passively placed through full range of motion from a foot position of full ankle plantar flexion, subtalar inversion, and first MTP and interphalangeal joint plantar flexion to a position of ankle dorsiflexion, subtalar eversion, and first MTP and interphalangeal joints extension.

Occasionally patients can demonstrate triggering of the hallux.

If there has been a recent partial rupture of the FHL tendon, there may be associated swelling and ecchymosis over the tendon.

- MRI may show FHL tendon tenosynovitis or tears along with other causes of posterior medial hindfoot pain including a symptomatic os trigonum, posterior ankle impingement, or retrocalcaneal bursitis, but normal ordering of this test to assess for FHL tenosynovitis should be deferred to a specialist.
- Treatment
  - Initial treatment consists of rest, limitation of FHL motion with a shoe with a stiff forefoot rocker or in more symptomatic cases a cam walker or posterior ankle splint, anti-inflammatory medication, and consideration of a corticosteroid injection into the FHL sheath, which can be more accurately done under ultrasound guidance.
  - Acute triggering of the toes usually eventually resolves, although it may be associated with some discomfort.
  - Recalcitrant FHL tenosynovitis or triggering of the hallux may require surgical release of the fibro-osseous sheath along with tenosynovectomy and tendon repair.

## *Diabetic Foot Disorders*

- General Considerations
  - Patients with diabetes mellitus may present to the emergency department with disorders of the foot including ulceration, infection, and Charcot arthropathy.
  - Charcot arthropathy is a disorder in which bone fragmentation and fracture or joint subluxation or dislocation may occur in patients with neuropathy.

    The bony changes are likely secondary to a combination of autonomically mediated hyperemia that leads to increased bone resorption and erosion and microfractures secondary to trauma in the presence of decreased proprioceptive feedback.

    These bony changes may lead to the disruption of the ligamentous attachments to bones causing joint instability.

    Diabetes mellitus is the most common cause of this associated neuropathy, but Charcot arthropathy may also occur in patients with rheumatoid arthritis, previous alcohol abuse, previous chemotherapy treatment, spinal disorders including syringomyelia, and idiopathic neuropathy.

The neuropathy may be significant or subtle, and some of these patients may not have a preexisting diagnosis of neuropathy or not realize that they have it.

- Although Charcot arthropathy may be minimally painful in some patients with neuropathy, it may be uncomfortable in other patients with neuropathy, although usually not to the same extent as in patients without neuropathy and with a similar acute fracture or dislocation.
- There is often, but not always, a history of previous injury, which can be a minor one such as an ankle sprain and may precede the onset of symptoms or physical findings up to a few weeks.
- Usually patients develop a warm, swollen, erythematous-appearing foot or ankle and may or may not initially present with deformity.

This appearance may lead to acute Charcot arthropathy being misdiagnosed as an acute infection, although sometimes the two disorders coexist, particularly because diabetes mellitus may be associated with changes in skin integrity, immune function, and vascular perfusion that increase the risk of infection developing and limit the body's ability to resolve it.

The deformity is most commonly noted within the midfoot followed by the hindfoot, ankle, and forefoot regions.

The presence of bony deformity increasing pressure on the skin and neuropathy may lead to concurrent ulceration.

- Other causes of neuropathic ulceration besides Charcot arthropathy include pressure from shoe wear on bony prominences such as bunions and hammer toes and increased weight-bearing forces on prominent metatarsal heads or sesamoids secondary to factors including anatomically long metatarsals, cavovarus feet increasing pressure over the sesamoids or fifth metatarsal head, and gastrocnemius or soleus contractures.
- Ulceration can also occur secondary to skin disruption from internal pressure buildup from a deep abscess or infection in the presence or absence of Charcot arthropathy.

The vascular status of the foot should be assessed as arterial insufficiency or significant venous stasis disease can negatively affect the patient's ability to fight infection and heal ulceration.

- In Charcot arthropathy, the foot is typically well perfused because the presence of significant arterial insufficiency limits the autonomically induced hyperemia thought to be necessary for Charcot arthropathy to develop.

The presence of significant neuropathy may be assessed by history or by decreased sensation to

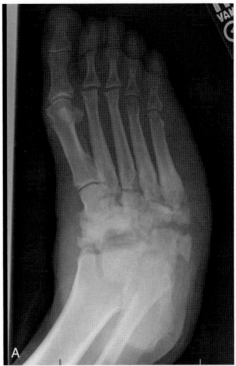

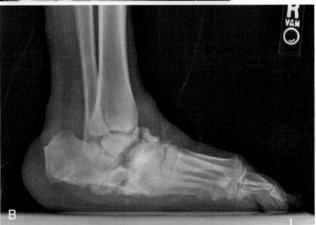

**FIGURE 16-52.** Charcot arthropathy of the hindfoot. Anteroposterior **(A)** and lateral **(B)** x-ray views.

light touch, vibration, or a Semmes-Weinstein 5.07 monofilament.

- Weight-bearing anteroposterior, lateral, oblique, and Cobey foot and ankle mortise x-rays should be obtained to assess for fracture, deformity, and joint subluxation. Charcot arthropathy may affect the ankle, the hindfoot (Fig. 16-52), the midfoot (Fig. 16-53), or less commonly the forefoot.
- MRI may show increased bone edema before plain x-ray changes are noted in acute Charcot arthropathy.
- MRI also shows bone fracture, fragmentation, deformity, and subluxation later in the Charcot process.

These findings may also be mistakenly thought to be diagnostic of osteomyelitis.

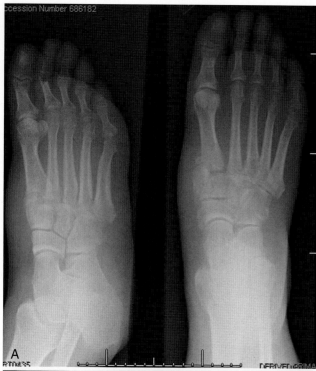

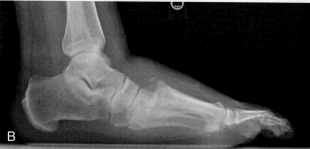

**FIGURE 16-53.** Charcot arthropathy of the midfoot. Anteroposterior **(A)** and oblique and lateral **(B)** x-ray views.

- The modified Eichenholz classification describes the radiographic and physical examination findings over the progression of the Charcot process.

    Stage 0—at the onset of Charcot arthropathy, there may be swelling, warmth, and erythema clinically and increased bone edema on MRI, but no bone deformity is noted on physical examination or plain x-rays

    Stage I (fragmentation)—clinically the foot is typically warm, swollen, erythematous, and deformed with x-rays showing osteopenia, bone fragmentation and dissolution, and joint subluxation or dislocation

    Stage II (coalescence)—clinically the edema and warmth begins to decrease, and the progression of bony deformity decreases

- X-rays show evidence of new bone formation.
- This stage typically does not begin until 3 to 9 months after the onset of the Charcot process.

    Stage III (consolidation)—clinically acute inflammation resolves, and deformity progression stops

- There is typically residual deformity and increased foot size secondary to the previous bone formation and soft tissue changes.
- Plain radiographs show residual deformity and evidence of fracture consolidation.

■ Treatment
- The presence of concurrent soft tissue infection or osteomyelitis may need to be ruled out.

    Systemic signs such as fever, recent-onset lack of glucose control, and elevated erythrocyte sedimentation rate or white blood cell count are suggestive of infection.

    Although hematogenous seeding occasionally may occur, the absence of foot ulceration or a recent history of a break in foot skin integrity argues against the presence of infection, particularly if radiographs show bony changes suggestive of an acute Charcot deformity.

    Elevation of the foot above the heart for several minutes typically leads to a decrease in the foot rubor associated with an acute Charcot foot but not of the erythema associated with cellulitis and infection.

    MRI and technetium-labeled bone scans are typically not helpful in distinguishing osteomyelitis from the bony changes seen in acute Charcot arthropathy, although MRI may show the presence of a soft tissue abscess.

    Indium-labeled white blood cell scan is typically positive in the presence of infection and negative in the presence of isolated Charcot arthropathy.

    Typically, a sulfur colloid scan is added to rule out a false-positive result secondary to appendicular marrow activation from chronic disease, although this is typically not seen in the bones of the foot.

- In the absence of infection or ulceration, initial treatment of Charcot arthropathy should involve making the patient non–weight bearing on the affected foot until he or she is evaluated by a specialist, preferably within a few days.

    Closed reduction of a neuropathic dislocation is difficult to maintain without internal or external fixation and should be deferred to a specialist.

    Although applying a compressive Jones cotton dressing or immobilizing the foot in a splint or cam walker to decrease edema and protect the foot from further injury can be considered, care needs to be taken to avoid excessive pressure on any bony prominences that may lead to ulceration.

    In patients without medical contraindications such as chronic renal disease, bisphosphonates such as alendronate may inhibit the increased osteoclast activity associated with Charcot arthropathy, potentially leading to decreased bone destruction

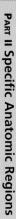

and a faster progression to Eichenholtz stage II and III.

Because of an increased risk of surgical complications including infection, wound problems, failure of fixation, and recurrent or progressive deformity with surgical intervention during Eichenholtz stage I, along with the fact that many resultant deformities can be effectively treated with orthoses, most patients with acute Charcot arthropathy are initially treated nonoperatively.

Nonoperative treatment consists of limited weight bearing or non–weight bearing and immobilization in a total contact cast or orthosis to limit further deformity, offload bony prominences to decrease the risk of ulceration, and decrease edema.

Potential indications for acute surgical intervention include deep infection, a reducible deformity in Eichenholtz stage 0 or early stage I, and a non-braceable deformity at significant risk for future ulceration and infection.

- Cellulitis and mild infections can often be treated with parenteral or intravenous antibiotics without surgical intervention.
- Significant deep infections with abscess formation, significant purulent drainage, or deep ulceration down to bone typically require semiurgent consultation with a specialist for surgical débridement.

    In the absence of significant septicemia, antibiotics should be withheld until the specialist evaluates the patient and determines whether more accurate deep intraoperative cultures should be obtained first.

    In the presence of significant septicemia, blood cultures and cultures of any purulent drainage or deep ulceration should be obtained ideally before empiric antibiotics are given.

- Noninfected ulcers that do not track down to bone are treated with offloading and referral to a specialist within a few days for additional offloading and wound care.
- Nonhealing ulcers may require surgery to decrease pressure on the ulcer by bone exostectomy, realignment of deformity, or tendon transfer or lengthening to redistribute weight-bearing forces.

    Gastrocnemius or Achilles tendon lengthening may be needed to offload forefoot or midfoot pressure ulcers, but this procedure should be avoided in calcaneal ulcers because it may increase heel weight-bearing pressures.

■ Common Pitfalls
- The clinician must have a high suspicion for Charcot arthropathy in patients with any degree of neuropathy to prevent or limit morbidity secondary to the development of additional deformity or ulceration or of an unnecessary surgical débridement for a misdiagnosis of osteomyelitis.

## Bibliography

Aronow MS: Joint preserving techniques for Lisfranc injury. Tech Orthop 26:43–49, 2011.

Banargee R, Nickisch F, Easley ME, et al: Foot Injuries. In Browner BD, Jupiter JB, Levine AM, et al, editors: Skeletal trauma: basic science, management, and reconstruction, ed 4, Philadelphia, 2008, Saunders.

Boack D, Manegold S: Peripheral talar fractures. Injury 35S:B23–BB35, 2004.

Buckely RE, Tough S: Displaced intra-articular calcaneal fractures. J Am Acad Orthop Surg 12:172–178, 2004.

Couglin MJ, Mann RA, Saltzman CL, editors: Surgery of the Foot and Ankle, ed 4, Philadelphia, 2007, Mosby.

De Clercq PFG, Bevernage BD, Leemrijse T: Stress fracture of the navicular bone. Acta Orthop Belg 74:725–734, 2008.

Digiovanni CW: Fractures of the navicular. Foot Ankle Clin N Am 9:25–63, 2004.

Boden BP, Osbahr DC: High-risk stress fractures: evaluation and treatment. J Am Acad Orthop Surg 8:344–353, 2008.

Early JS: Talar fracture management. Foot Ankle Clin N Am 13:635–657, 2008.

Essex-Lopresti P: The mechanism, reduction technique, and results in fractures of the os calcis. Br J Surg 39:395–519, 1952.

Manoli A: Compartment syndromes of the foot: current concepts. Foot Ankle 10:340–344, 1990.

Myerson MS, Fisher RT, Burgess AR, et al: Fracture dislocations of the tarsometatarsal joints: end results correlated with pathology and treatment. Foot Ankle 6:225–242, 1986.

Myerson MS, Cerrato RA: Current management of tarsometatarsal injuries in the athlete. J Bone Joint Surg 90:2522–2533, 2008.

Pinzur MS: Current concepts review: Charcot arthropathy of the foot and ankle. Foot Ankle Int 28:952–959, 2007.

Rammelt S, Zwipp H: Talar neck and body fractures. Injury 40:120–135, 2009.

Sanders DW: Fractures of the Talus. In Buckholz RW, editor: Rockwood and Green fractures in adults, ed 6, Philadelphia, 2006, Lippincott Williams & Williams, pp 2249–2292.

Sanders R: Intra-articular fractures of the calcaneus: present state of the art. J Orthop Trauma 6:252–265, 1992.

Sanders R: Displaced intra-articular fractures of the calcaneus. J Bone Joint Surg Am 82:225–250, 2000.

Sanders R, Clare MP: Fractures of the calcaneus. In Buckholz RW, editor: Rockwood and Green fractures in adults, ed 6, Philadelphia, 2006, Lippincott Williams & Williams, pp 2293–2336.

Sangeorzan BJ, Benirschke SK, Mosca V, et al: Displaced intra-articular fractures of the tarsal navicular. J Bone Joint Surg Am 71:1504–1510, 1989.

Swords MP, Schramski M, Sqitzer K, et al: Chopart fractures and dislocations. Foot Ankle Clin N Am 13:679–693, 2008.

Thompson MC, Mormino MA: Injury to the tarsometatarsal joint complex. J Am Acad Orthop Surg 11:260–267, 2003.

Van der Ven A, Chapman CB, Bowker JH: Charcot neuroarthropathy of the foot and ankle. J Am Acad Orthop Surg 17:562–571, 2009.

Chapter 17  # *Pelvis*

Bruce D. Browner, Michael Pensak, Alise Frallicciardi, and Andrew W. Ritting

## PELVIC RING INJURIES

### *Differential Diagnosis of Traumatic Complaints*

■ History

Disruption of the pelvic ring can be one of the most dangerous and life-threatening conditions encountered by emergency department physicians and orthopedic surgeons because of the potential for injury to the vital organs within the pelvis and the numerous nerves and vessels as they exit the torso and enter the lower extremities. It is essential for the responding provider to act in a calculated, yet prudent manner to stabilize the patient and prepare for definitive management. Despite advances in emergent care in pelvic trauma, mortality rates have been estimated to be 20% for unstable injuries and up to 50% for open fractures.[1,2] In a study by McMurtry et al. in 1980,[3] other musculoskeletal injuries and respiratory injury were the most commonly associated injuries with pelvic disruption, and gastrointestinal and major head injury had the highest mortality. If neurosurgery was required, mortality increased to 60%.

Two general populations of patients present to the emergency department with a pelvic injury: (1) individuals who have sustained high-energy trauma from motor vehicle accidents, falls, or crush injuries and (2) individuals who have sustained low-energy trauma resulting from simple falls. The second group commonly comprises elderly, osteoporotic individuals.[4]

The pelvic ring is composed of the pelvic bones (ischium, ilium, pubis) and the articulation with the posterior sacrum. The bony structures themselves have little inherent stability and rely on the ligamentous and soft tissue attachments to allow the pelvis to maintain its ringlike structure during activities of daily living. About 40% of ring stability arises from the anterior pubic symphysis and pubic rami, whereas the remaining 60% comes from the posterior sacroiliac

complex, including the anterior and posterior sacroiliac ligaments, the iliolumbar ligaments, and the pelvic floor (sacrospinous and sacrotuberous ligaments) (Fig. 17-1).

Another important consideration in pelvic fractures and pelvic disruption is the vast blood supply that exits the torso en route to the lower extremitites. The external iliac arteries exit anteriorly over the pelvic brim, and the internal iliac arteries course adjacent to the sacroiliac joint. These branch further into the superior gluteal artery, which exits the greater sciatic notch, and the lateral sacral, obturator, inferior gluteal, pudendal, vesical, umbilical, and hemorrhoidal arteries (Fig. 17-2). This massive blood supply is a major source for bleeding in polytrauma patients with pelvic disruption.

■ Mechanism of Injury

Owing to the ring shape of the pelvis, when there is disruption in one area of the ring, by definition, there must be disruption in another location of the ring. This concept is true even when apparent nondisplaced fractures through the pubic rami are present.[5] Complying with this rule, forces such as anteroposterior compression, lateral compression, vertical shearing, or any such combination, create fractures or ligamentous damage in more than one region of the pelvic ring. These forces have the potential to create instability and are the basis for the classification of pelvic ring fractures described by Young and Burgess (Fig. 17-3).[6] All vertical shear injuries are inherently unstable, whereas compression injuries have the potential for instability. The goal of this classification system is to allow the responder to provide appropriate counterforces to increase stability. Evaluation of the posterior displacement of the sacroiliac complex is a prognostic indicator for the general resuscitation of the patient.[7]

■ Timing

Pelvic ring injuries require urgent, and frequently emergent, evaluation, as outlined further on. The key to pelvic ring injuries is recognizing an unstable injury in an unstable patient and stabilizing the injury and patient in the fastest, most efficient manner possible.

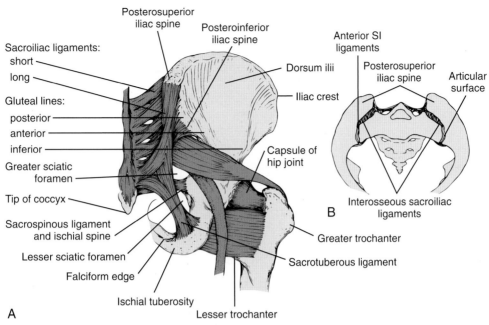

**FIGURE 17-1.** Ligamentous complexes of the pelvis. **A,** Posteriorly, the major ligaments in the region of the sacroiliac joint are the long and short posterior sacroiliac ligaments. The long ligaments blend with the sacrospinous and the sacrotuberous ligaments. **B,** In cross section, the orientation of the very thick posterior interosseous sacroiliac ligaments is noted. *(From Browner BD, Jupiter JB, Levine AM, et al, editors: Skeletal trauma: basic science, management, and reconstruction, ed 4, Philadelphia, 2008, Saunders.)*

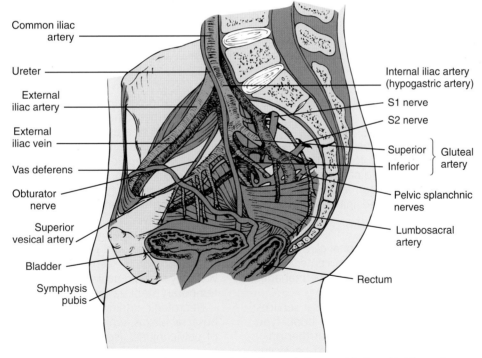

**FIGURE 17-2.** Internal aspect of the pelvis showing the great vessels, lumbosacral plexus, pelvic floor, bladder, and rectum. *(From Browner BD, Jupiter JB, Levine AM, et al, editors: Skeletal trauma: basic science, management, and reconstruction, ed 4, Philadelphia, 2008, Saunders.)*

■ Preexisting Illness
  • A full patient history is necessary to determine important medical and orthopedic comorbidities.
  • Medical comorbidities, such as cardiomyopathy, valvular disease, or arterial disease, may change resuscitation measures.
  • Orthopedic or surgical comorbidities, such as osteoporosis, bone disease, or metastatic disease to the bone, may require changes in the initial management of pelvic stabilization.

■ Pain
  • The physical examination should include as many of the common principles of inspection, palpation, neurovascular evaluation, and motion as possible in the acute trauma setting. The first finding in an awake, coherent patient is pain surrounding the pelvic area;

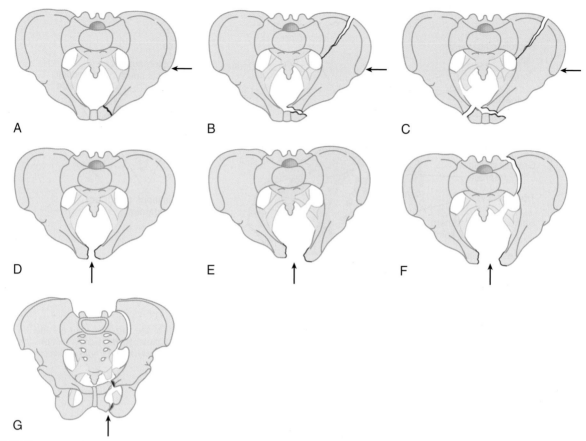

**FIGURE 17-3.** Young and Burgess classification of pelvic ring injuries. **A-C,** Lateral compression fracture patterns. **D-F,** Anterior-posterior compression fracture patterns. **G,** Vertical shear pattern.

additional findings may be present in a patient with polytrauma.

■ Dysfunction
  • Dysfunction in a patient with pelvic injury may be directly related to neurovascular compromise around the pelvis, splinting secondary to pain, mental status changes secondary to head trauma, or dysfunction related to any other associated injuries found on initial evaluation.

■ Prehospital Care
  • The most important part of prehospital care is emergent transfer to a designated trauma center where further stabilization, followed by definitive management, can occur.
  • Treatment rendered by emergency medical services personnel can include closure of open book–type pelvic injuries using devices as outlined further on.
  • Any obvious vascular compromise should be evaluated, a pressure dressing should be applied, and fluid resuscitation should commence as quickly as possible.

■ Physical Examination: Standard Focus Examination
Inspection of the position of the patient commonly can provide information regarding the type of injury or its mechanism. The hemipelvis may appear malrotated, the extremity may be shortened, and open fractures may be obvious. The anterior and superior iliac spines can be palpated to determine the pelvic rotation. Inspection should also include looking for signs of open

fracture and damage to adjacent structures that could indicate a pelvic fracture. Such signs include blood at the urethral meatus in men or at the meatus or vagina in women. These findings are indicative of an occult pelvic fracture. Posterior urethral rupture has been reported in 4% to 14% of pelvic fractures and almost exclusively in men.[8-10]

Palpation is essential to aid in the diagnosis of an unstable pelvis. Inward compression of the iliac crest can evoke changes in the pubic symphysis diastasis, whereas vertical and posterior displacement without a firm endpoint is seen with push-pull palpation in a vertically sheared pelvis.[11] These findings require urgent temporary stabilization, as outlined further on.

Neurologic findings include deficiencies of the lumbosacral plexus, which are seen in approximately 50% of pelvic injuries (see Fig. 17-2).[12,13] Vascular examination is imperative because hemodynamically unstable trauma patients or patients with vessels lacerated by pelvic fracture may have thready or nonpalpable pulses distally. Examination may require Doppler evaluation.

■ Diagnostic Testing
  • Imaging: X-ray, computed tomography (CT), and magnetic resonance imaging (MRI)
Radiographic information must be obtained to supplement physical examination findings. A plain film anteroposterior view of the pelvis should always be included in the initial trauma work-up. Additional films may be beneficial, depending on the stability of the patient.

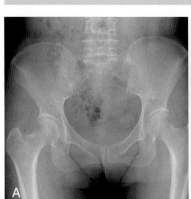
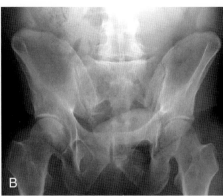
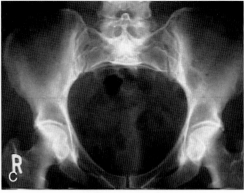

**FIGURE 17-4.** Normal anteroposterior **(A)**, outlet **(B)**, and inlet **(C)** views of the pelvis.

Inlet views, taken with the patient supine and the radiation beam directed from cranial to caudal, angled at 40 degrees, allow the viewer to gain information about the anteroposterior displacement of the pelvic ring. Outlet views, taken with the patient supine and the radiation beam directed from caudal to cranial, angled at 40 degrees, allow the viewer to gain information about the vertical displacement of the pelvis (Fig. 17-4).[7] Greater than 1 cm of vertical displacement, the presence of avulsion fractures from the sacrospinous ligaments, or L5 transverse fractures likely indicate an unstable pelvis.[11] The combination of anteroposterior, inlet, and outlet views can help the orthopedist classify the fracture type, although CT scan is more commonly used in the trauma setting at the present time because the patient may frequently require CT scan to evaluate for concurrent visceral and other bony injury.

Other studies that may be beneficial in polytrauma patient injuries include ultrasound, diagnostic peritoneal lavage, and arteriography, all of which may aid in identifying intra-abdominal bleeding in an unstable patient. CT scanning is now nearly commonplace in polytrauma patients, and CT scan can be used to identify the source of bleeding. In a study that compared contrast-enhanced CT scan with pelvic angiography, contrast-enhanced CT scan had a sensitivity of 84% and a specificity of 85% in locating the source for the bleeding and an accuracy of 90% for determining the presence or absence of bleeding (Fig. 17-5).[14]

• Serum studies

   Initial laboratory evaluation in the trauma bay should include a complete blood count, chemistry panel, coagulation studies (prothrombin time, partial thromboplastin time, and international normalized ratio), and type and screen (or crossmatch).

■ Differential Diagnosis

Care in the emergency department should always begin with the advanced trauma life support (ATLS) protocol, with focus first on airway, breathing, and circulation (ABCs). Patients with pelvic fractures frequently have polytrauma, and it is essential to follow these guidelines. As previously discussed, hemodynamic instability is very common in a patient with pelvic trauma or polytrauma. Biffl et al.[15] reported a 30% transfusion rate in emergency department patients in their review of

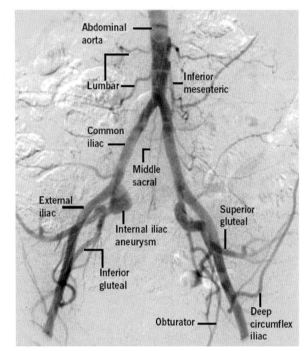

**FIGURE 17-5.** Normal pelvic angiography with important vascular structures identified.

pelvic trauma. In the previously mentioned study by McMurtry et al.,[3] survivors on average needed 7 units of blood, whereas nonsurvivors on average needed 24 units. Burgess et al.[16] found average blood requirements of 3.6 units in patients with lateral compression injuries, 8.5 units in patients with combined mechanism injuries, 9.2 units in patients with vertical shear, and 14.8 units in patients with anterior compression injuries. Both blood products and asanguineous products should be used because they can aid in decreasing blood viscosity and maintain renal blood flow.[17-19] In a hemodynamically unstable patient, closure of an open pelvic ring is an essential step in management of bleeding.

Pelvic ring closure can be accomplished by many methods, which are outlined further on. If stabilization methods fail or hemodynamic instability continues despite closure of the ring, angiographic stabilization may be warranted. In a study by Starr et al.,[20] 10% of patients with a pelvic fracture required angiographic embolization, with a trend toward embolization in older patients and patients with a higher Revised Trauma Score. Emergent angiography is indicated in patients with pelvic injuries who remain hemodynamically unstable; preemptive angiography can be considered in patients who are stable but have injuries that are likely to bleed.[21] Injuries with arteries found to be transected on angiography are at risk for delayed hemorrhage that can occur with clot lysis.[22] Other authors recommend nonselective embolization to control multiple bleeding sites and undetected injuries caused by vasospasm. Embolization is performed in the bilateral internal iliac arteries.[21] Embolization can effectively stop pelvic arterial bleeding, with success rates of 86% to 100% in some studies.[23-25] Agolini et al.[24] advocated embolization within the first 3 hours on arrival at the trauma center, whereas Balogh et al.[26] advocated embolization in the first 90 minutes.

From a bony perspective, the key to managing an unstable pelvic ring injury is to quickly make the diagnosis and temporarily restore as much stability as possible to the pelvis. Meighan et al.[27] reviewed the trauma management in Scotland and found that only 8 of 31 "major accident units" were able to make the distinction of stable versus unstable injury and diagnose an unstable pelvis in less than 60 minutes. The literature supports the establishment of a standardized protocol or treatment algorithm for polytrauma patients with pelvic fractures, and evidence shows that these measures can greatly increase the probability of rapid stabilization and survival.[28-30] Biffl et al.[15] described the implementation of a treatment algorithm involving the immediate presence of an orthopedic attending surgeon in the emergency department with pelvic wrapping followed by aggressive use of C-clamps. This measure decreased mortality from 31% to 15% (Fig. 17-6).

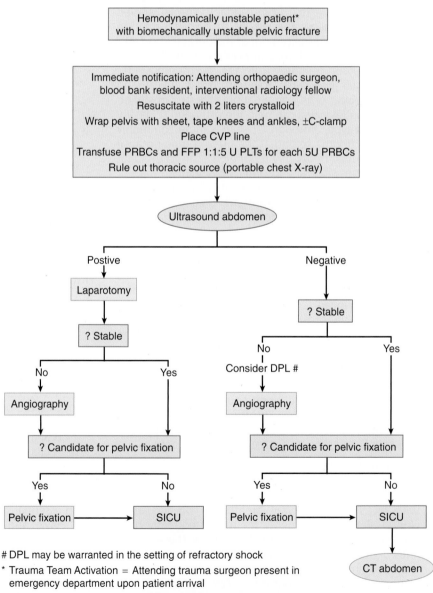

**FIGURE 17-6.** Algorithm described by Biffl et al.[15]

CVP, central venous pressure; PRBCs, packed red blood cells; FFP, fresh frozen plasma; PLTs, platelets; DPL, diagnostic peritoneal lavage; SICU, surgical intensive care unit.

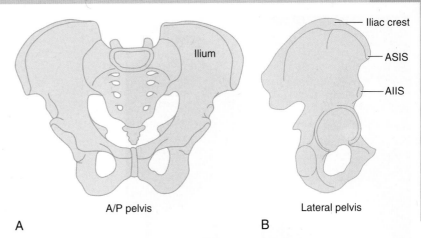

**FIGURE 17-25. A** and **B,** Anatomy of the iliac wing.   **A**                                **B**

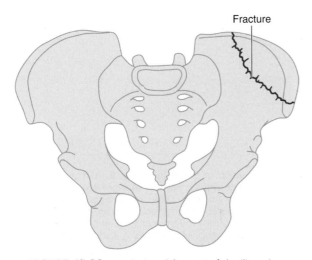

**FIGURE 17-26.** Nondisplaced fracture of the iliac wing.

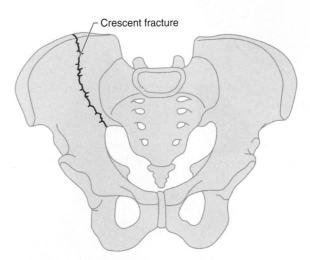

**FIGURE 17-27.** Crescent fracture.

notch. They can be associated with a dislocation of the anterior sacroiliac joint (Fig. 17-27).

Avulsion injuries of the pelvis often occur during athletic activities. They occur during a sudden, forceful muscular contraction and stress the attachment points on the pelvis. These injuries are often seen in children and teenagers when sports participation increases, but physes are not yet closed. They may also occur in adults most commonly when there is repetitive stress involving a tendon with underlying chronic tendinosis. The most common sites for avulsion injuries are the ischial tuberosity, anterior superior iliac spine (ASIS), and anterior inferior iliac spine.

The ischial tuberosity is the most common location in the pelvis for an avulsion injury. It is the point of origin for the semimembranosus, semitendinosis, adductor magnus, and long head of the biceps femoris tendons.

The ASIS is the origin of the sartorius tendon and the tensor fascia lata. The anterior inferior iliac spine is the origin of the rectus femoris tendon (Fig. 17-28).

■ Mechanism of Injury
Iliac wing fractures may be seen alone or in conjunction with other pelvic injuries or with polytrauma. Isolated iliac wing fractures are often caused by direct traumatic

application of a medially directed force. Crescent fractures of the posterior ilium occur commonly after laterally directed forces but also may occur with anterior and posterior forces.

Avulsion injuries occur when there is sudden forceful contraction of a muscle. The ischial tuberosity may be avulsed during strenuous contraction of the hamstrings, as occurs in hurdlers, pole-vaulters, cheerleaders, and any other athletes whose sport involves jumping.

The iliac crest may be avulsed by contraction of the abdominal muscles. The ASIS may be avulsed by forceful contraction of the sartorius muscle as seen in sprinters and soccer players when they forcefully extend the hip with the knee in flexion.

The anterior inferior iliac spine is often avulsed during a kicking motion that causes forceful contraction of the rectus femoris muscle.

■ Timing
● Pelvic fractures may occur in a polytrauma patient and often require emergent evaluation and management. Iliac wing and avulsion fractures may manifest later in the course of the trauma and may be seen in patients with distant history of trauma and subsequent chronic pain.

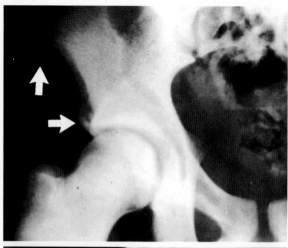

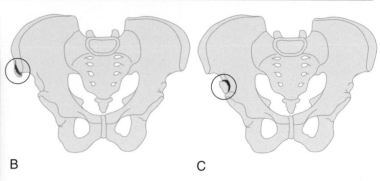

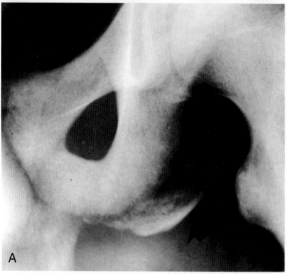

FIGURE 17-28. **A,** Avulsion of ischial tuberosity. **B,** ASIS avulsion fracture. **C,** Anterior inferior iliac spine avulsion fracture. (**A,** *From Rogers L, Taljanovic M, Boles C: Skeletal trauma. In Adam A, Dixon AK, Grainger RG, et al, editors: Grainger and Allison's diagnostic radiology, ed 5, Philadelphia, 2008, Churchill Livingstone;* **B,** *from Fiechtl J, Fitch R: Femur and hip. In Marx J, Hockberger R, Walls R, editors: Rosen's Emergency Medicine, ed 7, Philadelphia, 2009, Mosby;* **C,** *adapted from Fiechtl J, Fitch R: Femur and hip. In Marx J, Hockberger R, Walls R, editors: Rosen's Emergency Medicine, ed 7, Philadelphia, 2009, Mosby.)*

- Preexisting Illness
  - A complete history is necessary to determine important medical and orthopedic comorbidities in a patient with a pelvic injury.
- Pain
  - Abductors of the hip insert on the iliac wing; with isolated fractures of the iliac wing, there is pain on hip abduction or walking.
  - Generally, patients with avulsion injuries present with localized pain and swelling in the area of the injury. Pain is worse with use of the involved muscle.
  - Patients with avulsion injuries of the ischial tuberosity may have pain on palpation of the involved tuberosity.
  - Patients with avulsion injuries of the ischial tuberosity have pain on walking, especially in the posterior thigh and gluteal area.
  - Avulsion injury to the ASIS is associated with pain on flexion and abduction of the hip. There usually is point tenderness and swelling directly overlying the ASIS.
  - Patients with an ASIS avulsion have pain in the area of the avulsion.

- Dysfunction
  - The dysfunction in iliac wing and avulsion fractures is often related to the pain felt by the patient when walking.
  - The patient may experience difficulty in ambulation and lower extremity range of motion.
- Physical Examination: Standard Focus Examination
  - Any fracture of the pelvis warrants exploration for other injuries.
  - Patients with iliac wing fractures should have a thorough trauma evaluation, pelvic stability test, thorough distal neurovascular examination, genital examination, rectal examination, and back examination.
  - Patients with avulsion injuries often have an isolated injury, but a thorough examination should be performed to reveal any occult traumatic injuries.
  - As in any fracture of the pelvis, a thorough primary and secondary survey should be performed. Bowel, nerve, and arterial injuries may occur secondary or in addition to a fracture of the iliac wing.

- Diagnostic Testing
  - Imaging: X-ray, CT, and MRI

    In a trauma situation, a CT scan of the head, chest, abdomen, and pelvis should be obtained.

    An anteroposterior radiograph of the pelvis should be obtained specifically to evaluate the pelvis and may reveal the initial injury.

    Inlet, outlet, and Judet views and a CT scan of the pelvis should be obtained in the emergency department to evaluate the injury further.

    Avulsion injuries are usually detected on radiographs but may require a CT scan or MRI in the outpatient setting to identify subtle injury.

- Differential Diagnosis
  - Pelvic fractures may manifest in patients with polytrauma. It is important to have a wide differential diagnosis with multiple traumatic injuries in mind including other pelvis, spine, soft tissue, neurologic, and vascular injuries.
  - Soft tissue injury is common in patients with iliac wing fractures.
  - Other organs that may be injured include the bowel most commonly.
  - Arterial injuries involving the iliac and gluteal arteries may also be present.
  - Nerve injuries in the local area of injury may include the genitofemoral, lateral femoral cutaneous, and gluteal nerves.

## Treatment of Specific Injuries

- Analgesia, Anesthesia Block, and Sedation
  - Any fracture of the pelvis may be extremely painful and requires adequate analgesia while in the emergency department.
- Discharge or Admit as Inpatient
  - Isolated stable iliac wing fractures that are not associated with any other injuries can be treated conservatively but require a consultation with an orthopaedist to ensure that the fracture does not extend into the acetabulum.
  - Avulsion injuries are treated conservatively. In the case of an isolated avulsion injury, a phone consultation should be obtained to arrange follow-up care.
  - Occasionally, fragments displaced more than 2 cm are treated surgically, but disagreement exists. In this case, it would be important to obtain an orthopedic bedside consultation and referral.
  - Any iliac wing fracture that is open, severely displaced, involves the posterior segment or acetabulum, or involves other organ injury warrants an orthopedic bedside consultation.
  - Indications for operative management include open fractures, severely displaced or comminuted iliac wing fractures, unstable fractures, bowel incarceration or herniation, and fractures that are associated with unstable pelvic ring injuries.

- Discharge Care and Instruction—Timing for Follow-up
  - Most patients with uncomplicated iliac wing fractures do well with a short period of bed rest, analgesics, and weight bearing as tolerated. Patients should follow up with an orthopedist within 1 week after discharge from the emergency department.
  - Patients with avulsion fractures require analgesia and bed rest in a comfortable position and should follow up with orthopedics in 1 week.
- Common Pitfalls
  - A common pitfall in isolated iliac wing fractures is missing additional associated injuries, including injuries to other bones, bladder, bowel, nerves, or arteries.
  - Failure to recognize and treat avulsion injuries can lead to chronic pain syndromes.

## PUBIC RAMI FRACTURES

### Differential Diagnosis of Traumatic Complaints

- History
  Pubic rami fractures are common in patients with severe polytrauma with pelvic ring disruption; however, an isolated fracture of the superior or inferior pubic ramus is the most common pelvic fracture. They are considered stable fractures (Fig. 17-29). Fractures of the superior and inferior pubic rami on the same side are often seen after falls. These are also generally stable fractures (Fig. 17-30). Four-pillar injuries, or fractures to the pubic rami on both sides of the symphysis pubis, are produced by direct blows or straddle injuries (Fig. 17-31). These often involve the posterior pelvic arch and genitourinary trauma. These types of fractures are considered pelvic ring disruptions and are discussed elsewhere.
- Mechanism of Injury
  Pubic rami fractures are common in elderly patients after a fall. They can also be seen in younger patients as stress fractures secondary to exercise. Pregnant

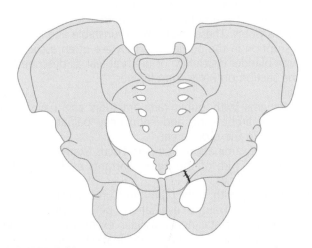

**FIGURE 17-29.** Nondisplaced unilateral single pubic ramus fracture.

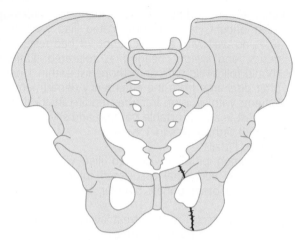

**FIGURE 17-30.** Unilateral fracture of both pubic rami. *(Redrawn from Canale ST, Beaty JH, editors: Campbell's operative orthopaedics, ed 11, Philadelphia, 2007, Mosby.)*

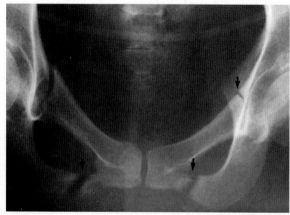

**FIGURE 17-31.** Pelvic ring disruption with bilateral pubic rami fractures. *(From Rogers L, Taljanovic M, Boles C: Skeletal Trauma. In Adam A, Dixon AK, Grainger RG, et al, editors: Grainger and Allison's diagnostic radiology, ed 5, Philadelphia, 2008, Churchill Livingstone.)*

women can have stress fractures of the pubic rami that manifest in the third trimester.

Straddle fractures are four-pillar injuries that refer to fractures of the pubic rami on both sides of the symphysis pubis. These fractures are unstable and indicate disruption in the pelvic ring. They are often associated with bladder disruption or urethral tear as described in the section on Pelvic Ring Injuries.

■ Pain
  ● Patients with pubic rami fractures can have pain while ambulating and upon deep palpation, especially in the groin area.
■ Physical Examination: Standard Focus Examination
  ● Any fracture of the pelvis warrants exploration for other injuries.
  ● Patients with pubic rami fractures should have a thorough trauma evaluation, pelvic stability test, thorough distal neurovascular examination, genital examination, rectal examination, and back examination.

  ● Any displacement of the pubic rami indicates a possible disruption in the pelvic ring and must be thoroughly explored as described earlier in the section on Pelvic Ring Injuries.
  ● Bowel, nerve, and arterial injuries may occur secondary or in addition to a fracture of the pubic rami.
■ Diagnostic Testing
  ● Imaging: X-ray, CT, and MRI

    In a trauma situation, a CT scan of the head, chest, abdomen, and pelvis should be obtained.

    An anteroposterior radiograph of the pelvis should be obtained specifically to evaluate the pelvis and may reveal the initial injury.

    Inlet, outlet, and Judet views and a CT scan of the pelvis should be obtained in the emergency department to evaluate the injury further.

## Treatment of Specific Injuries

■ When to Consult a Specialist
  ● Telephone consultation

    For isolated single and unilateral double rami fractures, a telephone consultation with an orthopedist is indicated to arrange follow-up. These are generally stable fractures and are treated conservatively.

    A bilateral pubic rami fracture requires consultation with an orthopedist because there may be disruption of the pelvic ring.

    Patients with nondisplaced unilateral pubic rami fractures can be discharged to home if they can ambulate.

    Patients with significant pain, inability to ambulate, or any displacement must be admitted for pain control.

■ Plan for Follow-up Care
  ● Most patients with pubic rami fractures that are considered stable do well with bed rest and analgesics.
  ● Patient can walk with the aid of crutches with weight bearing as tolerated.
  ● Normal activity can be resumed by 8 weeks or when otherwise instructed at the orthopedic follow-up visit.
■ Common Pitfalls
  ● Failure to diagnose a pelvic ring injury
  ● Failure to diagnose associated injuries

## Bibliography

Abrassart S, Stern R, Peter R: Morbidity associated with isolated iliac wing fractures. J Trauma Inj Infect Crit Care 66:200–203, 2009.

Amr S, Abdel-Meguid K, Kholeif A: Neurologic injury caused by fracture of the iliac wing: case report. J Trauma 52:370–376, 2002.

Burgess AR, Eastridge BJ, Young JW, et al: Pelvic ring disruptions: effective classification system and treatment protocols. J Trauma 30:848, 1990.

Coppola P, Coppola M: Emergency department evaluation and treatment of pelvic fractures. Emerg Med Clin North Am 18:1–27, 2000.

Choi S, Cwinn A: Pelvic trauma. In Marx J, Hockberger R, Walls R, editors: Rosen's Emergency Medicine, ed 7, Philadelphia, 2009, Mosby.

Dasgupta B, Shah N, Brown H, et al: Sacral insufficiency fractures: an unsuspected cause of low back pain. Br J Rheumatol 37:789–793, 1998.

Day A, Kinmont C, Bircher M, et al: Crescent fracture-dislocation of the sacroiliac joint. J Bone Joint Surg Br 89:651–658, 2007.

Denis F, Davis S, Comfort T: Sacral fractures: an important problem. Retrospective analysis of 236 cases. Clin Orthop Relat Res 227:67–81, 1988.

Dunn W, Morris H: Fractures and dislocations of the pelvis. J Bone Joint Surg Am 50:1639–1648, 1968.

Fardon D: Sacral fractures. J Neurosurg 48:316, 1978.

Gibbons K, Soloniuk D, Razack N: Neurological injury and patterns of sacral fractures. J Neurosurg 72:889–893, 1990.

Gotis-Graham I, McGuigan L, Diamond T, et al: Sacral insufficiency: fractures in the elderly. J Bone Joint Surg Br 76:882–886, 1994.

Hill R, Robinson C, Keating J: Fractures of the pubic rami: epidemiology and five year survival. J Bone Joint Surg Br 83:1141–1144, 2001.

Hunt T, Gruen G: Sacral fractures. Curr Opin Orthop 8:2–6, 1997.

Jerrard D: Pelvic fractures. Emerg Med Clin N Am 11:147–163, 1993.

Levine A: Fractures of the sacrum. In Browner BD, Jupiter JB, Levine AM, et al, editors: Skeletal trauma: basic science, management, and reconstruction, ed 4, Philadelphia, 2008, Saunders.

Mehta S, Auerbach J, Born C, et al: Sacral fractures. J Am Acad Orthop Surg 14:656–665, 2006.

Routt M, Simonian P, Swiontkowski M: Stabilization of pelvic ring disruptions. Orthop Clin North Am 28:369–388, 1997.

Sabiston CP, Wing PC: Sacral fractures: classification and neurologic implications. J Trauma 26(12):1113–1115, 1986 Dec.

Sanders T, Ziatkin M: Avulsion injuries of the pelvis. Semin Musculoskel Radiol 12:42–53, 2008.

Schmidek H, Smith D, Kristiansen T: Sacral fractures. Neurosurgery 15:735–745, 1984.

Stover M, Mayo K, Kellam J: Pelvic ring disruptions. In Browner BD, Jupiter JB, Levine AM, et al, editors: Skeletal trauma: basic science, management, and reconstruction, ed 4, Philadelphia, 2008, Saunders.

Switzer J, Nork S, Routt M: Comminuted fractures of the iliac wing. J Orthop Trauma 14:270–276, 2000.

Vaccaro AR, Kim D, Brodke D, et al: Diagnosis and management of sacral spine fractures. Inst Course Lect 53:375–385, 2004.

# References

1. Rothenberger DA, Fisher RP, Strate RG, et al: The mortality associated with pelvic fractures. Surgery 84:356–361, 1978.

2. Perry JF, Jr: Pelvic open fractures. Clin Orthop 151:41–45, 1980.

3. McMurtry R, Walton D, Dickinson D, et al: Pelvic disruption in the polytraumatized patient: a management protocol. Clin Orthop Relat Res 151:22–30, 1980.

4. Gansslen A, Pohlemann T, Paul CH, et al: Epidemiology of pelvic ring injuries. Injury 27(Suppl 1):S-A-13, 1996.

5. Gertzbein SD, Chenowith DR: Occult injuries of the pelvic ring. Clin Orthop 128:202, 1977.

6. Young JW, Burgess AR, Brumback RJ, et al: Pelvic fractures: value of plain radiography in early assessment and management. Radiology 160:445–451, 1986.

7. Pennal GF, Tile M, Waddell JP, et al: Pelvic disruption: assessment and classification. Clin Orthop 151:12–21, 1980.

8. Holdsworth FW: Injury to the genito-urinary tract associated with fractures of the pelvis. Proc R Soc Med 56:1044, 1963.

9. McCague EJ, Semans JH: The management of traumatic rupture of the urethra and bladder complicating fracture of the pelvis. J Urol 52:36, 1994.

10. Mitchell JP: Injuries to the urethra. Br J Urol 40:649, 1968.

11. Tile M: Acute pelvis fractures: II. principles of management. J Am Acad Orthop Surg 4:152–161, 1996.

12. Slatis P, Huittinen VM: Double vertical fractures of the pelvis: a report on 163 patients. Acta Chir Scand 138:799–807, 1972.

13. Scheid DK, Kellam JF, Tile M: Open reduction and internal fixation of pelvic fractures. Presented at the Annual Meeting of the Orthopaedic Trauma Association, Toronto, November 7-10, 1990.

14. Cerva DS, Jr, Mirvis SE, Shanmuganathan K, et al: Detection of bleeding in patients with major pelvic fractures: value of contrast-enhanced CT. AJR Am J Roentgenol 166:131–135, 1996.

15. Biffl WL, Smith WR, Moore EE, et al: Evolution of a multidisciplinary clinical pathway for the management of unstable patients with pelvic fractures. Ann Surg 6:843–850, 2001.

16. Burgess AR, Eastridge BJ, Young JW, et al: Pelvic ring disruptions: Effective classification system and treatment protocols. J Trauma 30:848–856, 1990.

17. Shoemaker WC: Comparison of relative effectiveness of whole blood transfusion and various types of fluid therapy in resuscitation. Crit Care Med 4:71, 1976.

18. Shoemaker WC, Monson DD: The effect of whole blood and plasma expanders on volume flow relationships in critically ill patients. Surg Gynecol Obstet 137:453, 1973.

19. Carey JS, Brown RS, Woodward NW, et al: Comparison of hemodynamic responses to whole blood and plasma expanders in clinical traumatic shock. Surg Gynecol Obstet 121:1059, 1965.

20. Starr AJ, Griffin DR, Reinert CM, et al: Pelvic ring disruptions: prediction of associated injuries, transfusion, requirement, pelvic arteriography complications, and mortality. J Orthop Trauma 16:553–561, 2002.

21. Velhamos GC, Toutouzas KG, Vassiliu P, et al: A prospective study on the safety and efficacy of angiographic embolization for pelvic and visceral injuries. J Trauma Inj Infect Crit Care 2:303–308, 2002.

22. Ben-Menachem Y, Coldwell DM, Young JW, et al: Hemorrhage associated with pelvic fractures: causes, diagnosis, and emergent management. AJR Am J Roentgenol 157:1005–1014, 1991.

23. Mucha P, Jr, Farnell MB: Analysis of pelvic fracture management. J Trauma 24:379–386, 1984.

24. Agolini SF, Shah K, Jaffe J, et al: Arterial embolization is a rapid and effective technique for controlling pelvic fracture hemorrhage. J Trauma 43:395–399, 1997.

25. Eastridge BJ, Starr A, Minei JP, et al: The importance of fracture pattern in guiding therapeutic decision-making in patients with hemorrhagic shock and pelvic ring disruptions. J Trauma 53:446–451, 2002.

26. Balogh Z, Caldwell E, Heetveld M, et al: Institutional practice guidelines on management of pelvic fracture-related hemodynamic instability: do they make a difference? J Trauma 58:778–782, 2005.

27. Meighan A, Gregori A, Kelly M, et al: Pelvic fractures: the golden hour. Injury 29:211–213, 1998.

28. Croce MA, Magnotti LK, Savage SA, et al: Acute mortality associated with injuries to the pelvic ring: the role of early patient mobilization and external fixation. J Am Coll Surg 204:935–942, 2007.

29. Riemer BL, Butterfield SL, Diamond DL, et al: Acute mortality associated with injuries to the pelvic ring: the role of early patient mobilization and external fixation. J Trauma 44:454–459, 1993.

30. Miller PR, Moore PS, Mansell E, et al: External fixation or arteriogram in bleeding pelvic fracture: initial therapy guided by markers of arterial hemorrhage. J Trauma 54:437–443, 2003.

31. Flint LM, Jr, Brown A, Richardson JD, et al: Definitive control of bleeding from severe pelvic fractures. Ann Surg 189:709–716, 1979.

32. Routt ML, Jr, Falicov A, Woodhouse E, et al: Circumferential pelvic antishock sheeting: a temporary resuscitation aid. J Orthop Trauma 16:45–48, 2002.

33. Bottlang M, Krieg JC, Mohr M, et al: Emergent management of pelvic ring fractures with use of circumferential compression. J Bone Joint Surg Am 84(Suppl 2):43–47, 2002.

34. Ganz R, Krushell RJ, Jakob RP, et al: The antishock pelvic clamp. Clin Orthop Relat Res 267:71–78, 1991.

35. Archdeacon MT, Hiratzka J: The trochanteric C-clamp for provisional pelvic stability. J Orthop Trauma 20:47–51, 2006.

36. Grimm MR, Vrahas MS, Thomas KA: Pressure-volume characteristics of the intact and disrupted pelvic retroperitoneum. J Trauma 44:454–459, 1998.

37. Tile M: Pelvic ring fractures: should they be fixed? J Bone Joint Surg Br 70:1–2, 1988.

38. Pohlemann T, Bosch U, Gansslen A, et al: The Hannover experience in management of pelvic fractures. Clin Orthop Relat Res 305:69–80, 1994.

39. Nerlich M, Maghsudi M: Algorithms for early management of pelvic fractures. Injury 27(Suppl 1):S-A29-37, 1996.

40. Baumgaertner MR, Wegner D, Booke J: SSEP monitoring during pelvic and acetabular fracture surgery. J Orthop Trauma 8:127–133, 1994.

41. Judet R, Judet J, Letournel E: Fractures of the acetabulum: classification and surgical approaches for open reduction—preliminary report. J Bone Joint Surg Am 46:1615–1646, 1964.

42. Smith W, Williams A, Agudelo J, et al: Early predictors of mortality in hemodynamically unstable pelvis fractures. J Orthop Trauma 21:31–37, 2007.

43. Letournel E, Judet R, Elson RA (trans-ed): Fractures of the Acetabulum, ed 2, Berlin, 1992, Springer-Verlag.

44. Middlebrooks ES, Sims SH, Kellam JF, et al: Incidence of sciatic nerve injury in operatively treated acetabular fractures without somatosensory evoked potential monitoring. J Orthop Trauma 11:327–329, 1997.

45. Colapinto V: Trauma to the pelvis: Urethral injury. Clin Orthop Relat Res 151:46–55, 1980.

46. Mucha P, Jr, Farnell MB: Analysis of pelvic fracture management. J Trauma 24:379–386, 1984.

47. Bosch U, Pohlemann T, Haas N, et al: Classification and management of complex pelvic trauma [German]. Unfallchirurg 95:189–196, 1992.

48. Dalal SA, Burgess AR, Siegel JH, et al: Pelvic fracture in multiple trauma: classification by mechanism is key to pattern of organ injury, resuscitative requirements, and outcome. J Trauma 29:981–1002, 1989.

49. Velmahos GC, Toutouzas KG, Vassiliu P, et al: A prospective study on the safety and efficacy of angiographic embolization for pelvic and visceral injuries. J Trauma 53:303–308, 2002.

50. Helfet DL, Anand N, Malkani AL, et al: Intraoperative monitoring of motor pathways during operative fixation of acute acetabular fractures. J Orthop Trauma 11:2–6, 1997.

51. Flint LM, Jr, Brown A, Richardson JD, et al: Definitive control of bleeding from severe pelvic fractures. Ann Surg 189:709–716, 1979.

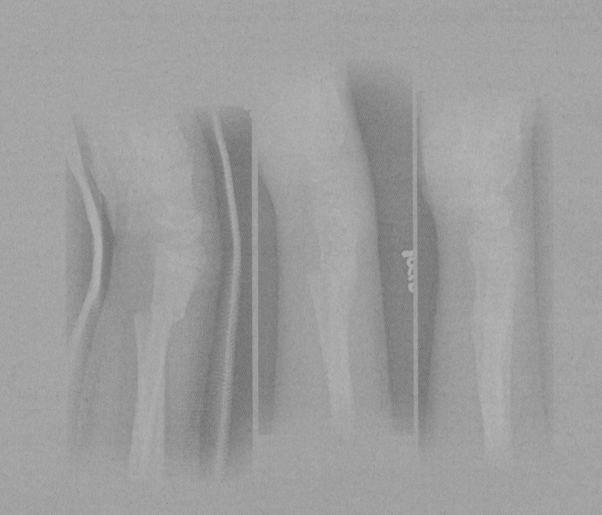

# PART III
# Pediatrics

## Chapter 18

# *Introduction to Pediatric Trauma*

Mark C. Lee, Silas Marshall,
and John C. Brancato

**OVERVIEW**
**EPIDEMIOLOGY**
**BIOLOGY OF PEDIATRIC BONE**
**GENERAL MANAGEMENT OF PEDIATRIC MUSCULOSKELETAL**
**COMPLAINTS**

**TECHNIQUES OF CAST AND SPLINT APPLICATION**
**COMPARTMENT SYNDROME**
**OSTEOMYELITIS**
**SEPTIC ARTHRITIS AND LYME ARTHRITIS**

## OVERVIEW

- Intrinsic differences distinguish musculoskeletal injuries in children from injuries in adults.
- Pediatric bones are continuously growing in length, through growth plates (physes) at either end of the bone, and width, through bony apposition from a biologically active layer of periosteum that surrounds the bone.
- Remodeling, or the ability of bone to reshape a deformity spontaneously, is robust in the pediatric skeleton and is a reflection of its active growth.
- Pediatric bones are more flexible than adult bone. Fracture patterns in which the bone deforms plastically are unique to pediatric patients.
- Healing is far more rapid in children compared with adults with the same fracture; this is likely a reflection of the richer endosteal and periosteal blood supply of the bone.
- Children have a much greater tolerance for prolonged periods of immobilization and generally regain range of motion quickly. As a result, more musculoskeletal injuries can be successfully treated nonoperatively in children than in adults.
- Evaluation of a pediatric patient with a musculoskeletal injury markedly differs from evaluation of an injured adult.
- Communication with the patient may be limited for numerous reasons and interfere with the acquisition of an appropriate history. The patient may have an absent or limited vocabulary. Even if able to communicate, the willingness to communicate may be limited. Patience, judicious use of distraction, and indirect examination techniques are often required.
- Treatment decisions and treatment success depend greatly on both the parent or caretaker. The physician must understand and be comfortable with the idea that a third party—the caretaker—will make all treatment decisions for the patient. Compliance with the treatment regimen and subsequent follow-up are dictated by the interest and understanding of this third party.
- The possibility that musculoskeletal injury is not accidental and a product of inflicted trauma is a sobering aspect of caring for a pediatric patient. However, it is imperative that the physician identify incongruous injury mechanisms and recognize common musculoskeletal patterns of child abuse to protect the child from further harm.

## EPIDEMIOLOGY

- Incidence
  Multiple socioeconomic, temporal, and environmental variables affect the incidence of fractures in children.
  Galano et al.[1] estimated that approximately 84,000 children were admitted to the hospital for fractures in 1997 in the United States.
  These admissions resulted in almost $1 billion in hospital charges.
  More than 70% of these fractures were treated at nonpediatric hospitals, emphasizing the importance of a basic understanding of the management of pediatric musculoskeletal injuries for all emergency medicine physicians.
  Rennie et al.[2] evaluated all children presenting to a hospital in Edinburgh, Scotland, over a 1-year period and found the overall incidence to be 20.2 per 1000 children per year. Other studies show similar incidences.
  Of fractures, 61% occur in boys; this percentage increases in older age groups.
  Overall incidence shows a bimodal distribution with a peak at 6 to 8 years of age and another at 12 to 14 years of age.
  Incidence varies with season and time of day. More fractures occur in the summer months when school is out and children are participating in outdoor activities. In addition, fracture incidence increases in the evening with a peak around 6 P.M.; this correlates with the period of time between the end of the school day and sunset.[3]

■ Etiology
There are three main causes of pediatric fractures.
• Accidental trauma
Accidental trauma is the most common cause of fractures in children.

Injuries in the home environment are common and are usually due to a fall from a height, such as a fall from furniture, an open window, or a tree.

Injuries related to school activities are usually due to sporting activities or accidents involving playground equipment.

Injuries associated with recreational activities include falls from a height (i.e., trampolines or monkey bars), bicycle or skateboard crashes, and skiing or snowboarding injuries.

Motor vehicle crashes can cause significant injury. Child passengers in motor vehicle crashes sustain a relatively greater proportion of pelvic and spinal injuries compared with adults. The varying range of pediatric heights and weights also influences the fracture pattern. For example, children struck by cars frequently sustain femur fractures, whereas adults sustain tibia fractures; this is dictated by which bone is at the level of the car bumper.[3]

• Nonaccidental trauma
Nonaccidental trauma (child abuse) is less common but should be considered in patients with skeletal injury patterns that are incongruous with the injury mechanism, age-inappropriate fracture patterns (i.e., femur fractures in nonambulators), or multiple fractures at various stages of healing.

The incidence of child abuse is approximately 4.9 per 1000 children; 55% of abused children sustain fractures.[3]

Child abuse reporting laws are specific to each state. Nevertheless, it is important always to document findings carefully.

If child abuse is suspected, a skeletal survey should be ordered to rule out other fractures, and child protective services should be involved.

• Pathologic fractures
Pathologic fractures are fractures that result from a process that weakens or disrupts the integrity of the bone; these are discussed later.

## BIOLOGY OF PEDIATRIC BONE

■ General Considerations
The highly metabolic cartilaginous growth plate or physis is unique to pediatric bone. It sits between metaphysis, adjacent to the shaft of the long bone, and epiphysis, the section of the long bone closer to the joint (Fig. 18-1).

The physis is separated histologically into four separate zones of cartilage cell or chondrocyte activity (Fig. 18-2).
• Zone of resting—the source of stem cells for production of chondrocytes in the subsequent layers
• Zone of proliferation—a zone of high mitotic activity where chondrocytes divide and produce a noncollagenous protein matrix integral to the mineralization process

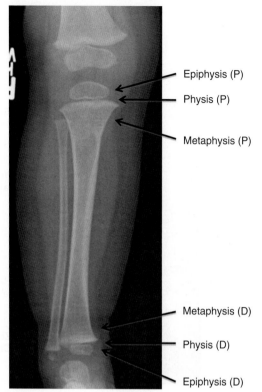

**FIGURE 18-1.** Example of tibial physes. The proximal *(P)* and distal *(D)* tibial epiphyses, physes, and metaphyses are marked.

- Epiphysis (P)
- Physis (P)
- Metaphysis (P)
- Metaphysis (D)
- Physis (D)
- Epiphysis (D)

• Zone of hypertrophy or maturation—chondrocytes increase in size and begin to produce collagen X
• Zone of calcification—chondrocytes undergo apoptosis, releasing calcium stores into the extracellular matrix, and the extracellular matrix ossifies
Growth plates also exist at the site of insertion of a tendon or ligament. An apophysis, analogous to an epiphysis, is a cartilaginous cap overlying such a growth plate that ossifies with growth (Fig. 18-3).

As a child matures, the ossification of each cartilaginous epiphysis or apophysis occurs at predictable times during skeletal development. With further growth, the growth plates slow in function and ultimately close as all residual cartilage ossifies. Each growth plate closes at a predictable time, typically earlier in girls than boys, unless closure is accelerated or delayed by injury or metabolic disease. A clinician must have knowledge of the order of ossification of the epiphyses and apophyses and the timing of closure of the physes to interpret pediatric radiographs accurately.

The six ossification centers around the elbow serve as a good example of this concept. The chronologic sequence of the appearance of the secondary centers of ossification around the elbow may be remembered with the mnemonic *CRMOTL* (capitellum, radial head, medial epicondyle, olecranon, trochlea, and lateral epicondyle) (Table 18-1). The capitellum ossifies at 1 year of age, the radial head and medial epicondyle ossify almost 4 years later, the trochlea

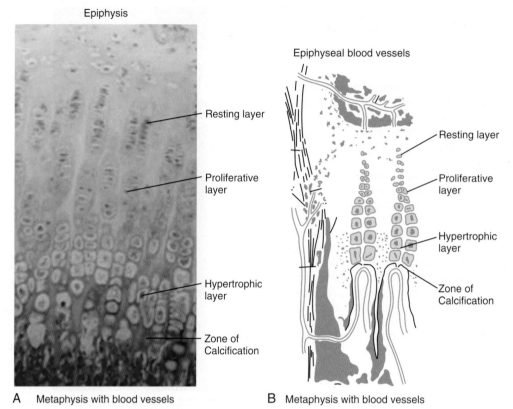

Epiphysis

Resting layer

Proliferative layer

Hypertrophic layer

Zone of Calcification

A    Metaphysis with blood vessels

Epiphyseal blood vessels

Resting layer

Proliferative layer

Hypertrophic layer

Zone of Calcification

B    Metaphysis with blood vessels

**FIGURE 18-2. A,** Zones of the physis as seen on histology. **B,** Diagrammatic representation of the zones of the physis. *(From Green N, Swiontkowski M, editors: Skeletal trauma in children, ed 4, Philadelphia, 2008, Saunders.)*

**TABLE 18-1** Order of Appearance of Secondary Ossification Centers Around the Elbow

| Secondary Ossification Center | Girls (yr) | Boys (yr) |
| --- | --- | --- |
| Capitellum | 1 | 1 |
| Radial head | 5 | 6 |
| Medial epicondyle | 5 | 7.5 |
| Olecranon | 8.7 | 10.5 |
| Trochlea | 9.0 | 10.7 |
| Lateral epicondyle | 10 | 12 |

Adapted from Cheng JC, Wing-Man K, Shen WY, et al: A new look at the sequential development of elbow-ossification centers in children. J Pediatr Orthop 18:161–167, 1998.

and olecranon ossify 4 years after the radial head and medial epicondyle, and the lateral epicondyle ossifies 2 years after the trochlea and olecranon.

The growth plate is relatively weaker than the surrounding bone and is prone to injury. However, the metabolic activity of the growth plate provides for rapid healing and remodeling when an injury is sustained.

If the growth plate is traumatized and ceases to function, either partially or completely, limb length discrepancies or angular deformities may result.

A physeal fracture is a fracture that extends through a growth plate. Microscopically, failure of

the bone occurs at the level of the hypertrophic zone. Physeal fractures are classified according to the Salter-Harris classification (Fig. 18-4).[4]

- Type I—pure physeal fracture without involvement of the metaphysis or epiphysis; may be detectable only by tenderness over the physis on examination (with negative x-rays) or may involve complete physeal separation
- Type II—physeal fracture with extension into the metaphysis
- Type III—physeal fracture with extension into the epiphysis
- Type IV—fracture extending from the metaphysis, through the physis and into the epiphysis
- Type V—crush injury to the physis with a high risk of growth arrest (not shown in Fig. 18-4).

■ Stress/Strain Relationships in Pediatric Bone

Pediatric bone has greater vascularity and a thicker periosteum than adult bone. Biomechanically, the modulus of elasticity is lower for pediatric bone than it is for adult bone. For any given stress, more strain is experienced in pediatric bone, and pediatric bone can absorb a greater amount of energy before failure.

Although children do sustain many of the fracture patterns seen in adults, the different biomechanical properties of pediatric bones yield several types that are unique to children (Fig. 18-5).

- Plastic deformity—failure of the bone at the microscopic level with resultant deformity. Although there is no discrete fracture line on x-ray, deformity remains

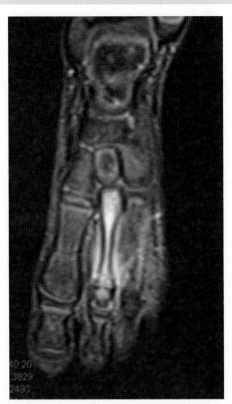

**FIGURE 18-8.** T2-weighted coronal section through the left foot shows increased marrow signal in the second metatarsal with surrounding periosteal edema, suggesting acute osteomyelitis with likely periosteal abscess.

such as in an intra-articular distal tibia fracture, to assist in operative decision making.

Magnetic resonance imaging (MRI)

MRI is useful for identifying soft tissue pathology including ligament and tendon ruptures, cartilaginous insults, or infections. Although MRI avoids the radiation exposure of CT, the examination is long, and children younger than 8 years often have to be sedated for the duration of the examination. MRI is most commonly ordered in the emergency department to evaluate osteomyelitis, septic arthritis, or occult spinal cord injury (Fig. 18-8). All other MRI studies are typically performed on an outpatient basis after appropriate splintage in the emergency department.

Ultrasound

Ultrasound can be used to look for fluid collections such as soft tissue abscesses or joint effusions. In addition, with ultrasound guidance, therapeutic and diagnostic aspirations of fluid collections can be performed. Ultrasound is an extremely useful modality in pediatric patients. There is no radiation exposure, and the patient rarely needs to be sedated for the examination. However, it is not effective in examining bone architecture.

Electromyography (EMG)

EMG is used to evaluate for disruption or impingement of nerves. EMG is rarely used in the acute setting.

- Blood tests
  In the acute setting, blood tests are used mainly to rule out infection. In addition, for patients who are to undergo extensive surgery, preoperative laboratory tests help to screen for bleeding disorders or anemia before surgery.

  Laboratory tests performed to exclude infection include complete blood count with differential and erythrocyte sedimentation rate (ESR) and C-reactive protein (CRP) levels. Normal values help to rule out infection.

  Preoperative laboratory tests are not usually necessary in pediatric patients unless there is potential for significant blood loss or a long operative time. These tests include complete blood count, Chem-7 blood panel, partial thromboplastin time, prothrombin time, international normalized ratio, and a type and screen if a need for transfusion is anticipated.

- Joint fluid analysis is performed in cases of suspected infection.

  Cell count with differential

  Generally, a white blood cell (WBC) count of 50,000 cells/mL or greater and 75% or greater polymorphonuclear cells is indicative of septic arthritis; however, lower WBC counts with a high percentage of polymorphonuclear cells (≥90%) are highly concerning for infectious etiology.

  Crystal analysis

  Gout (sodium urate crystals) and pseudogout (calcium pyrophosphate crystals) are extremely uncommon in pediatric patients.

  Gram stain and culture should be sent to determine the appropriate antibiotic therapy for the infection.

■ Fracture Description
Several features of a fracture influence the treatment plan. These features must be communicated to the orthopedist on call when consultation is sought.

- Open or closed
  A fracture is considered open when the soft tissue envelope over the fracture has been disrupted and the fracture now communicates with the environment. This communication leaves the patient at higher risk of wound infection and subsequent osteomyelitis. In addition, if there is significant soft tissue damage, there is an increased risk of nonunion or delayed union. All open fractures warrant consultation with the orthopedist on call.

- Location of the fracture
  The appropriate initial management is dictated in part by the bone involved in the injury. For example, clavicle fractures tend to be nonoperative injuries. Even when surgical fixation is indicated, clavicle fractures are almost always treated on an outpatient

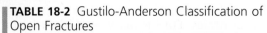
**TABLE 18-2** Gustilo-Anderson Classification of Open Fractures

| Type | Description |
|------|-------------|
| I | Clean wound <1 cm |
| II | Wound >1 cm, without extensive soft tissue damage |
| III | Massive soft tissue damage, compromised vascularity, severe wound contamination |
| IIIA | Adequate soft tissue coverage present |
| IIIB | Extensive soft tissue loss (requiring flaps), usually associated with massive contamination |
| IIIC | Associated arterial injury |

Adapted from Gustilo RB, Mendoza RM, Williams DN, et al: Problems in the management of type III (severe) open fractures: a new classification of type III open fractures. J Trauma 24:742–746, 1984.

basis and rarely necessitate orthopedic consultation in the emergency department.

- Fracture site within the involved bone
  Generally, shaft and metaphyseal fractures can heal rapidly and yield predictably good results. However, injuries at the growth plate level and intra-articular injuries must be identified early because these require more aggressive and timely treatment to avoid undesirable late sequelae.
- Degree of deformity
  Displacement, or how far apart the fracture ends lie, and angulation, the degree of angular deformity of the bones, dictate initial and definitive management. Markedly deformed extremities that are threatening the soft tissue envelope may need emergent reduction by the emergency department staff.
- Classification
  Accurate classification of fractures allows for appropriate emergency management and efficient communication between providers. However, for most fractures, a specific classification system is unnecessary to convey the severity of an injury accurately. The Gustilo-Anderson classification is useful for the description of an open fracture (Table 18-2).
- Specific bones are discussed in the following chapters; however, nondisplaced fractures can generally be treated with appropriate immobilization by emergency department staff. These patients can see an orthopedic surgeon for follow-up on an outpatient basis.
- Appropriate initial management of displaced fractures varies from bone to bone and from patient to patient. Generally, the more displaced the fracture and the older the patient, the more likely it will be necessary to consult an orthopedist on call to perform a formal closed reduction.
- Even in bones that can tolerate significant amounts of deformity, formal closed reduction can be beneficial for patient comfort, time to healing, and long-term function.
- If the degree of deformity is so great that either the skin or the neurovascular structures are at risk, immediate closed reduction via inline traction should be performed by the emergency department staff or

first responders followed by immobilization of the bone involved and the joints above and below the affected bone.

- Treatment
  Initial management of open fractures includes irrigation, gross débridement of foreign material at the site of the wound, wound coverage and splinting, administration of appropriate antibiotics, tetanus prophylaxis, and orthopedic consultation.

  There has been a paradigm shift in regard to operative management in recent years. Previously, operative management of all open fractures within 6 hours of injury was recommended with the belief that this approach decreases the ultimate risk of osteomyelitis. However, convincing evidence has emerged to suggest that delaying treatment of an open fracture without neurovascular compromise until the following day, after appropriate initial management, produces similar or better outcomes.[7]

  Depending on the amount of contamination of the wound, more recent evidence in the pediatric orthopedic literature suggests that grade I open fractures may not need an operative irrigation and débridement.

  Risk of infection in children with grade I open fractures treated only with appropriate emergency department management is 2.5%. Deep infection in grade I open fractures in children younger than 12 years is rare.[7]

  However, scattered cases exist describing horrific complications from infections that developed in otherwise benign-appearing wounds. Often, the soft tissue injury fails to describe the degree of bony contamination. Thorough surgical débridement should still be offered for this group of patients.

  Regardless of the surgical treatment approach, all open fractures require discussion with and close follow-up by an orthopedist.

## TECHNIQUES OF CAST AND SPLINT APPLICATION

- General Considerations
  - Splinting and casting are basic tools in the initial stabilization or definitive treatment of a patient with a musculoskeletal injury to the extremity.
  - Proper application and knowledge of appropriate indications is paramount to ensure patient comfort and to provide the best environment for healing of the injured extremity.
  - Splint and cast application is an art and is best learned through practice.
- Indications
  - Splint
    A splint can be applied as temporary stabilization for most injuries of the extremities. The splint affords the patient improved comfort, portability for transfers, and rest to the soft tissues. The typical absence of a hard circumferential shell is ideal when there is concern for increasing intracompartmental pressures. The splint can also be easily removed for repeated evaluation without the need for a specialized saw.

**TABLE 18-3** Typical Splints and Casts Used for Specific Fracture Types

| Fracture Type | Splint Type | Cast Type | Note |
|---|---|---|---|
| **Upper Extremity** | | | |
| Proximal humerus | NA | NA | Sling immobilization is sufficient |
| Humeral shaft | Coaptation | NA | More permanent treatment may be Sarmiento functional bracing |
| Supracondylar or condylar humerus fracture | Long arm | Long arm | |
| Radial neck or olecranon | Long arm | Long arm | |
| Forearm | Long arm | Long arm | |
| Distal radius or ulna | Short arm | Short arm | |
| Hand and wrist | Short arm with hand extension | Short arm with hand extension | Immobilize fingers with flexion at the metacarpals and extension at the interphalangeal joints |
| **Lower Extremity** | | | |
| Hip or proximal femur fracture | NA | Spica cast | Initial splintage for this injury to facilitate patient transport is to put a small pillow between the legs and bind the legs with a sheet<br>Splints are ineffective at controlling this fracture |
| Femoral shaft | NA | Spica cast | Initial splintage for this injury to facilitate patient transport is to put a small pillow between the legs and bind the legs with a sheet<br>Splints are ineffective at controlling this fracture |
| Distal and supracondylar femur | Long leg | Long leg | For patients < 8 years old, a spica cast may allow better control of this fracture type |
| Proximal tibia | Long leg | Long leg | |
| Tibial and fibular shaft | Long leg | Long leg | |
| Distal tibia, ankle, and foot | Short leg | Short leg | |

*NA,* Not applicable.

A splint can be transitioned to permanent stabilization, if well applied, after discharge by overwrapping the splint with permanent casting material.

Specific splints are indicated for specific fracture patterns (Table 18-3).

• Cast

A cast is typically applied as definitive treatment for a skeletal injury to an extremity after consultation with an orthopedic specialist.

Specific casts are indicated for specific fracture patterns (see Table 18-3).

■ Splinting and Casting Prerequisites

Before a cast or a splint is applied to a pediatric patient, appropriate plain radiographic evaluation of the extremity should be performed and the injury should be clearly delineated.

Generally, before definitive immobilization, the injury should be discussed with an orthopedic specialist, and a consensus should be reached on the treatment plan. This simple communication between the evaluating physician and the specialist obviates repeated work, multiple trips to radiology, and the need for unnecessary repeated rounds of sedation or attempted pain control.

However, if multiple distracting injuries exist, a splint can be initially applied in the absence of an orthopedic consultation to facilitate continued trauma evaluation and to provide initial protection of the injured extremities.

The correct type of splint must be applied for the specific fracture. Proximal femoral and femoral shaft fractures should not be splinted with long leg splints. The splint would invariably end at the fracture site or just proximal to the fracture, creating a lever arm for fracture movement (Fig. 18-9). In this case, skeletal traction or binding to the contralateral leg is more effective.

■ Materials

• Fiberglass or plaster casting material

Fiberglass is popular at the present time for casting because of its lighter weight and enhanced durability compared with plaster.

• Fiberglass or plaster premade slabs for splinting

• Cotton padding

• Waterproof padding

Waterproof padding has no significant role in the emergency department treatment of a pediatric patient. Application of this padding is a unique technique and is best reserved for outpatient treatment to minimize potential complications.

■ Techniques

• Application of cotton padding

Cast padding should be applied evenly over the surface of the extremity with slight tension. The cast

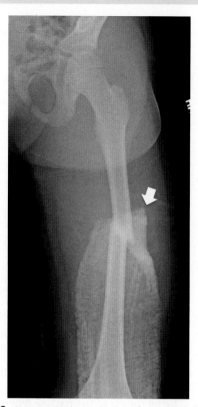

**FIGURE 18-9.** Anteroposterior projection of a midshaft femur fracture in a 9-year-old boy. The posterior splint ends at the fracture site *(arrow)*, creating a lever arm for the distal fragment and contributing to fracture instability.

padding should overlap itself by 50% during each roll around the extremity.

Wrapping the cast padding from one end of the planned casting limit to the other may be considered creating a single "sheet" of padding. No more than three sheets of casting material are necessary. However, all bony prominences (i.e., elbow, knee, heel) should be reinforced with three to four additional layers of cast padding.

The edges of the padding should extend well past the planned limits of the cast to allow the cast material to protect the skin from the cast edge. Additional casting material may be applied to these edges.

- Application of the splint or cast material

Upper extremity splint

- Long arm splint
  The elbow is usually kept at 90 degrees of flexion, and the wrist is maintained in neutral position. A premade fiberglass or plaster slab (10 plaster layers thick) can be applied posteriorly and end at the metacarpal. The slab should extend to the level of the shoulder because short pediatric arms always cause the humeral component of the splint to be shorter than is optimal. Reinforcing struts may be made across the medial and lateral aspects of the elbow joint. Elastic bandage wrap is applied loosely over the premade slab, taking care to leave the fingers and thumb free (Fig. 18-10).

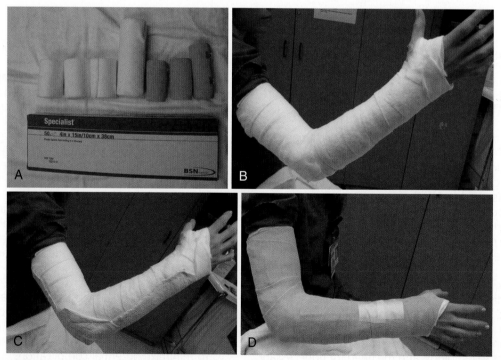

**FIGURE 18-10.** Sequential application of a long arm splint. **A,** Typical splint supplies consist of cotton cast padding, elastic bandages, and precut slabs of plaster or fiberglass. **B,** The cast padding is applied in overlapping layers with extra layers of padding applied around the proximal and distal extents of the splint and the bony prominence of the elbow. The elbow is held in 90 degrees of flexion. **C,** A posterior plaster slab has been applied with a small lateral bridge of plaster across the elbow for additional support. **D,** An elastic bandage has been applied. Tape has been used instead of metal clips because metal clips can fall off and cause injury.

- Short arm splint

  The slab of plaster or fiberglass may be applied volarly and end at the elbow. The remainder of the procedure remains the same as a long-arm splint.

Upper extremity cast

- Long arm cast

  The elbow is usually maintained at 90 degrees of flexion, and the wrist is in neutral position. Fiberglass casting rolls are rolled in sheets, similar to cotton padding. No more than two sheets of fiberglass are required, with two to three additional layers for reinforcement of convexities along the extremity (i.e., posterior surface of the elbow). The cast should also be rolled as proximal as possible because pediatric arms cause the proximal limb of the cast to be short. Care should be taken to ensure that the fingers and thumb are free. The distal end of the cast should stop dorsally at the metacarpal heads and volarly at the distal palmar flexion crease.

- Short arm cast

  Cast application is similar to a long arm cast except that the casting material stops at the level of the elbow.

Lower extremity splint

- Long leg splint

  The ankle is kept at 90 degrees of flexion. This application may be performed with an assistant or, for stable injuries, with the use of a foot rest. A premade fiberglass or plaster slab (10 plaster layers thick) can be applied posteriorly and should extend past the plantar surface of the toes. A separate U-shaped slab may be placed around the heel and along either side of the leg to reinforce the splint. Elastic bandage wrap is wrapped loosely over the premade slab, and the splint is held in position. A neutral position for the ankle is desirable.

- Short leg splint

  The same procedure as described for the long leg splint is performed except that the posterior slab stops short of the knee (Fig. 18-11).

Lower extremity cast

- Long leg cast

  The ankle is maintained in neutral position, and cast padding is applied with double the number of layers of cast padding over the posterior heel. Fiberglass casting rolls are rolled in sheets, similar to cotton padding. No more than two sheets of fiberglass are required except for the convexity of

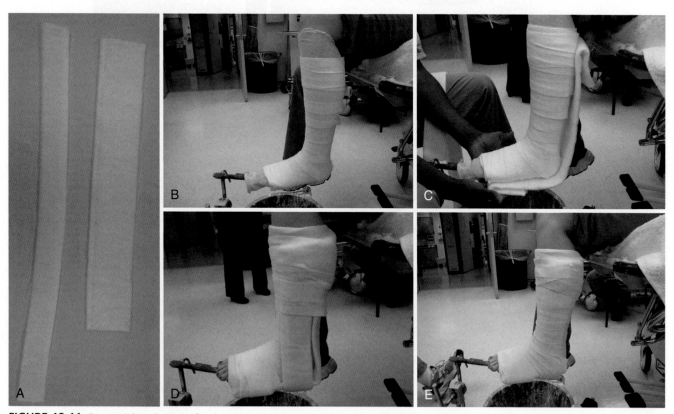

**FIGURE 18-11.** Sequential application of a short leg splint. **A,** Typical fiberglass slabs that may be used for application of a short leg splint. **B,** The ankle is placed in a neutral position with no dorsiflexion and no plantar flexion. Cast padding is applied in layers with extra padding applied to the proximal and distal extents of the splint and over the heel. A leg support casting aid is very helpful for application of the splint. Alternatively, if tolerated, the patient may be placed prone with the knee bent and the ankle held in neutral. **C,** The fiberglass slab is applied posteriorly. **D,** A U-shaped slab is placed around the medial and lateral aspects of the ankle for extra reinforcement and held in position with cast padding. **E,** The elastic bandage wrap is applied with tape to secure the edges of the bandage.

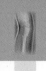

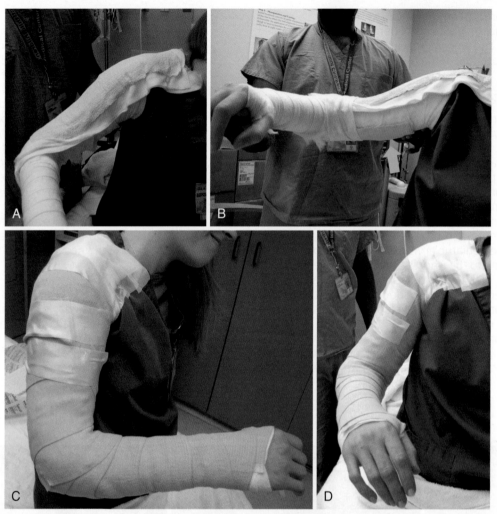

**FIGURE 18-12.** Sequential application of a coaptation splint. **A,** Cast padding is applied for the length of the arm. A plaster slab is created on a four-layer section of cast padding. The cast padding and plaster slab unit is applied to the lateral surface of the arm. The plaster and cast padding extend well over the acromion process and sit along the midclavicle. **B,** A separate, smaller medial plaster slab *(arrow)* is applied to the medial humerus and secured with cast padding. **C** and **D,** An elastic bandage is placed around the arm. The proximal portion of the splint is covered and secured to the skin of the shoulder with tape.

the heel, which requires reinforcement with at least two or three layers of casting material because this area is the quickest to wear down. The distal end of the cast should stop distal to the metatarsal heads plantarly.

Coaptation splint

A coaptation splint is used for provisional stabilization of humeral shaft fractures.

A premade fiberglass or plaster slab (10 plaster layers thick) is measured to the length of the lateral border of the arm, including a length to be placed over the acromion. A shorter slab is used for the medial aspect of the arm, extending from the elbow to just short of the level of the axilla. Five layers of cast padding are cut to the length of the fiberglass or plaster slabs and placed on the slabs. The slabs are placed on lateral and medial borders of the arm. An elastic bandage wrap is placed loosely from the hand to the arm. The proximal portion of the lateral

slab remains exposed. This portion is secured to skin of the shoulder with adhesive tape (Fig. 18-12).

Molding of the splint or cast is performed according to the specific fracture. Generally, the apex of the cast mold should be concentrated over the apex of the deformity and reverse the identified deformity.

■ Casting and Splinting Pearls
  • There is always a paucity of padding along the convexities of extremities, whereas an abundance of padding exists in the concavities.
  • Apply elastic wrap or bias wrap loosely when creating splints.
  • For long arm splints, the splint should end in the axilla of pediatric patients because the proximal segment tends to be short.
  • Cast indices measuring the quantity of excess padding visible on radiographs to hold a fracture reduction have been correlated with the risk of fracture redisplacement.[8]

## COMPARTMENT SYNDROME

■ General Considerations
Edema or hemorrhage into a closed myofascial space leads to an increase in pressure in that space. Compartment syndrome occurs when this pressure exceeds the perfusion pressure of the tissue, leading to tissue death. Compartment syndrome can occur with any fracture but occurs most commonly in high-energy injuries, fractures with significant initial displacement, and fractures of the tibia or forearm.

■ Diagnosis
- Diagnosis of compartment syndrome is primarily clinical.
- Signs and symptoms include the six "P's"—pain, pallor, paresthesias, paralysis, pulselessness, and poikilothermia.
- The five "P's" other than pain tend to be late findings.
- The most sensitive findings include increasing narcotic requirements, pain out of proportion to the injury, and pain with passive stretch of muscles within the compartment of concern (i.e., significant pain with passive dorsiflexion of the great toe may indicate a developing compartment syndrome in the posterior compartment of the leg).
- Compartment pressures can be measured with a pressure monitoring device such as the Stryker STIC device (Kalamazoo, MI) (Fig. 18-13).
- When diagnosing compartment syndrome, the difference between the compartment pressure and the diastolic blood pressure ($\Delta$P) is a more sensitive measurement than the absolute compartment pressure.[9]
- Pressures should be measured at the level of the fracture.
- A $\Delta$P of 30 mmHg or less is indicative of compartment syndrome.
- In trauma patients who are in hypotensive shock, compartment pressures should be re-evaluated after the blood pressure is stabilized.

■ Treatment
Compartment syndrome is a surgical emergency. When compartment syndrome is suspected, the orthopedist on call should be notified in anticipation of surgical decompression via fasciotomy. In cases of compartment syndrome without an underlying fracture, the general surgery team may be contacted first, depending on the institutional policies.

Nonoperative management is relevant for worsening compartment syndromes and is useless in the definitive treatment of compartment syndromes. Loosening or removal of potentially constrictive dressings is primary. Elevation of the extremity should be avoided in patients with developing compartment syndromes because this reduces an already inadequate blood flow further.

## OSTEOMYELITIS

■ General Considerations
Osteomyelitis is infection of the bone, usually with bacteria. Patients with varying degrees of immunocompromise may also be affected by fungi and mycobacteria.

The incidence is unknown, although more recent studies in Scotland and Norway reported incidences of 3 to 13 cases per 100,000. It is more common in younger ages; more than half of all patients are younger than 5 years. The incidence in males is approximately twice that of females.[10]

The predominant mechanism of inoculation is acute hematogenous spread, although direct inoculation may also occur, such as after penetrating trauma (animal bites and other puncture wounds) or surgery. Inoculation can also occur from local spread of infection, such as sinusitis.

The most common sites are in long bones, with more than half of all cases involving the femur, tibia, or fibula. Approximately 20% of cases occur in other areas such as bones of the pelvis, vertebrae, and calcaneus.[10]

Animal models show osteomyelitis is more likely after bacteremic animals sustain some kind of trauma. These models may provide an explanation for the approximately 30% of children with osteomyelitis who have a history of preceding trauma to the affected area.

■ Anatomic Considerations
The metaphysis is the most highly vascularized area of growing bone. Bacteria lodge in the juxtaphyseal blood vessels and replicate, adhering to the cartilage/bone matrix (Fig. 18-14).

In the neonatal and early infant periods, the bony cortex is thinner and more easily allows the spread of infection from its origin in the metaphyseal marrow space to adjacent soft tissues. As infants and toddlers become older, the bony cortex and periosteum thicken resulting in more localized infections.

Concomitant joint involvement is thought to be more likely in the youngest infants for two reasons. The first reason is the presence of transphyseal blood vessels that can allow infection to develop and spread from marrow space, across physis, to epiphysis and then into the joint. The second reason is the extension of the joint capsule (especially in the shoulder, hip, and knee) to the metaphysis so that spread from the adjacent marrow through the cortex can lead directly into the joint space.

■ History
The most common symptoms and findings in children with osteomyelitis are fever, localized pain, and decreased mobility, each found in approximately 50% to 85% of patients.[11]

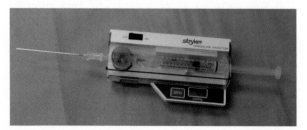

**FIGURE 18-13.** Stryker STIC pressure monitoring device (Kalamazoo, MI).

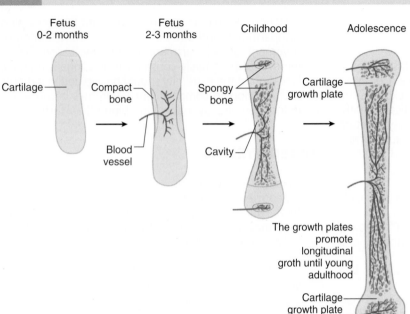

Fetus
0-2 months

Fetus
2-3 months

Childhood

Adolescence

Cartilage

Compact
bone

Blood
vessel

Spongy
bone

Cavity

Cartilage
growth plate

The growth plates
promote
longitudinal
groth until young
adulthood

Cartilage
growth plate

**FIGURE 18-14.** The vascular channels invade the cartilaginous bony anlage and establish an intraosseous metaphyseal circulation. The circulation to the epiphysis is provided by separate vessels, and the physis acts as a relative barrier to vascular flow from metaphysis to epiphysis.

An Australian review of 102 patients with hematogenous osteomyelitis found that 44% of patients had symptoms for at least 3 days with 22% having symptoms for 1 week or more.[11]

■ Physical Examination

Localized tenderness, swelling, and erythema become more common with advancing duration of illness.

Younger children with vertebral osteomyelitis may present with difficulty walking or a limp, whereas older children more commonly report back pain. Patients with diskitis may be younger than patients with vertebral osteomyelitis.

Patients with pelvic osteomyelitis may present with signs and symptoms suggestive of other pathologies in that area, such as appendicitis, septic arthritis of the hip, and urinary tract infection.

■ Microbiology

The most common bacterial cause of osteomyelitis is *Staphylococcus aureus*; methicillin-resistant *S. aureus* (MRSA) strains are the cause of an increasing percentage of all cases.

Other organisms implicated as infecting agents vary with patient age. *Escherichia coli* and group B streptococcus are prevalent in the neonatal period, whereas group A streptococcus and *Streptococcus pneumoniae* are more prevalent in older children. The effects of polyvalent pneumococcal immunization on the incidence of osteomyelitis are unknown. However, immunization with the *Haemophilus influenzae* type B (Hib) vaccine has resulted in a marked decline in cases caused by *H. influenzae* type B.

*Kingella kingae*, a gram-negative coccobacillus present in the throat flora of young children, is being increasingly recognized as a cause of osteomyelitis and septic arthritis owing to improved culture techniques. A cluster of cases of osteomyelitis in a Minnesota daycare center in 2003 was linked to *K. kingae*, and another study reported the application of polymerase chain reaction testing to culture-negative specimens from cases of osteomyelitis and septic arthritis showed that *K. kingae* was the leading cause of infection.

Patients with underlying sickle cell disease who develop osteomyelitis are more commonly infected with *Salmonella* species and other gram-negative organisms. A review of the literature published in 1998 reported a ratio of cases caused by *Salmonella* and *S. aureus* as 2.2 : 1.[12] Osteomyelitis of the foot caused by foreign body penetration through a sneaker is commonly due to *Pseudomonas aeruginosa*.

Osteomyelitis is less frequently due to fungal agents, although coccidioidomycosis, common in the Southwest, may infect the long bones and vertebral bodies. *Aspergillus* osteomyelitis, described in immunocompetent patients, is more likely in patients with chronic granulomatous disease. The rate of *Mycobacterium tuberculosis* infection in the United States is at its lowest level since the early 1950s, but this organism should be in the differential diagnosis of any indolent osteomyelitis, especially in foreign-born children.

■ Diagnosis

Definitive diagnosis rests on associating an appropriate clinical picture with positive bone aspirate examination or culture, blood culture, and radiographic findings.

Laboratory findings are highly variable. A review of 44 patients found an elevated WBC count in 35%, but ESR was elevated in 92% and CRP was elevated in 98%.[13]

Blood cultures are positive in approximately 30% to 60% of cases. Bone aspirates from the suspected site are positive in 45% to 85% of cases. In contrast to blood cultures, aspirate cultures may remain positive for several days after initiation of antibiotic therapy. Negative initial cultures should prompt consideration of *K. kingae*.[11]

Plain radiography is often negative early in the course of infection because bony destruction and periosteal

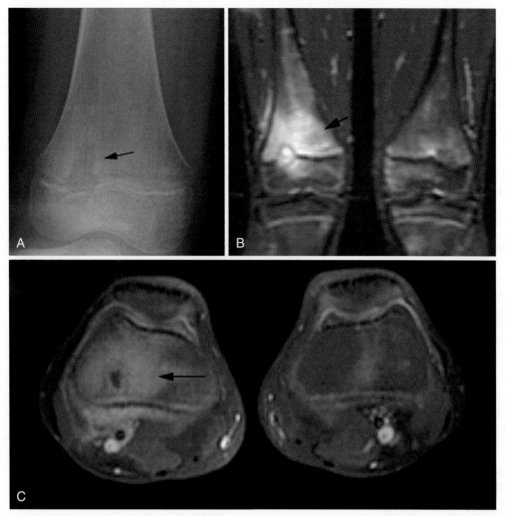

**FIGURE 18-15.** Distal femur osteomyelitis in a 10-year-old girl. **A,** Anteroposterior projection of the distal femur shows a lucency *(arrow)* adjacent to the distal femoral physis. **B,** T2-weighted MRI shows edema in the distal femur *(arrow)* with a walled-off high signal region corresponding to the radiographic lucency. **C,** Axial T1 section shows bony edema *(arrow)* with a necrotic nidus corresponding to the lucency on radiographs.

changes may take 1 to 2 weeks to become visible. However, x-rays remain the initial imaging modality of choice to exclude other diagnoses, such as fracture or tumor.

As infectious involvement of the cortex develops, swelling of the adjacent soft tissues results in displacement of the normal soft tissue planes in 3 or 4 days. Further swelling of muscle and soft tissues may lead to loss of normal tissue planes.

Technetium-99m bone scan takes advantage of increased metabolic activity of the bone in areas of infection or fracture. Triple-phase scans provide images taken over several hours. Sensitivity and specificity may be 90%, although neonates may have false-negative lesions in 22% to 68% of cases.

Gallium scans localize the nuclear material in polymorphonuclear cells, in contrast to technetium-99m scans, which localize it in metabolically active bone. Sensitivity is also in the range of 90%. Gallium scans are reserved for difficult cases because of a higher amount of radiation than in technetium-99m scans.

MRI is rapidly becoming the imaging modality of choice. Because most patients with acute hematogenous osteomyelitis are younger than 5 years, testing usually requires sedation. Sensitivity and specificity are reported to be 90% to 99% (Fig. 18-15).

Use of gadolinium enhancement may be helpful in cases that show adjacent bone marrow or soft tissue edema to identify early abscess formation.

■ Treatment

Recovery of the specific organism involved is essential for the ultimate choice of appropriate therapy. Aspiration of affected bone marrow, periosteal fluid collection, or adjacent soft tissue abscess should be performed whenever possible.

Treatment of osteomyelitis is usually with parenteral antibiotics guided by likely or identified organisms. Nafcillin, ampicillin/sulbactam, and ceftriaxone are common initial choices for infants and young children, especially individuals in daycare settings, who are at higher risk for infection with *K. kingae*. Clindamycin and vancomycin should also be considered for older children at risk for infection with group A streptococcus and MRSA. Vancomycin is the preferred agent in communities that have a higher clindamycin resistance rate (>15%) among MRSA isolates.

There is little prospective evidence to guide the duration of antibiotic therapy, although shorter courses have been associated with higher rates of complications. Standard therapy is considered to be 4 to 6 weeks. Parenteral antibiotics may be administered for 2 weeks with 2 to 4 additional weeks of oral antibiotics (sequential antibiotic therapy). Oral antibiotics suffice for the entire treatment course as long as the organism shows sensitivity and adequate serum levels are achievable.

# SEPTIC ARTHRITIS AND LYME ARTHRITIS

■ General Considerations

Septic arthritis is the inflammation of a joint caused by infection. With increasing use of artificial joint replacement, cases caused by the external introduction of bacteria directly into the joint space are increasing in adults. However, in children, most cases are due to hematogenous spread.

Septic arthritis is most frequently seen in children younger than 3 years. In this age group, osteomyelitis may spread under the joint capsule to involve the joint space.

The most frequently involved joint in children is the hip. However, the knee and, to a lesser extent, the shoulder may also be affected. Although more than 90% of cases involve only a single site, infants may develop multiple joint infections.

The immune response to the infection results in neutrophil migration and inflammation within the joint capsule. The inflammatory reaction and increased pressure within the closed space are responsible for the clinical features of septic arthritis.

■ History

Because the hip and knee are most commonly affected, children with septic arthritis are likely to present with gait-related symptoms such as limp or other gait abnormality or a refusal to bear weight.

In one review of 47 cases of septic arthritis in children, 58% of children were younger than 2 years, and 72% had symptoms for 3 days or less. Although all patients had a painful joint and 90% had restricted movement of the affected joint, only 72% had fever, 59% had local swelling, and only 28% had overlying erythema. In this study, the hip and knee together accounted for almost two thirds of cases.[14]

A septic joint is not likely if a nearly full and easy range of motion of the joint in question can be obtained on examination.

Infants may present with more obscure symptoms, such as paradoxical irritability—being calmer when left still than when being held.

The septic hip is often held in a flexed, abducted, and externally rotated position.

Neisseria gonorrhoeae causes dermatitis-arthritis syndrome, characterized by dermatitis, migratory polyarthritis, and tenosynovitis, in approximately 60% of patients. Upper extremity joints are more frequently involved, especially the wrists and elbows, but ankles and knees are also affected. In the remaining 40%, N. gonorrhoeae infection leads to a focal septic arthritis.[15]

■ Microbiology

Organisms vary with the age of the patient. In infants and young children, S. aureus and group B streptococcus are most common. Since the introduction of the Hib vaccine, H. influenzae type B is less frequently a pathogen. N. gonorrhoeae is the most frequent pathogen identified among sexually active adolescents with S. aureus close behind.

Other pathogens need to be considered in specific situations. P. aeruginosa must be considered in the differential diagnosis of septic arthritis following a nail puncture of the foot through a sneaker sole. Similarly, Salmonella species are often the offending agents in patients with sickle cell anemia who contract septic arthritis. Borrelia burgdorferi (the causative agent in Lyme disease) is frequently involved in cases of arthritis in endemic areas. Other occasional pathogens include K. kingae and Fusobacterium necrophorum.

M. tuberculosis is an infrequent cause but may result in a chronic joint infection.

■ Diagnosis

Maxim: "The sun should never rise or set on a septic hip." In other words, a delay in diagnosis and treatment for septic arthritis will yield predictably bad outcomes.

The differential diagnosis of septic arthritis includes transient synovitis, osteomyelitis, adjacent soft tissue infection, and occult fracture.

Diagnostic algorithms have been developed to aid in the differentiation of septic arthritis of the hip from transient synovitis. Most algorithms include factors such as fever, elevated ESR or CRP, elevated WBC count, and non–weight bearing status. Patients with all of these features have a greater than 99% probability of having septic arthritis.[16]

Arthrocentesis and evaluation of the joint fluid is necessary to make a definitive diagnosis of septic arthritis. A specimen should be obtained before initiation of antibiotic therapy whenever possible.

Normal synovial fluid is clear and slightly viscous. Cloudy fluid recovered from a joint in question should be treated as presumptive evidence of infection. The color may range from yellow to greenish.

Gram staining should be performed on aspirated fluid, although actual organisms are often not identified.

A synovial WBC count of greater than 50,000/mm$^3$ with a predominance of polymorphonuclear cells supports the diagnosis with higher counts providing stronger evidence. However, a WBC count of less than 50,000/mm$^3$ does not rule out septic arthritis.

Fluid culture is positive in most cases, although it is positive in only 25% of cases caused by N. gonorrhoeae. Obtaining blood cultures increases the likelihood of identifying the organism. If clinical suspicion exists for N. gonorrhoeae, urethral or cervical specimens or both should be obtained for culture or polymerase chain reaction testing.

ESR and CRP are both commonly (92% to 98%) elevated in septic arthritis. ESR is often greater than 30 mm/hr, and CRP is greater than 10 mg/L.

Plain radiographs may show an increase in the joint space, consistent with an effusion. Radiographs are also

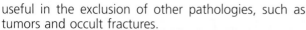
useful in the exclusion of other pathologies, such as tumors and occult fractures.

Ultrasound is most sensitive for identification of a joint effusion, although the false-negative rate is reported to be 5%.

- Treatment

An attempt should be made in all patients with suspected septic arthritis to obtain synovial fluid for microscopy and culture. Commonly, synovial fluid is obtained through needle aspiration of the joint space, with or without ultrasound guidance.

When the hip is the joint in question, diagnostic and management procedures overlap. Needle aspiration may be performed under ultrasound guidance to confirm the diagnosis. However, the hip joint is at the highest risk of poor outcome from bacterial infection owing to the tenuous nature of blood flow to the femoral head and its easy compromise from the elevated intracapsular pressures associated with infection. There is also an increased risk of subsequent femoral head subluxation. When clinical suspicion is high, arthrotomy and lavage has long been held as the standard of care. There are no studies directly comparing needle aspiration with arthrotomy. However, arthroscopic drainage and irrigation has been shown in small studies to be just as effective as open arthrotomy with shorter hospital stays.

Empiric antibiotic therapy should be initiated as soon as possible after recovery of blood and synovial fluid specimens for culture.

Choice of antibiotic should be based on the most likely offending organisms, which varies slightly with patient age. For all ages, *S. aureus* (including MRSA strains) is the most common cause of septic arthritis. Cefazolin and vancomycin are both good initial choices, depending on local incidence of methicillin resistance.

Young infants should also receive empiric coverage for the organisms commonly involved in neonatal or infant sepsis, including group B streptococcus and *E. coli*. Cefotaxime and ceftriaxone are appropriate initial choices.

Older infants and children should receive empiric antibiotic therapy to cover other likely agents, such as *K. kingae,* group A streptococcus, and *S. pneumoniae*. Ampicillin, cefotaxime, and ceftriaxone are such agents.

The standard duration of therapy is 3 weeks. Initial parenteral therapy for 1 to 2 weeks often may be successfully completed with high-dose oral therapy.

- Lyme Arthritis

In endemic areas, Lyme arthritis is prominent in the differential diagnosis of septic arthritis. Approximately 60% of untreated patients with Lyme disease develop arthritis as a secondary manifestation between 2 months and 2 years after initial infection. Because patients with erythema migrans frequently receive testing and therapy, most patients with Lyme arthritis provide no history of the rash.

In a review of 391 children from an endemic area with joint effusion aspirations, 123 (31%) were diagnosed with Lyme arthritis, whereas 51 (13%) had culture-positive septic arthritis. Multivariate analysis showed that a complete refusal to bear weight was the strongest predictor of septic arthritis over Lyme arthritis.[17]

More than 90% of cases involve the knee, although the hip, ankle, wrist, and elbow may also be affected. Fever is present in 25% to 50% of children with Lyme arthritis. In contrast to patients with septic arthritis, children with Lyme arthritis usually have a normal WBC count and only modestly elevated ESR (approximately two thirds or ≤60 mm/hr). Synovial WBC count tends to be lower than with other bacterial etiologies.

We have noted a milder restriction of movement in many patients with Lyme arthritis compared with patients with septic arthritis.

Correlation of clinical findings of a milder infectious arthritis with positive serology for *B. burgdorferi* or positive synovial polymerase chain reaction is adequate for the diagnosis because successful culture of the organism is difficult.

Treatment is with oral amoxicillin or cefuroxime for 28 days. Doxycycline may be used for patients older than 8 years.

## References

1. Galano GJ, Vitale MA, Kessler MW, et al: The most frequent traumatic orthopaedic injuries from a national pediatric inpatient population. J Pediatr Orthop 25:39–44, 2005.
2. Rennie L, Court-Brown CM, Mok JY, et al: The epidemiology of fractures in children. Injury 38:913–922, 2007.
3. Landin LA: Fracture patterns in children: analysis of 8682 fractures with special reference to incidence, etiology and secular changes in a Swedish urban population 1950-1979. Acta Orthop Scand Suppl 202:1–109, 1983.
4. Salter R, Harris W: Injuries involving the epiphyseal plate. J Bone Joint Surg Am 45:35, 1963.
5. Wilkins K, Aroojis A: Incidence of fractures in children. In Beaty J, Kasser J, editors: Rockwood and Wilkins' Fractures in Children, Philadelphia, 2006, Lippincott Williams & Wilkins.
6. Sairyo K, Henmi T, Kanematsu Y, et al: Radial nerve palsy associated with slightly angulated pediatric supracondylar humerus fracture. J Orthop Trauma 113:227–229, 1997.
7. Stewart DG, Jr, Kay RM, Skaggs DL: Open fractures in children: principles of evaluation and management. J Bone Joint Surg Am 87:2784–2798, 2005.
8. Alemdaroglu KB, Iltar S, Cimen O, et al: Risk factors in redisplacement of distal radial fractures in children. J Bone Joint Surg Am 906:1224–1230, 2008.
9. Olson SA, Glasgow RR: Acute compartment syndrome in lower extremity musculoskeletal trauma. J Am Acad Orthop Surg 137:436–444, 2005.
10. Blyth MJ, Kincaid R, Craigen MA, et al: The changing epidemiology of acute and subacute haematogenous osteomyelitis in children. J Bone Joint Surg Br 83:99–102, 2001.
11. Riise OR, Kirkhus E, Handeland KS, et al: Childhood osteomyelitis—incidence and differentiation from other acute onset musculoskeletal features in a population-based study. BMC Pediatr 8:45, 2008.
12. Burnett MW, Bass JW, Cook BA: Etiology of osteomyelitis complicating sickle cell disease. Pediatrics 101:296–297, 1998.
13. Unkila-Kallio L, Kallio MJ, Eskola J, et al: Serum C-reactive protein, erythrocyte sedimentation rate, and white blood cell count in acute hematogenous osteomyelitis of children. Pediatrics 93:59–62, 1994.
14. Kang SN, Sanghera T, Mangwani J, et al: The management of septic arthritis in children: systematic review of the English language literature. J Bone Joint Surg Br 91:1127–1133, 2009.
15. Rice PA: Gonococcal arthritis (disseminated gonococcal infection). Infect Dis Clin North Am 19:853–861, 2005.
16. Kocher MS, Zurakowski D, Kasser JR: Differentiating between septic arthritis and transient synovitis of the hip in children: an evidence-based clinical prediction algorithm. J Bone Joint Surg Am 81:1662–1670, 1999.
17. Milewski MD, Cruz AI, Jr, Miller CP, et al: Lyme arthritis in children presenting with joint effusions. J Bone Joint Surg Am 93:252–260, 2011.

| Chapter 19 | *Pediatric Pathologic Fractures* |
| --- | --- |
| | Mark C. Lee, Silas Marshall, and John C. Brancato |

## INTRODUCTION

■ A pathologic fracture is a fracture through abnormal bone.
■ Bone can become abnormal in its structural properties as a result of local or generalized processes that weaken the bone.
■ The spectrum of pathologic processes is broad and ranges from benign local phenomena such as simple bone cysts to global collagen abnormalities such as osteogenesis imperfecta (OI). Causes of pathologic fractures in pediatric patients are listed in Box 19-1.
■ Any fracture that occurs with an incongruous mechanism of injury, such as a femoral shaft fracture from a simple twist, must be evaluated for the possibility of a pathologic process.

## GENERAL APPROACH TO A PEDIATRIC PATIENT WITH A PATHOLOGIC FRACTURE

■ A thorough history and physical examination are required. The information provided by the patient and the patient's family allows the clinician to narrow the differential diagnosis considerably.
  • Age of patient—certain lesions are more common in certain age groups (e.g., Wilms' tumor occurs in children <5 years old)
  • Location of symptoms—different diseases are more common in different areas of specific bones
  • Pain characteristics—specifically, duration of pain symptoms, timing, and alleviating and worsening factors

  • Associated signs—erythema or fevers may suggest infection
■ Plain radiographs of the fracture and the bone provide invaluable diagnostic information.
  • Size of the lesion—big lesions suggest aggressive behavior; smaller lesions suggest less aggressive behavior
  • Location of the lesion—different bony processes have a preference for specific bone regions (Figs. 19-1 and 19-2)
  • Bony response to the lesion—the response of the bone to the presence of the lesion may indicate the aggressiveness of the lesion; if the bone establishes thick cortical walls around the lesion, a slow process is suggested; thinned and expansile walls suggest a rapid, aggressive process
  • Effect of the lesion on bone—distinguishing between an osteolytic, osteoblastic, or mixed process can narrow the diagnosis
  • Associated soft tissue mass—a concurrent soft tissue mass suggests a malignant process
■ In all cases, it is useful to rule out bone infection as a cause of the pathologic fracture with additional laboratory studies (white blood cell count, C-reactive protein). Serum vitamin D levels may be useful for evaluating patients with suspected rickets. Additional imaging studies such as magnetic resonance imaging (MRI) and computed tomography scan may help to narrow the diagnosis further and distinguish malignant from benign processes.
■ In all pathologic fractures, it is necessary to understand that the fracture is a symptom of a primary diagnosis. The treating physician not only must treat the fracture but also understand the cause of the fracture and treat the inciting process as well.

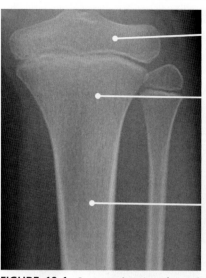

**FIGURE 19-1.** Common locations for pathologic lesions in pediatric long bones.

Brodie's abscess
Chondroblastoma
Giant cell tumor

Almost all tumors

Adamnatinoma
Fibrous dysplasia
Eosinophilic granuloma
Ewing's sarcoma
Lymphoma/leukemia

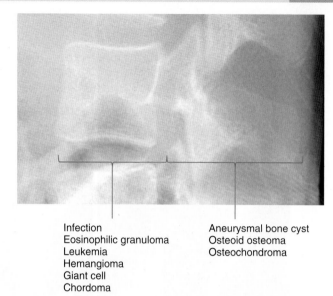

Infection
Eosinophilic granuloma
Leukemia
Hemangioma
Giant cell
Chordoma

Aneurysmal bone cyst
Osteoid osteoma
Osteochondroma

**FIGURE 19-2.** Common location of pediatric pathologic lesions in the spine.

## Box 19-1 Common Causes of Pathologic Fractures in Pediatric Patients

**Benign Bony Lesions\***
Unicameral bone cyst
Aneurysmal bone cyst
Nonossifying fibroma
Fibrous dysplasia
Chondroblastoma
Giant cell tumor
Brown tumor (hyperparathyroidism)
Langerhans cell histiocytosis and eosinophilic granuloma
Osteomyelitis and Brodie's abscess
Enchondroma

**Malignant Bony Lesions**
Metastatic tumors (neuroblastoma, Wilms' tumor)
Leukemia
Ewing's sarcoma
Osteogenic sarcoma

**Generalized Causes**
Neuromuscular disease (cerebral palsy, muscular dystrophy)
Neurofibromatosis
Osteogenesis imperfecta
Rickets and dietary deficiencies
Iatrogenic fractures

\*The listed diagnoses in this group share plain radiographic features and should be considered jointly in the differential of a lytic bony lesion.

## UNICAMERAL BONE CYST

- Unicameral bone cyst (UBC) is a benign solitary cystic lesion that occupies the metaphysis or metadiaphysis of long bones.
- Although the etiology is unclear, theories range from a developmental process in which there is an obstruction to the drainage of bony interstitial fluid to a true synovial neoplastic process with associated genetic alterations.[1,2]

- The proximal humerus and proximal femur are the site of UBCs in 40% to 80% of cases.[3] However, cysts may be found in almost any bone, including the calcaneus and ilium.
- Of cysts, 90% are found in patients younger than 20 years old with a 2:1 male-to-female ratio.[1,4]
- In 70% of cases, patients initially present with a pathologic fracture after minor trauma.[5]
- UBCs are classified as "active" or "latent" according to their relationship with the growth plate. Active cysts are closely opposed to the growth plate and may affect growth, whereas latent cysts tend to migrate away from the growth plate with growth.
- Plain radiographs are typically sufficient to make a diagnosis. UBCs are well-defined, centrally located lytic lesions surrounded by a sclerotic margin with a narrow zone of transition from normal bone to cyst (Fig. 19-3). On MRI, which is required in rare cases, UBCs typically appear as homogeneous bright signal on T2-weighted images and intermediate signal on T1-weighted images.
- Most UBCs persist into adulthood. However, most active UBCs stabilize and migrate away from the growth plate, and a few spontaneously regress by puberty.[3]
- Lesions with a typical radiographic appearance do not require biopsy and simply need serial radiographic evaluation.
- Lesions that involve more than 50% to 80% of the bone diameter on plain radiographs are at high risk for fracture and require prophylactic surgical treatment, especially UBCs that are painful or are in weight-bearing bones such as the hip.[6]
- Only 15% of UBCs resolve spontaneously after fracture. Complications from fracture through UBC include malunion, growth arrest, and proximal femoral osteonecrosis.[6]

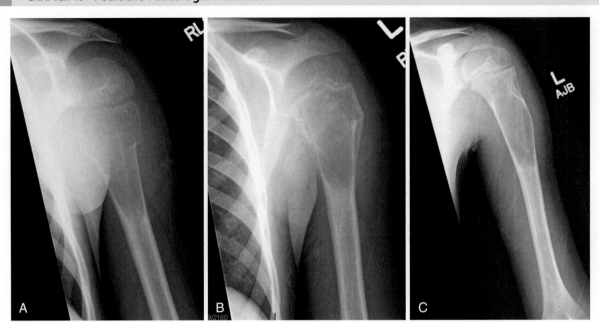

**FIGURE 19-3. A,** Large, proximal humeral UBC in a 6-year-old boy who sustained a minimally displaced pathologic fracture after a fall. **B,** At 4 weeks from injury, the fracture shows some healing. **C,** At 1.5 years after injury, the cyst has migrated from the proximal humeral physis but persists with its original dimensions.

## ANEURYSMAL BONE CYST

- Aneurysmal bone cysts (ABCs) are benign, locally aggressive bone tumors consisting of fibrous tissue and blood-filled spaces that typically occur in the metaphysis of long bones or the posterior elements of the spine.[7]
- The lesion is most likely a neoplastic process with evidence of a constitutive activation of a benign protease (ubiquitin protease 6).[8]
- The incidence of ABCs is on the order of 1.4 per 100,000, and ABCs represent 1.5% of all primary bone tumors.[9]
- Of ABCs, 75% are seen in patients younger than 20 years old; 50% are seen in patients 10 to 20 years old.[4]
- The long bones are involved in approximately 65% of patients, with the femur, tibia, and humerus most commonly involved. The vertebrae are involved in 12% to 27% of patients, with the lumbar vertebrae most commonly affected.[9,10]
- ABCs appear as eccentric bone lesions on radiographs with a thin, sometimes disrupted overlying cortex. The cystic spaces are septated, with a "soap bubble" appearance. Lesions near the growth plate tend to expand beyond the width of the adjacent epiphysis. Lesions in short tubular bones such as the metacarpals are typically more central, and spine lesions are typically in the posterior elements. Sometimes an involved vertebra has collapsed through the ABC, and the lesion manifests as a vertebra plana.[10]
- Although not pathognomonic, MRI can show a double-density fluid level with low signal on T1 images and high signal on T2 images.[11]
- Pathologic fractures occur in 11% to 35% of patients with ABCs of the long bones; most fractures occur in the femur and humerus (Fig. 19-4).[12]

- Simple immobilization as definitive treatment for fractures through ABCs is inadequate because recurrence is high, especially in pediatric patients.[12]
- The typical surgical approach is curettage with bone graft and surgical adjuvant therapy, such as cryotherapy, phenol, or laser ablation. The reported recurrence rate after this approach is approximately 10%.[13]

## NONOSSIFYING FIBROMA AND FIBROUS CORTICAL DEFECT

- Nonossifying fibromas (NOFs) and fibrous cortical defects (FCDs) are the most common bone tumors or tumor-like conditions seen in growing children. FCD differs from NOF only in that FCD is typically less than 2 cm in size and is mostly intracortical, whereas NOF is greater than 4 cm in size and can involve the entire extent of the long bone.[14]
- FCDs and NOFs can be seen in 25% of lower extremity radiographs of pediatric patients.[15] The actual incidence may be higher because most cases are asymptomatic.
- Most lesions are located in the distal femur, proximal tibia, and fibula.
- Histologically, these lesions consist of fibrous tissue, foam cells, and multinucleated giant cells.
- Radiographically, these are lytic lesions with a thick, sclerotic rim that are usually intracortical. Larger lesions extend across the diameter of the bone and along the intramedullary space.
- FCDs and NOFs spontaneously regress over time.[16] However, large lesions may cause pathologic fractures, typically in boys 6 to 14 years old.[15]
- No specific size criteria absolutely predict the likelihood of pathologic fracture. Given the benign natural history, most patients with large lesions may simply be observed.

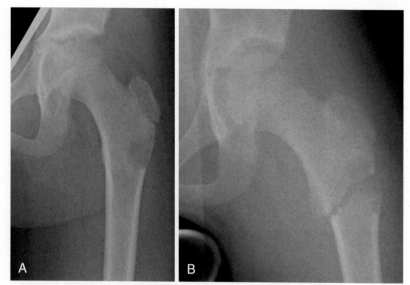

FIGURE 19-4. **A,** ABC in the proximal femur of a 9-year-old girl. **B,** The patient presented several months later with a pathologic fracture.

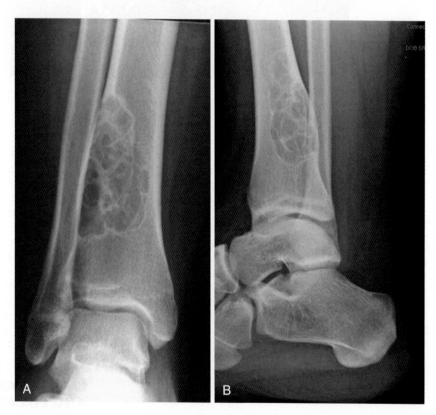

FIGURE 19-5. Anteroposterior **(A)** and lateral **(B)** projections of the ankle in a 13-year-old boy with activity-related pain. A large, septated, eccentric nonossifying fibroma is apparent in the distal tibia.

Relative indications for prophylactic treatment include a large lesion (>50% cortical diameter) in an active patient or a patient with pain.[17]

- Pathologic fractures through NOFs or FCDs may be managed with simple immobilization because healing is typically predictable, and repeat fractures are rare.[18] Surgery is necessary when there is concern of pathologic repeat fracture through a very large lesion, when the nature of the lesion is unclear, and in displaced distal femoral lesions (Fig. 19-5).[17]

## GIANT CELL TUMOR

- Giant cell tumors (GCT) are benign, aggressive tumors that involve the epiphysis of long bones after closure of the growth plate.
- GCTs are rarely identified in patients with persistent growth plates. The diagnosis is considered in pediatric patients 14 to 18 years old.[19]
- The incidence of pathologic fracture has been reported to be 30%.[20]

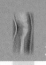
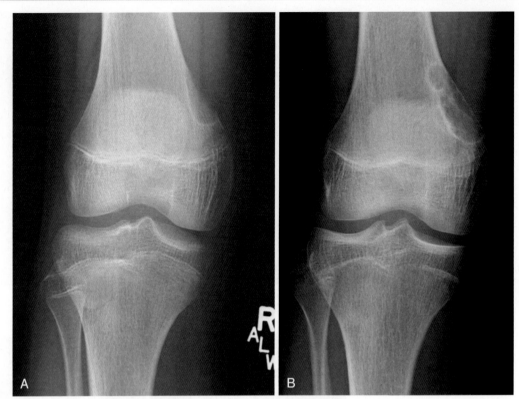

**FIGURE 19-6. A,** Anteroposterior projection of a well-circumscribed, eccentric, lytic lesion along the distal femur in a 15-year-old boy. **B,** The lesion has grown significantly 1 year later with a multiloculated appearance, inconsistent with NOF. Biopsy revealed GCT in an atypical location.

- Radiographically, GCTs are lytic epiphyseal lesions with well-defined borders that begin eccentrically but can extend into the metaphysis after physeal closure or across the entire epiphysis. Little sclerosis is present at the borders of these lesions (Fig. 19-6).
- GCTs associated with fracture typically require a biopsy to rule out other potential malignant diagnoses. The typical treatment involves extended curettage with adjuvant chemotherapy and cementation for structural support. Minimally to moderately displaced fractures are typically treated with operative reduction and fixation, although increasing displacement increases the complexity of the procedure and decreases the likelihood of restoring a functional joint.[21]

## ENCHONDROMA

- Enchondromas are benign cartilaginous tumors that are typically multiple in pediatric patients and may be part of a syndrome (Ollier syndrome and Maffucci syndrome).
- The most common sites of involvement are the phalanges, metacarpals, metatarsals, humerus, and femur.
- The most common presentation is pathologic fracture in the phalanges of the hands or feet.[22] Pathologic fracture in other locations is rare.
- Radiographically, enchondromas are central intramedullary lesions composed of cartilage with spotty calcification. Larger lesions cause cortical expansion, thinning, and fracture.

- Patients with Ollier syndrome may have concurrent growth disturbances in the lower extremities. With Maffucci syndrome, multiple hemangiomas are present in the setting of multiple enchondromas. Pathologic fractures occur in 30% of patients with Maffucci syndrome and are prone to nonunion or delayed union. Sarcomatous degeneration can occur in both conditions but is more commonly identified in Maffucci syndrome, with an incidence of 15%.[23]
- Symptomatic lesions without fracture are treated well with curettage and bone grafting.[24] Displaced fractures may be treated either with simple immobilization or internal fixation, depending on fracture characteristics.

## LANGERHANS CELL HISTIOCYTOSIS AND EOSINOPHILIC GRANULOMA

- Langerhans cell histiocytosis (LCH) comprises a rare group of disorders linked by the common pathologic finding of the Langerhans cell, a large, dendritic cell with characteristic tennis racket–shaped cytoplasmic organelles termed *Birbeck granules*. When an isolated bony lesion is noted, present terminology calls this condition eosinophilic granuloma (EG).
- LCH and EG are primarily disorders of childhood; 50% of cases occur in children younger than 15 years. The annual incidence of LCH and EG is 6 per 1 million children per year, with a peak incidence between 1 and 4 years old.[25]

- The disease course and presentation are highly variable. The disease may be isolated to a single bone or may involve multiple osseous locations and organ systems. Symptoms depend on the location of the lesion. In osseous involvement, bone pain occurs with night pain symptoms in 50% to 90% of patients.[26] Spinal LCH can manifest with aching neck or back pain or, with more extensive involvement, produce vertebral collapse with kyphosis. Mastoid lesions can cause diminished hearing and otitis media. LCH can involve soft tissue organ systems, contributing to symptoms such as diabetes insipidus, pituitary deficiency, hepatosplenomegaly, thrombocytopenia, and anemia. Letterer-Siwe disease is a LCH syndrome with autosomal recessive transmission that causes lymphadenopathy and hepatosplenomegaly and has a mortality rate of 50% in children.[27]
- The radiographic presentation is highly variable, and the disease has been called the "great imitator." Skeletal lesions may be solitary or multiple. Lesions typically occur in the diaphysis or metaphysis but may rarely occur in the epiphysis. Lesions typically have a lytic appearance with well-defined borders but can have varying degrees of sclerosis with periosteal reaction if a fracture has occurred. Vertebral involvement may manifest as a collapsed vertebra (vertebra plana) with notable preservation of the adjacent disk spaces.[28]
- Standard fracture care is adequate for the uncommon pathologic fracture through LCH or EG because fracture healing is not impaired. However, a biopsy is necessary to differentiate the lesion from more malignant bony processes. When the diagnosis is established, small lesions may be observed because the natural history of these lesions is typically one of gradual regression. For larger lesions, a range of treatment options has been reported to result in lesion healing including curettage, curettage and bone grafting, irradiation, and steroid injection. Chemotherapy is sometimes indicated in cases of multiple bone involvement or visceral involvement.[27]

## FIBROUS DYSPLASIA

- Fibrous dysplasia (FD) is a developmental abnormality of bone in which expansile fibrous lesions with metaplastic woven bone develop. These fibro-osseous lesions have no clear etiology, although the disease may be related to the autosomal dominant transmission of proto-oncogenes.[29]
- FD may involve only one bone (monostotic) or involve multiple bones (polyostotic). Associated endocrine abnormalities may be identified with either variety, including hyperparathyroidism, growth hormone excess, and hypercortisolism.[30]
- The diagnosis is most commonly made in patients 5 to 15 years old, although younger and older patients have been reported.[31] Most patients with polyostotic FD are diagnosed before age 10 years with limp, deformity, or pathologic fracture.[32]
- Most lesions are asymptomatic. However, pain may develop in the setting of subtle microfractures with associated progressive bony deformity or a complete pathologic fracture.
- Unilateral involvement of a single extremity is the typical pattern, although polyostotic FD may involve the spine and is frequently associated with limb length discrepancy.
- The most common fracture sites are the proximal femur, humerus, radius, ribs, and bones of the face. The severity of the bony metabolic disturbance is reflected in the number of fractures, the age at first fracture, and the fracture rate.
- Healing in pathologic fractures is typically not compromised in the monostotic form but may be delayed in the polyostotic variety.
- FD lesions have a 0.5% incidence of sarcomatous degeneration, which occurs approximately 15 years after the initial diagnosis.
- On radiographs, FD generally appears as a mixed sclerotic and lytic diaphyseal lesion with a ground-glass appearance that is a product of metaplastic woven bone (Fig. 19-7). Associated bowing and angular deformity may exist. Bone scan and skeletal survey are helpful to distinguish monostotic from polyostotic forms.
- Treatment for diaphyseal fractures through small lesions is simple cast immobilization because healing potential is not compromised. Proximal femoral pathologic fractures and fractures through large areas of diseased bone, as found in the polyostotic form, may require curettage, bone grafting, and internal fixation. Internal fixation provides better maintenance of fracture alignment in patients younger than 18 years old.[33]

## OSTEOMYELITIS

- Bone infections in children are discussed in more detail in Chapter 18.
- Pathologic fracture at the site of an infection is rare in the developed world and is typically a product of neglected or chronic osteomyelitis, neonatal osteomyelitis, or septic arthritis.
- When pathologic fracture occurs through a site of infection, treatment may be challenging and can be complicated by nonunion, malunion, and growth arrest.[34,35]
- Initial management of pathologic fractures through infected bone centers on immobilization. Definitive surgical treatment is focused on aggressive débridement of the sequestrum, with or without bone autograft and supplemental internal fixation, and extended antibiotic therapy.[36]

## SICKLE CELL DISEASE

- Sickle cell disease (SCD) is an autosomal recessive disease in which a mild alteration in the protein structure of hemoglobin causes sickling of red blood cells in low oxygen tension environments, resulting in ischemic injury to multiple tissues including bone.
- Pathologic fractures in patients with SCD are relatively common; the range is from 20% to 25%.[37,38]

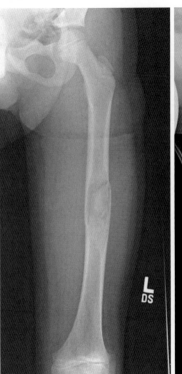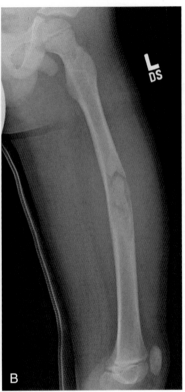

**FIGURE 19-7.** Anteroposterior **(A)** and lateral **(B)** projections of the femur in an 8-year-old boy with inability to bear weight. The ground glass appearance of the lesion in the midshaft of the femur with associated fracture is classic for fibrous dysplasia.

■ The exact mechanism of pathologic fracture in SCD is unclear. Although the fracture is often associated with a bony infarct, the fracture itself does not typically occur through the site of infarct. Overlying osteomyelitis may often be the contributing factor to fracture. In addition, there may be an intrinsic predisposition to fracture from a combination of whole body mineral content deficits in children with SCD and marrow hyperplasia with resultant cortical thinning.[39,40]

■ Pathologic fractures in SCD are typically displaced despite a history of minimal trauma. Definitive management of fractures typically is nonoperative, and healing is not impaired.

■ Operative fixation is indicated for proximal femoral fractures or fractures of the femoral shaft.

■ If operative intervention is considered, it is critical to minimize the sickle hemoglobin concentrations before surgical intervention to prevent perioperative systemic complications. The patient's hemoglobin concentration should be maintained at greater than 10 g/dL with transfusions and aggressive intravenous hydration.

## NEUROFIBROMATOSIS

■ Neurofibromatosis (NF) is an autosomal dominant condition with variable penetrance that involves the hypertrophy and hyperplasia of numerous tissues, including nerves, vessels, skin, and bones.

■ NF occurs in 1 in 3000 live births. NF-1 is the form with multiple orthopedic manifestations including pseudarthrosis of long bones and kyphoscoliosis.

■ Pseudarthrosis, a painless but mobile nonunion at the site of a fracture, most commonly occurs in the tibia in patients with NF-1 (Fig. 19-8). However, pseudarthroses may occur in various alternative locations, including the radius, ulna, femur, clavicle, and humerus.[41,42]

■ Tibial pseudarthrosis in NF-1 is termed congenital, but the actual pseudarthrosis does not develop until 1 year of life. However, tibial deformity may be noted earlier.[43]

■ Radiographically, pseudarthrosis in the tibia initially appears as a diaphyseal cyst or persistent fracture line in a section of sclerotic, thinned bone that commonly has an associated anterolateral bowing deformity. With complete fracture and displacement, the fracture ends appear markedly atrophic, with a smaller shaft diameter than the more proximal or distal tibial segments.

■ Definitive treatment for tibial pseudarthrosis is typically surgical, although functional bracing may be used for short intervals. The historical results of surgery have been poor, and amputation is a common end result after multiple attempts at surgical salvage. More recent data suggest promising results with the use of bone morphogenetic proteins.[44]

## NEUROMUSCULAR DISEASE

Diseases in the category of neuromuscular disease are varied and include pathologies such as myelomeningocele, cerebral palsy (CP), muscular dystrophy, and spinal cord injury. However, these diseases share in common the disturbance of the neuromotor unit with resultant skeletal fragility from disuse and osteoporosis. The following

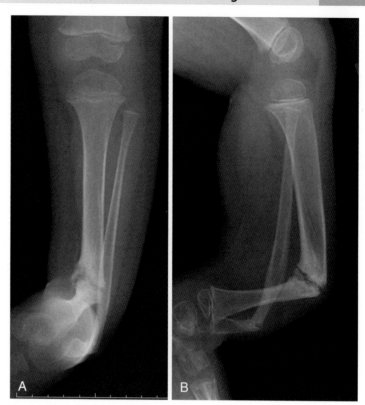

**FIGURE 19-8.** Anteroposterior **(A)** and lateral **(B)** projections of the tibia in a 3-year-old boy shows significant angular deformity at the site of a tibial pseudarthrosis in the setting of NF type 1.

sections briefly summarize each disease process and describe management options for the associated pathologic fractures.

## Myelomeningocele

■ Myelomeningocele is the abnormal failure of the neural sac to close in utero. The congenital defect results in a motor and sensory deficit that typically can be localized to the level of the closure defect. Patients can have minimal involvement with mild bladder control issues (sacral level) or be wheelchair bound with limited control of upper and lower extremities (cervical level).

■ Fractures in patients with myelomeningocele result from multifactorial causes and include disuse osteopenia in nonambulators, immobilization from reconstructive procedures, and increased urinary calcium loss.[45]

■ The incidence of fractures in children with myelomeningocele is 12% to 31%.[46] Most fractures occur in the lower extremity, most commonly in metaphyseal and diaphyseal locations from minor trauma, and typically consist of minimally displaced fractures that heal rapidly.

■ Lower extremity injuries in ambulatory patients are treated with standard approaches to fracture care.

■ Most lower extremity fractures in nonambulatory patients may be treated with minimal immobilization, such as with a bulky Ace wrap dressing or a splint, and predictably heal within 3 to 4 weeks.

■ Physeal fracture is an unusual subtype of fracture that occurs in patients with myelomeningocele and often presents a diagnostic and treatment challenge. The fracture may manifest as massive swelling with erythema and an elevated white blood cell count, mimicking infection. Radiographically, the fracture appears initially as physeal widening with irregularity and may progress to a striking picture of massive periosteal reaction. In contrast to diaphyseal and metaphyseal fractures, treatment is typically with casting for 8 to 12 weeks with non–weight bearing precautions because delayed healing is observed in the absence of less stringent treatment.[47]

## Cerebral Palsy

■ CP is an anatomically nonprogressive neonatal encephalopathy that results in spasticity and associated movement disorders with variable involvement of the extremities. Affected patients range from fully functional patients with mild weakness in one ankle to nonambulatory, nonverbal patients with a severe seizure disorder.

■ Risks associated with pathologic fracture in children with CP include nonambulatory status, anticonvulsant therapy, feeding gastrostomy tube, elevated body mass index, and history of previous fracture.[48,49]

■ Most fractures occur with low-energy mechanisms. However, fractures may also occur without a history of trauma in nonambulatory patients, simply from routine positioning activities or transfers.[48,50] A combination of disuse osteopenia, nutritional deficiencies (particularly vitamin D), and preexisting joint contractures predisposes patients with severe CP to these fractures (Fig. 19-9).

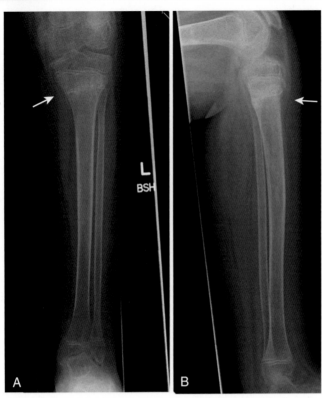

**FIGURE 19-9.** Anteroposterior **(A)** and lateral **(B)** projections of the tibia in an 11-year-old boy with spastic quadriplegia. Diffuse osteopenia is noted with an insufficiency fracture of the proximal tibia *(arrow)*.

- The goal of fracture treatment in patients with CP is restoration of baseline function.
- Ambulatory patients require anatomic alignment with conventional forms of surgical and nonsurgical treatment. Surgical options are desirable to allow early mobilization because patients with CP often require more time to recover from short periods of immobilization.
- For nonambulatory children, the goal should be the preservation of the ability to transfer. It is acceptable to sacrifice fracture alignment to prevent the complications of further disuse osteopenia, skin breakdown with immobilization, and interference with daily care. Casts for immobilization should be applied with abundant padding over bony prominences. The distal femoral buckle fracture, a common fracture variant in these patients, is easily treated with a bulky, well-padded Ace wrap from thigh to ankle.

### Duchenne Muscular Dystrophy

- Duchenne muscular dystrophy (DMD) is a sex-linked disorder of muscle characterized by progressive muscular degeneration. Clinically, patients deteriorate from ambulatory in juvenile years to nonambulatory in adolescence. Life expectancy is typically to the mid-20s.
- Risk factors for fractures in DMD include age older than 9 years, nonambulatory status, and history of steroid treatment.[51,52] Fractures are a product of a global

osteoporosis, most profound in the lower extremities, that develops before loss of ambulatory ability.[53]

- Fractures are most commonly located in the femur and proximal humerus.[51]
- Fracture management in ambulatory patients with DMD focuses on not causing the premature loss of ambulatory function with the proposed treatment. Walking ability is typically tenuous in patients with fractures, and small periods of immobilization can permanently destroy ambulatory function. In one report, 25% of ambulatory patients lost the ability to walk after fracture.[54]
- Although treatment should be individualized, prolonged rigid casting should be limited. Upper extremity fractures generally may be managed in a sling. Lower extremity fractures may be treated in light walking casts or braces. Physical therapy and routine activities should be initiated as soon as tolerable.[54]
- Operative fracture intervention is rarely considered in nonambulatory patients because medical comorbidities, such as a significantly limited pulmonary reserve and baseline cardiomyopathy, effectively preclude all procedures that are not critical to subsequent function.

### Spinal Cord Injury

- Spinal cord injury in childhood is uncommon.
- The etiology of fracture is osteoporosis in a denervated limb.[55]
- The most common fractures are along the distal femur and tibia.[56]
- Fractures should be managed according to the treatment recommendations for patients with myelomeningocele.

## OSTEOGENESIS IMPERFECTA

- Osteogenesis imperfecta (OI) comprises a heterogeneous group of inherited disorders resulting from an abnormality in the structure and function of type I collagen.
- Incidence is 1 in 20,000 births, with a prevalence of 16 per 1 million.[57,58]
- The disorder is genetically heterogeneous, with more than 150 mutations described.
- The spectrum of clinical presentations is diverse and reflects the variability in the specific genetic abnormality (Figs. 19-10 and 19-11). Some patients are nonambulatory with a short-trunked dwarfism, marked limb deformity with fractures in various stages of healing, and associated kyphoscoliosis. Other patients are morphologically and functionally normal with a limited number of long bone fractures over a lifetime.[57]
- Radiographic findings are also variable. Patients with severe OI have old fractures with residual angular deformity, marked osteoporosis, and gracile long bones with cystic foci. Vertebral compression deformities (codfish vertebra) may be identified on spine radiographs of patients with severe OI. Patients with mild OI have

**TABLE 20-1** Musculoskeletal Examination of the Upper Extremity

| Nerve | Motor | Sensory | Result of Injury |
|---|---|---|---|
| Axillary | Deltoid muscle | Lateral aspect shoulder | Weak shoulder abduction |
| Musculocutaneous | Biceps and brachialis muscle | Lateral aspect forearm | Weak elbow flexion |
| Median | Finger and wrist flexors | Volar forearm and radial half of palm | Weak wrist and finger flexion, decreased sensation in first palmar web space |
| Ulnar | Interosseous muscle | Ulnar side of hand | Weak finger abduction, loss of sensation along small finger |
| Radial | Finger and wrist extensors | Dorsal forearm and radial half of dorsum of hand | Weak wrist and finger extension, loss of sensation in first dorsal web space |

secondary to pain. Loss of active and passive range of motion is more indicative of dislocation or loose bodies within the joint.

- Neurologic Examination
  - The upper extremity is innervated by nerves arising from the brachial plexus. Brachial plexus injury is a rare but serious complication of clavicle fractures, shoulder dislocations, and proximal humerus fractures.
  - However, brachial plexus injury rarely warrants emergent management and is often treated with observation.
  - Every musculoskeletal examination of the upper extremity must include evaluation of both motor and sensory input from each of the five branches of the brachial plexus (Table 20-1).
- Vascular Examination
  - A vascular examination is imperative for all injuries of the upper extremity. There is potential for occlusion or disruption of the vessels in the upper extremity at multiple points in the vascular tree.
  - Vascular compromise with reduced or absent perfusion to the extremity is an emergency.
  - Evaluation of adequate perfusion requires several points of inspection.

The axillary artery pulse can be palpated in the axilla.

The brachial artery pulse can be palpated just proximal to the elbow, posterior and medial to the biceps muscle (Fig. 20-5).

The radial artery pulse can be palpated at the wrist just radial to the flexor carpi radialis tendon (Fig. 20-6).

The ulnar artery pulse can be palpated just radial to the pisiform bone at the wrist (see Fig. 20-6).

Capillary refill in the fingers should be less than 2 seconds.

Signs of poor perfusion in the upper extremity include blue or dusky color in the fingers or hand.

## DIAGNOSTIC STUDIES

- X-ray (Fig. 20-7)
  - An anteroposterior shoulder film is obtained relative to the plane of the scapula. The AP film is used to

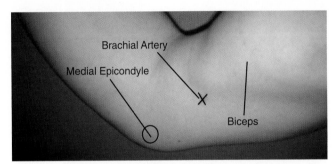

**FIGURE 20-5.** Anatomic locations for palpation of the brachial artery pulse.

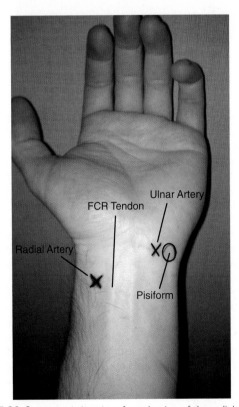

**FIGURE 20-6.** Anatomic locations for palpation of the radial and ulnar artery pulses.

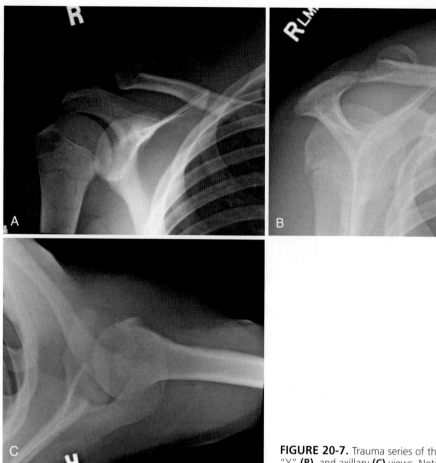

**FIGURE 20-7.** Trauma series of the shoulder, including anteroposterior **(A)**, scapular "Y" **(B)**, and axillary **(C)** views. Note the distal clavicle fracture identified in this series.

evaluate for shoulder dislocation, clavicle fractures, acromioclavicular joint separations, proximal humeral fractures, and scapular fractures.

- A scapular "Y" view is taken parallel to the scapular body and can be used to visualize scapular fractures. However, this view is unhelpful when evaluating traumatic shoulder injuries.
- The axillary view is a mandatory view for all traumatic shoulder injuries. It is used to evaluate for shoulder dislocations and glenoid or acromial fractures.
- A Velpeaux view is an acceptable option for a patient who cannot abduct the shoulder secondary to pain (Fig. 20-8).

■ Computed Tomography (CT) Scan
- CT scan is necessary to evaluate scapular fractures, intra-articular proximal humerus fractures, or glenohumeral dislocation when an axillary or modified axillary view is not possible because of patient discomfort. In addition, CT is the study of choice to evaluate medial third clavicle fractures.

■ Magnetic Resonance Imaging (MRI)
- MRI is rarely used in the acute setting but can be used to evaluate for osteomyelitis or septic sternoclavicular, acromioclavicular, or glenohumeral joint arthritis. In the outpatient setting, MRI is used to look for ligament, tendon, labral, and muscle injury.

■ Ultrasound
- Ultrasound can be used to look for sternoclavicular, acromioclavicular, and glenohumeral joint effusions.
- In infants, ultrasound can be used to make the diagnosis of clavicle fracture, proximal humeral epiphyseal separation, or shoulder dislocation.

■ Joint Aspiration
- Definitive diagnosis of joint sepsis can be accomplished with aspiration of the affected joint.
- The shoulder should be aspirated 2 cm distal and 2 cm medial to the posterolateral corner of the acromion (Fig. 20-9). The needle should be directed toward the coracoid process anteriorly.
- Aspirated fluid should be sent for Gram stain, culture, cell count with differential, and crystal analysis.

■ Laboratory Tests
- In cases of suspected septic glenohumeral, acromioclavicular, or sternoclavicular joints or osteomyelitis, appropriate laboratory work should be sent as outlined in Chapter 18.

## DIFFERENTIAL DIAGNOSIS

■ Cervical spine injury should always be considered in the differential diagnosis.

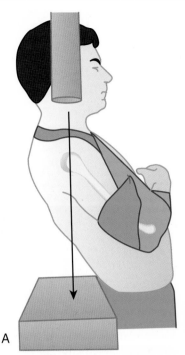 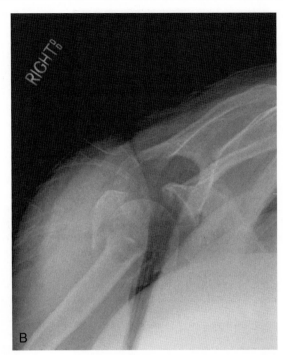

**FIGURE 20-8. A,** Velpeau axillary lateral technique. **B,** Comminuted proximal humerus fracture in a skeletally mature individual imaged with the Velpeau technique. *(From Cuomo F, Zuckerman JD: Proximal humerus fracture. In Browner BD, editor: Techniques in orthopaedics, vol 9. New York, 1994, Raven Press, p 143.)*

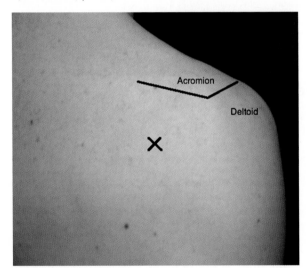

**FIGURE 20-9.** Posterior view of the right shoulder showing the appropriate position for needle aspiration and injection of the glenohumeral injection (2 cm distal and 2 cm medial to the posterolateral corner of the acromion).

- Clavicle fracture
- Proximal humeral physeal fracture
- Humeral shaft fracture
- Shoulder dislocation
- Brachial plexus palsy
- Septic shoulder
- Hemiplegia
- Stroke
- Child abuse

## TREATMENT OF SPECIFIC INJURIES

- Shoulder (Glenohumeral) Dislocation (Fig. 20-10)
  - Dislocations of the glenohumeral joint are very rare in patients with open growth plates, and descriptions typically exist as small case series.[1] With the mechanism of injury for a glenohumeral dislocation, pediatric patients more frequently sustain a fracture through the proximal physis.
  - Shoulder dislocations are classified and treated similarly to shoulder dislocations in adults (see Chapter 9).
  - Classification of pediatric shoulder dislocations should also include any bony deformity (glenoid dysplasia) or syndromic hyperlaxity (e.g., Ehlers-Danlos syndrome). Similarly, a distinction should be made between traumatic and atraumatic dislocations.
  - Risk of recurrence in pediatric and adolescent patients is significantly higher than in adults. Risk of recurrence is typically related to age of first dislocation. Overall, the risk of recurrent dislocation in younger patients approaches 90%.[1,2]
- Clavicle Fracture
  - Fracture of the clavicle is one of the most common childhood fractures, constituting 8% to 15% of all

- Distal and medial third clavicle fractures may mimic sternoclavicular joint and acromioclavicular joint dislocations in pediatric patients.
- Infections involving the shoulder include septic sternoclavicular, acromioclavicular, or glenohumeral joints and osteomyelitis (rare in the upper extremity).
- Pathologic fractures, especially involving benign cystic lesions along the proximal humerus, should be distinguished from fracture through normal bone.
- A broad differential diagnosis needs to be considered in infants with pseudoparalysis of one extremity.

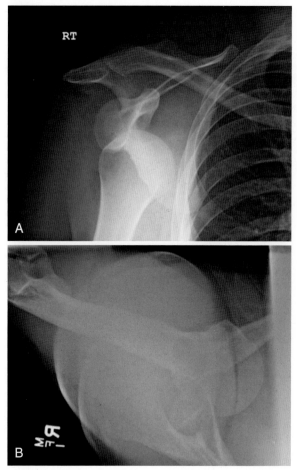

**FIGURE 20-10.** Anteroposterior **(A)** and axillary **(B)** views of an antero-inferior shoulder dislocation in an 18-year-old boy. Note the anterior position of the proximal humerus relative to the glenoid on the axillary lateral view.

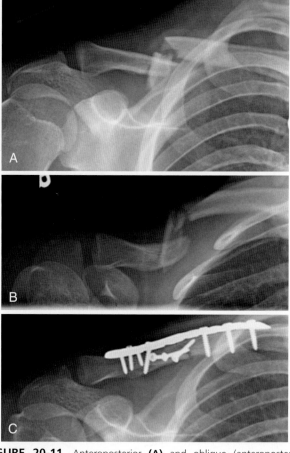

**FIGURE 20-11.** Anteroposterior **(A)** and oblique (anteroposterior with beam angled 30 degrees cephalad) **(B)** views of the right clavicle. A segmental clavicle fracture is noted. Operative fixation was performed for this clavicle fracture **(C)**.

fractures, and accounts for 90% of obstetric fractures.

- Clavicle fractures are caused either by a fall onto the lateral aspect of the shoulder or by a direct blow. Obstetric fractures are caused by a medial-to-lateral pressure on the clavicle, most commonly as an unavoidable consequence of the anatomic constraints of the vaginal birthing process.
- Symptoms in newborns are typically manifested as pseudoparalysis of the limb.
- Symptoms in older children include pain at fracture site, visible deformity, and inability to abduct the arm. Numbness, paresthesias, or weakness may be present if the brachial plexus is involved. Respiratory distress may be a feature of medial clavicular fractures with mediastinal involvement.
- Anteroposterior plain radiographs typically show superior and inferior displacement, but their utility is limited by the fact that the scapula and ribs can obscure visualization. An x-ray obtained with the beam angled 30 degrees cephalad minimizes this overlap (Fig. 20-11). Evaluation of distal clavicle fractures may require an axillary lateral projection. CT scan has replaced a serendipity view (an x-ray with

the beam angled 40 degrees cephalad) for evaluation of medial clavicle fractures.

- Ultrasound can be used to make the diagnosis in neonates.
- CT scan is useful for delineating distal clavicular fractures or medial clavicular fracture dislocations. CT is the study of choice for physeal level medial clavicular fractures.
- Fractures may be classified according to anatomic location: middle third, medial third, and distal third. Most clavicle fractures are middle third (76% to 85%).

Distal third fractures—because distal clavicular epiphyseal ossification does not occur until 18 years of age, the apparent acromioclavicular joint separation in a child is typically a fracture through the distal clavicular metaphysis or physis. True acromioclavicular joint separations in children are rare.

Medial third fractures—most are Salter-Harris type I or type II fractures through the medial physis classified according to the direction of displacement, either anterior or posterior.

- Treatment is dictated by the location of the fracture, displacement, and age.

Middle third fractures

- Most middle third fractures are treated with a short period of immobilization. In infants, the shirt sleeve can be safety-pinned to the shirt for 2 weeks. In older children, a sling may be used for a short time. A figure-of-eight brace is of historical interest because this form of immobilization often contributes to shoulder edema or impairs venous return.
- Surgical indications include open fractures, neurovascular compromise, multiple trauma, or a "floating shoulder" (a clavicle fracture with associated scapular or proximal humeral fracture). Fractures in a dominant arm with more than 2 cm of shortening in young, active adolescents may have better functional results if treated operatively (see Fig. 20-11).[3]

Distal third fractures

- Most authors agree that minimally displaced distal third fractures can be treated with sling immobilization.
- Controversy exists regarding the treatment options for displaced distal third clavicle fractures in pediatric patients, with some authors suggesting no functional deficits despite wide ranges of displacement.[4]
- Most orthopedists agree that displaced distal clavicle fractures in children older than 13 years should be managed with operative reduction and stabilization, either with hardware or with suture repair.
- A follow-up visit should be scheduled for within 1 week from the emergency department visit for further management planning.

Medial third fractures

- Minimally displaced medial third clavicular fractures may be treated with a short period of sling immobilization.
- Anteriorly displaced medial third fractures may be treated with simple sling immobilization because the residual deformity has no bearing on shoulder function. A closed reduction may be attempted but is often difficult to maintain without fixation.
- Posteriorly displaced medial third fractures require immediate evaluation with CT scan secondary to potential danger to mediastinal structures. Closed reduction of the dislocation should be performed in the operating room with the assistance of a thoracic surgeon, and operative fixation typically with wire or suture fixation should be performed.

■ Scapula Fracture
- Fractures of the scapula are very rare. They are most commonly associated with high-energy blunt trauma and have a high incidence of associated injuries such as hemothorax or pneumothorax, rib fractures, flail chest, brachial plexus injury, and injury to major vessels. Associated injuries to the clavicle can result in a "floating shoulder."[5]

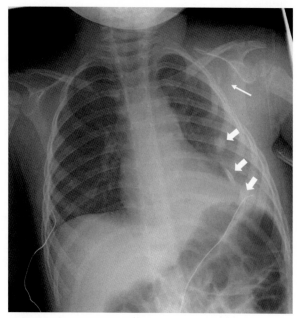

**FIGURE 20-12.** A 1.5-year-old girl was struck by a car. Chest radiograph shows a comminuted scapular body fracture *(thin arrow)* with multiple anterior rib fractures *(broad arrows).*

- Physical examination should be preformed of the upper extremity as described earlier after advanced trauma life support protocol has ruled out any intrathoracic or intra-abdominal injuries.

  The examiner should also look for evidence of clavicle or proximal humerus fractures.

  Although neurovascular injury directly related to the scapular fracture is rare, a thorough neurovascular examination should be preformed.

- Plain chest radiographs are typically the first imaging modality to reveal a scapula fracture (Fig. 20-12). Radiographs should be scrutinized for associated rib fractures or hemothorax or pneumothorax.

  Anteroposterior and scapular "Y" views of the shoulder can provide more fracture detail.

  CT scan is ultimately needed if there is concern for intra-articular involvement.

- Most closed scapula fractures can be treated with sling immobilization.
- Operative indications include the following conditions:

  Open fracture

  Associated clavicle fracture resulting in a "floating shoulder"

  Intra-articular involvement (glenoid fracture)

■ Proximal Humerus Fracture
- Proximal humerus fractures account for less than 5% of all pediatric fractures.

- Excellent remodeling potential exists in this region because the injury is through or at the level of a rapidly elongating physis.
- The mechanism of injury resulting in physeal separation in infants is birth canal trauma in vaginal deliveries, typically associated with breech presentation or large gestational size.
- For adolescents, fractures can be transphyseal or juxtaphyseal, resulting from sports or motor vehicle crashes.
- Pathologic fractures may occur in this region from malignant or benign tumors, radiation therapy, or shoulder joint neuropathy from spinal cord syrinx or myelomeningocele.
- Infants with this injury refuse to move the arm, giving the impression of a pseudoparalysis.
- Older children present with a traumatic history, pain in the shoulder, and swelling around the shoulder with loss of the normal anatomic contours.
- Injuries are classified according to the location of the fracture relative to the physis.

  Salter-Harris type I fractures are seen in patients younger than 5 years.

  Salter-Harris type II injuries are seen in patients older than 11 years with the fracture line through the metaphysis (Fig. 20-13).

  Salter-Harris type III fractures are rare and may occur with a concomitant glenohumeral dislocation.

  Salter-Harris type IV injuries have not been reported in children.

- Growth arrest is rare in these fractures.
- Metaphyseal proximal humerus fractures occur in children 5 to 12 years old.
- Treatment in patients younger than 11 years is generally conservative, despite the degree of displacement, because remodeling of the fracture results in a restoration of function. An infant with an epiphyseal level fracture generally requires simple immobilization of the sleeve to the shirt with no attempts at reduction.
- Patients older than 11 years have less remodeling capacity. Although some controversy exists regarding appropriate management for this age group, most pediatric orthopedists agree that patients in this age range with greater than 50% displacement and 20 degrees of angulation require closed reduction with or without internal fixation.

■ Humeral Shaft Fractures
- Humeral shaft fractures account for 2% to 5% of all fractures in children.
- There is a bimodal distribution with greatest frequency in patients younger than 3 years and older than 12 years.
- Humeral shaft fractures can occur as a result of the following conditions:

  Birth trauma—commonly from vaginal delivery in breech presentations or infants large for gestational age

  Child abuse—constitute 12% of all fractures in victims of child abuse

  Motor vehicle accidents, sports injuries, and penetrating trauma

  Stress injury—fracture may follow a throwing motion as a result of repetitive stresses or from poor mechanics

  Pathologic lesion—benign or malignant bone lesions or overriding conditions such as osteogenesis imperfecta may weaken the humerus

- Plain radiographs (anteroposterior and lateral or transthoracic lateral projections) typically show the

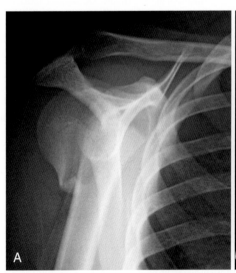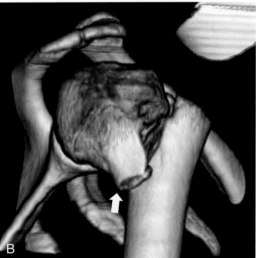

**FIGURE 20-13.** A 13-year-old girl with Salter-Harris type II proximal humerus fracture. **A,** Scapular "Y" projection of the proximal humerus shows the fracture. **B,** Three-dimensional CT reconstruction shows the fracture line at the level of the physis and the residual Thurston-Holland fragment (*arrow*).

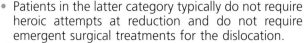

- Patients in the latter category typically do not require heroic attempts at reduction and do not require emergent surgical treatments for the dislocation.
- Clavicle Fractures
  - Patients with clavicle fractures should be examined to ensure that no sternoclavicular or acromioclavicular joint injury exists. Combined injuries more often may require surgical treatment and an orthopedic consultation.
  - Distal third fractures are typically metaphyseal or transphyseal in pediatric patients, and good healing and functional outcomes result in even widely displaced fractures.
  - Apparently painless right-sided clavicle fracture in an infant should raise the suspicion of a congenital clavicular pseudarthrosis and not an acute traumatic injury.
- Scapula Fractures
  - The clinician may fail to recognize the high-energy mechanism of injury and the potential for significant associated chest wall injury.
- Proximal Humerus Fracture
  - Most proximal humerus fractures can be treated with sling immobilization.

- Patients with less than 2 years of growth should be treated more aggressively because remodeling can be variable, and functional deficits may remain if the fracture is left significantly displaced.
- Humeral Shaft Fracture
  - Child abuse should be one of the differential diagnoses in a patient younger than 3 years old with a humeral shaft fracture, especially in combination with an unwitnessed accident or other fracture.

## References

1. Marans HJ, Angel KR, Schemitsch EH, et al: The fate of traumatic anterior dislocation of the shoulder in children. J Bone Joint Surg Am 74:1242–1244, 1992.
2. Rowe CR: Anterior dislocations of the shoulder: prognosis and treatment. Surg Clin North Am 43:1609–1614, 1963.
3. Canadian Orthopaedic Trauma Society: Nonoperative treatment compared with plate fixation of displaced midshaft clavicular fractures: a multicenter, randomized clinical trial. J Bone Joint Surg Am 89:1–10, 2007.
4. Black GB, McPherson JA, Reed MH: Traumatic pseudodislocation of the acromioclavicular joint in children: a fifteen year review. Am J Sports Med 19:644–646, 1991.
5. Goss TP: Scapular fractures and dislocations: diagnosis and treatment. J Am Acad Orthop Surg 3:22–33, 1995.
6. Beaty JH: Fractures of the proximal humerus and shaft in children. Instr Course Lect 41:369–372, 1992.

## Chapter 21 *Pediatric Elbow*

Mark C. Lee, Silas Marshall,
and John C. Brancato

## INTRODUCTION

- Upper extremity fractures account for 65% to 75% of all fractures in children, and elbow injuries constitute 7% to 9% of these injuries.[1]
- Supracondylar fractures are the most frequent elbow injuries in children, occurring in 55% to 75% of patients with elbow fractures, followed by lateral condyle fractures and medial epicondylar fractures.
- Elbow injuries are much more common in children and adolescents compared with adults. The peak age for elbow injuries is 5 to 8 years.[1]
- Reserved or delayed treatment of elbow injuries in children yields unsatisfactory results. More aggressive treatment is often required to avoid complications and to optimize function.

## ANATOMIC CONSIDERATIONS

- Bones (Fig. 21-1)
  - The elbow joint consists of the distal humerus and its articulation with the proximal ulna and proximal radius.
  - The distal humerus comprises the medial epicondyle, lateral epicondyle, trochlea, and capitellum.
  - The proximal radius comprises the radial head and neck and the bicipital tuberosity.
  - The proximal ulna comprises the olecranon, trochlear notch, and coronoid.
- Physes and Ossification (Fig. 21-2)[2]
  - The humeral shaft, radial shaft, and ulnar shaft begin ossification in utero.
  - Ossification of the lateral condyle begins at 1 to 2 years of age. Ossification of the remainder of the distal humerus and elbow proceeds in a predictable pattern, with ossification of the lateral epicondyle, occurring at age 10 years (see Chapter 18).
  - The distal humeral epiphysis includes all the secondary ossification centers of the distal humerus before age 6 years in girls and before age 8 years in boys. In older children, the epiphysis no longer includes the medial epicondyle because the medial epicondyle lies proximal to the distal humeral physeal line.
  - Just before the completion of growth, the capitellum, lateral epicondyle, and trochlea form to fuse one epiphyseal center. The distal humeral epiphysis fuses with the metaphysis. The medial epicondyle may not fuse with the distal humerus until the late teens.
  - Fusion of the proximal radial and olecranon epiphyseal centers occurs at the same time as distal humeral epiphyseal fusion, between 14 and 16 years of age.
  - The medial epicondylar apophysis is the attachment site for the forearm flexor mass and the primary medial stabilizing ligament of the elbow, the ulnar collateral ligament.
  - Ossification of the olecranon metaphysis gradually progresses proximally such that by 6 years of age, 75% of the semilunar notch is visible radiographically. Secondary centers of ossification are visible at the olecranon tip by age 9 years, and these typically fuse to themselves and to the olecranon metaphysis by 14 years.
- Joints
  - The ulnohumeral joint is the main articulation at the elbow.

    The primary stabilizers of the joint are the ulnar collateral ligament, the lateral collateral ligament, and the bony constraint of the trochlear notch.

    The secondary static stabilizers of the joint are the radiocapitellar articulation and the joint capsule. The surrounding muscles provide dynamic stability.

    Elbow dislocation requires a high-energy trauma and results in significant damage to the primary and secondary stabilizers.

  - The radiocapitellar joint allows for pronation and supination of the forearm. Dislocation of this joint is

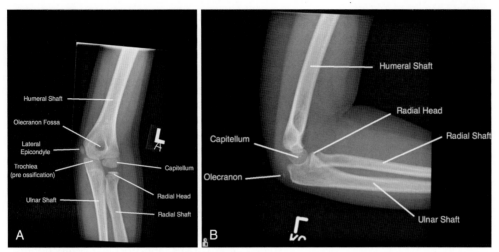

**FIGURE 21-1.** Bony anatomy of the elbow. Anteroposterior **(A)** and lateral **(B)** radiographs.

commonly missed as a second component of a more obvious fracture (Fig. 21-3).

- Muscles
  - The triceps and anconeus contribute to elbow extension. The anconeus also contributes to forearm pronation.
  - The brachialis is the strongest elbow flexor, but the biceps brachii and brachioradialis also contribute to forearm flexion.
  - The biceps brachii and supinator contribute to forearm supination.
  - As its name implies, the pronator teres is a forearm pronator.
  - The wrist and finger flexors (flexor carpi radialis, flexor digitorum superficialis, palmaris longus, and flexor carpi ulnaris) originate as a common flexor tendon at the medial epicondyle and contribute to its displacement in cases of medial epicondylar fractures.
  - The wrist and finger extensors (extensor carpi radialis longus and brevis, extensor digitorum, extensor digiti minimi, extensor carpi ulnaris) originate as a common extensor tendon at the lateral epicondyle and contribute to its displacement in cases of lateral epicondylar fractures.
- Vascular Structures (Fig. 21-4)
  - The vascular supply of the elbow in children is limited. The physis acts as a barrier between the intraosseous circulation and the extraosseous circulation. The vessels have limited access to the epiphyseal cartilage because they do not penetrate the articular capsule or articular surface except at the interface of the capsule with the bone. The limited points of entry into the epiphyseal cartilage may explain the irregularity of ossification observed at the trochlea and capitellum.
  - The brachial artery crosses the elbow in the cubital fossa. The pulse may be palpated just medial and posterior to the biceps brachii muscle and tendon. This artery is at risk with supracondylar humerus fractures and elbow dislocations. There is a rich

collateral circulation around the elbow, which may preserve viability of the arm in the case of a brachial artery occlusion.
  - The radial and ulnar arteries are branches of the brachial artery and are at risk with displaced fractures of the radius or ulna and lacerations to the forearm.
  - The basilic and cephalic veins are the main vascular outflow of the upper extremity. Thrombosis after elbow dislocation is a rare complication of this injury.
- Neurologic Structures Crossing the Elbow
  - The median nerve crosses in the cubital fossa with the brachial artery and is at risk with displaced supracondylar humerus fractures leading to flexion weakness at the wrist and proximal interphalangeal joints and loss of sensation of the radial side of the palm and palmar surface of the thumb, index, and middle fingers.
  - The anterior interosseous nerve (AIN) branches off of the median nerve just distal to the elbow. AIN neurapraxia is common with posterior or posterolateral dislocations of the elbow, leading to flexion weakness at the interphalangeal joint of the thumb and distal interphalangeal joints of the index and middle fingers. No sensory loss is associated with AIN palsy.
  - The ulnar nerve crosses just posterior to the medial epicondyle and is at risk with anterior dislocations of the elbow and displaced fractures of the medial epicondyle, leading to weakness in finger abduction, flexion weakness of ring and small finger distal interphalangeal joints, and loss of sensation in the small finger and ulnar side of the hand.
  - The radial nerve crosses anterior to the lateral epicondyle. Injury to the radial nerve at the elbow is rare.
  - The posterior interosseous nerve (PIN) branches from the radial nerve just distal to the elbow and passes around the radial neck. PIN neurapraxia is common with displaced radial neck fractures and radiocapitellar dislocations, leading to extensor weakness in wrist and fingers. No sensory loss is associated with PIN injury.

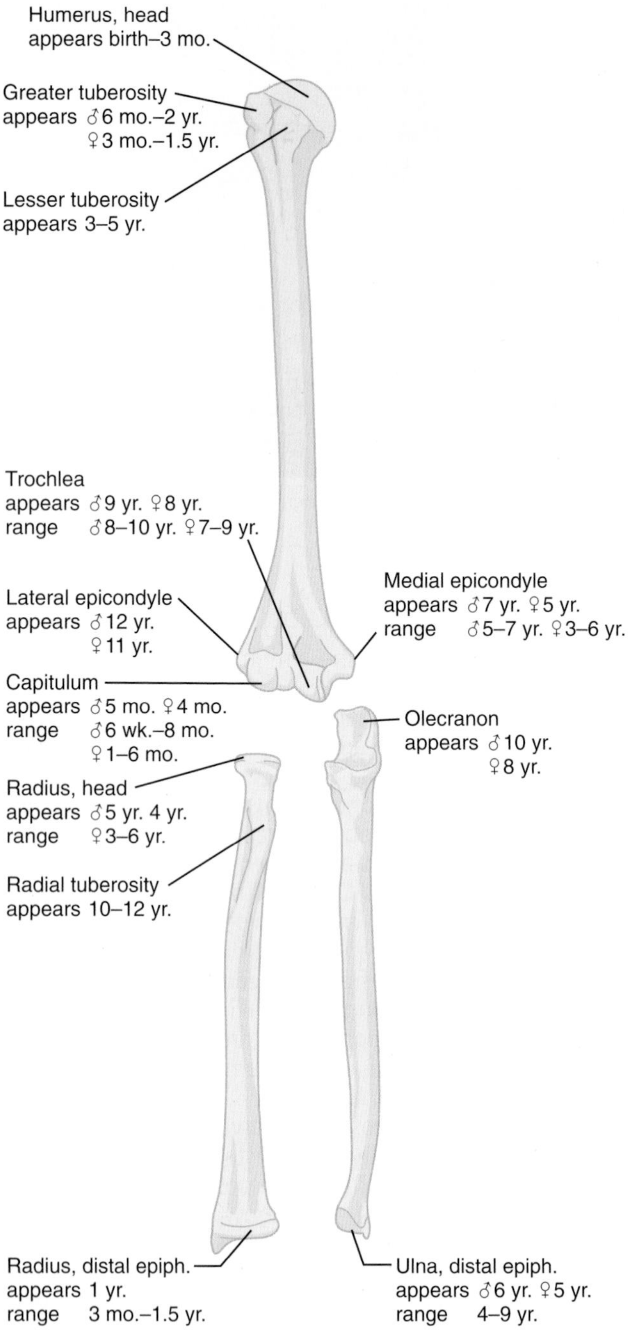

Humerus, head
appears birth–3 mo.

Greater tuberosity
appears ♂6 mo.–2 yr.
♀3 mo.–1.5 yr.

Lesser tuberosity
appears 3–5 yr.

Trochlea
appears ♂9 yr. ♀8 yr.
range     ♂8–10 yr. ♀7–9 yr.

Lateral epicondyle
appears ♂12 yr.
♀11 yr.

Capitulum
appears ♂5 mo. ♀4 mo.
range     ♂6 wk.–8 mo.
♀1–6 mo.

Radius, head
appears ♂5 yr. 4 yr.
range     ♀3–6 yr.

Radial tuberosity
appears 10–12 yr.

Medial epicondyle
appears ♂7 yr. ♀5 yr.
range     ♂5–7 yr. ♀3–6 yr.

Olecranon
appears ♂10 yr.
♀8 yr.

Radius, distal epiph.
appears 1 yr.
range     3 mo.–1.5 yr.

Ulna, distal epiph.
appears ♂6 yr. ♀5 yr.
range     4–9 yr.

**FIGURE 21-2.** Average age of appearance of centers of ossification of epiphyses in the arm and forearm. *(Adapted from von Lanz, et al: Praktische Anatomie, Berlin, 1938, Julius Springer, p 28.)*

## HISTORY

- Mechanism of Injury
  - A direct blow is a common mechanism for olecranon injuries.
  - Traction to the elbow can lead to nursemaid's elbow (radial head subluxation), medial or lateral epiphyseal avulsion injuries, and anterior elbow dislocation (less common).
  - A fall on an outstretched hand is the most common mechanism for supracondylar humerus fractures and

posterior elbow dislocations. It can also lead to radial head or neck fractures.
  - During a fall, a child is more likely to have the elbow in an extended posture, secondary to ligamentous laxity, as opposed to an adult, in whom the elbow assumes a semiflexed posture. This unique anatomic aspect makes children more likely to sustain supracondylar fractures and results in different olecranon fracture patterns than seen in adults.
- Pain
  - Injuries causing lateral elbow pain include lateral condyle fractures, radial head or neck fractures, radial head dislocations, lateral collateral ligament sprains, and capitellar osteochondral lesions.
  - Injuries causing medial elbow pain include medial epicondyle fractures, medial collateral ligament sprains, and trochlear osteochondral lesions.
  - Injuries causing generalized elbow pain include supracondylar humerus fractures, elbow dislocations, and elbow infections.
- Dysfunction
  - Joint dislocations place a limb in a characteristic fixed position. In posterior elbow dislocations, the elbow tends to be extended, whereas in anterior elbow dislocations, the elbow tends to be flexed.
  - Loose bodies can cause catching or locking of the joint. Both medial epicondyle fragments and radial head fragments can be trapped within the joint.

## PREHOSPITAL CARE AND MANAGEMENT

Children with elbow injuries should be evaluated by advanced trauma life support protocol in the field for other distracting injuries. If the elbow injury is isolated, adequate immobilization in the field consists of a sling with a swathe. It is often difficult to place well-fitting, appropriate-length upper extremity splints on small children, and the actual process may result in more discomfort than aid.

## PHYSICAL EXAMINATION

- A cervical spine examination should be performed routinely for patients presenting with elbow pain.
- The injured elbow should be compared with the contralateral elbow, and any differences should be noted.
- Edema, ecchymosis, open wounds, or deformity should be identified in the injured elbow.
- Palpate the olecranon, medial and lateral epicondyles, and cubital fossa for deformity and tenderness.
- Check active and passive range of motion of the elbow joint, and compare it with the contralateral side.
  - As in the shoulder, loss of active range of motion could indicate dislocation, neurologic dysfunction, or patient hesitation secondary to pain.
  - Loss of active and passive range of motion is more indicative of dislocation or loose bodies within the joint.

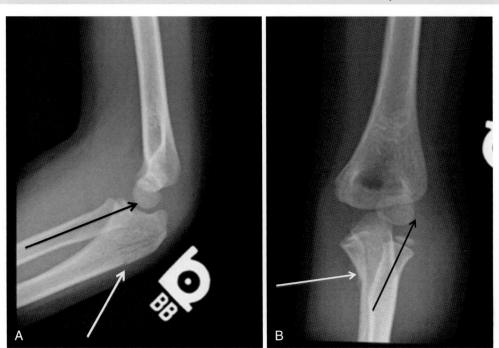

**FIGURE 21-3.** Monteggia fracture in a 6-year-old boy. **A,** Lateral radiograph of the elbow. A line drawn perpendicular to the radial head bisects the capitellum *(black arrow)*. Note the olecranon fracture *(white arrow)*. **B,** Anteroposterior radiograph of the elbow. A line drawn perpendicular to the radial head does not bisect the capitellum *(black arrow)*, suggesting lateral subluxation of the radial head.

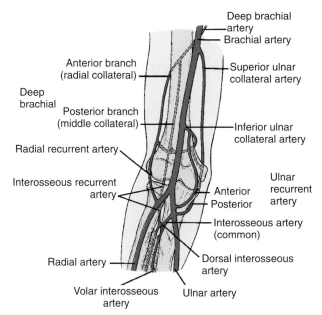

**FIGURE 21-4.** The vascular supply around the elbow is rich, with excellent collateral circulation. The collateral circulation is usually sufficient to maintain viability of the extremity in the event of occlusion of the brachial artery. *(From Green N, Swiontkowski M: Skeletal trauma in children, ed 4, Philadelphia, 2008, Saunders.)*

- In a child or adolescent, loss of active elbow motion compared with the opposite arm is 100% sensitive for fracture or effusion. Preservation of motion is 97% specific for absence of a fracture.[3]
- The neurologic examination should include an evaluation of the three main brachial plexus branches crossing the elbow (radial, ulnar, and median), paying close attention to the ulnar nerve, PIN, and AIN. Evaluation of these nerves was previously outlined.
- An upper extremity vascular examination should be performed as previously outlined.

## DIAGNOSTIC STUDIES

- X-ray
  - An anteroposterior view is obtained with the elbow in full extension and the forearm in supination. The anteroposterior view is used to evaluate the medial and lateral epicondyles, supracondylar region, ulnohumeral and radiocapitellar joints, and radial head and neck.
  - A true anteroposterior view is sometimes difficult to obtain in the setting of injury. The beam should be oriented perpendicular to the humeral shaft or the forearm, depending on the area of interest.
  - The lateral view is obtained with the elbow at 90 degrees of flexion and the forearm in the neutral position. The lateral view is used to evaluate the supracondylar region (degree of displacement), ulnohumeral and radiocapitellar joints, radial head and neck, olecranon, and fat pads.
  - With an occult fracture of the elbow, intra-articular hematoma forces the anterior and posterior fat pads out of the coronoid and olecranon fossae.

    The anterior fat pad is often visible on a normal lateral view of the elbow.

    The posterior fat pad is normally completely hidden in the confines of the olecranon fossa and specific

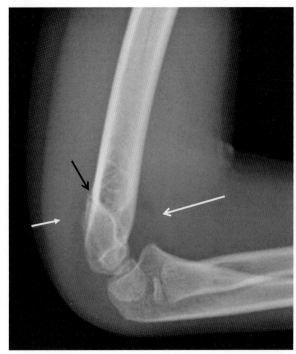

**FIGURE 21-5.** Lateral radiograph of a minimally displaced supracondylar humerus fracture *(black arrow)*. Note the lucent areas representing the anterior and posterior fat pads *(white arrows)*. Intra-articular hematoma pushes the posterior fat pad *(short white arrow)* out of the coronoid fossa, making it visible on the x-ray.

for intra-articular fluid when identified on radiographs (Fig. 21-5).

- The external oblique view is obtained with the elbow extended and externally rotated 45 degrees relative to the x-ray beam and is used to evaluate the radial head and neck, radiocapitellar joint, and proximal radioulnar joint.
- The internal oblique view is obtained with the elbow extended and forearm pronated. The elbow should be internally rotated 45 degrees relative to the x-ray beam. The internal oblique view is useful for assessing the true displacement of lateral condyle fractures and for evaluating the coronoid process and medial epicondyle.[4]
- Special attention should be paid to the radiocapitellar articulation because subluxation or dislocation of the radiocapitellar articulation is commonly found with other injuries. The radial head should line up with the capitellum on all x-ray views (see Fig. 21-1).

■ Computed Tomography (CT)
- CT is used to evaluate intra-articular fractures around the elbow better. However, CT is not part of the usual evaluation of these injuries without bedside consultation with an orthopedist for surgical decision making and planning.

■ Magnetic Resonance Imaging (MRI)
- MRI, similar to CT, is rarely used in the acute setting, but it can be used to evaluate for osteomyelitis, septic arthritis, and septic olecranon bursitis.
- MRI is used more commonly in the outpatient setting to look for ligament, tendon, and muscle injuries.

■ Aspiration
- The elbow can be aspirated from the lateral side through the center of the triangle formed by the radial head, tip of the olecranon, and lateral epicondyle.
- The fluid should be analyzed as described previously.

■ Laboratory Tests
- In cases of suspected septic elbow, septic bursitis, or osteomyelitis, appropriate laboratory work should be sent as outlined in Chapter 18.

## DIFFERENTIAL DIAGNOSIS OF ELBOW PAIN AND DYSFUNCTION

■ Cervical spine injury (C8-T1)
■ Brachial plexus injury (lower plexus injury)
■ Elbow fracture
■ Fracture or injury proximal or distal to the elbow joint
■ Infection—osteomyelitis, septic elbow, olecranon bursitis
■ Joint dislocation or subluxation—nursemaid's elbow, elbow dislocation
■ Overuse injury—traction apophysitis or physeal strain from repetitive activities, most commonly sports in an adolescent
■ Pathologic fracture through a benign or malignant lesion
■ Congenital dislocation of the elbow or radial head

## SPECIFIC INJURIES AND TREATMENT

■ Distal Humeral Epiphyseal Separation (Fig. 21-6)
- Distal humeral epiphyseal separation occurs when the entire distal humerus separates from the humerus through the physeal line.
- Although thought to be rare, this injury is recognized with increasing frequency.
- Most fractures occur before age 6 or 7 years. The younger the child, the greater the volume of the distal humerus occupied by the distal humeral epiphysis and the more likely the injury.
- These are believed to be strictly hyperextension injuries, although the exact mechanism of injury is unclear.
- Child abuse must be suspected in an infant with this injury, and the appropriate evaluation must be undertaken.
- Classification is based on the presence of the lateral condyle ossification.[5]

  Group A fractures—occur in infants younger than 12 months without lateral condyle ossification

  Group B fractures—occur in children 12 months to 3 years old with some lateral condyle ossification

  Group C fractures—occur in children 3 to 7 years old and result in a large metaphyseal fragment

- Radiographic findings may be subtle, especially in an infant. However, the radius and ulna maintain an

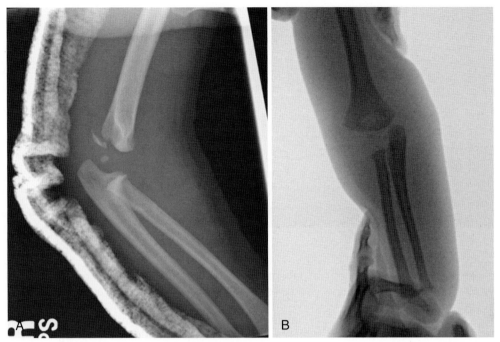

**FIGURE 21-6. A,** Distal humeral epiphyseal separation with a small Salter-Harris component, as evidenced by the corresponding metaphyseal fragment. **B,** Stress views obtained in the operating room show complete translation of the distal humerus and proximal radius and ulna medially.

anatomic relationship to each other, while the two bones are displaced posteromedially relative to the distal humerus. This appearance is to be distinguished from an elbow dislocation, where the distal fragment is primarily posterolateral, and a lateral condyle fracture, where the relationship of the radius to the capitellum is disrupted.

If additional information is needed, ultrasound or MRI can assist with the diagnosis.

- In very small infants, treatment involves arm immobilization in a figure-of-eight splint. In larger infants and children with acute injuries, a closed reduction with pin fixation is performed.

If the diagnosis is delayed, the arm is simply immobilized with the thought that an open reduction would endanger the physis and later deformity can be corrected with an osteotomy.

■ Supracondylar Humerus Fracture
- Supracondylar humerus fractures are the most common elbow fractures in children.
- The peak age range is 5 to 6 years.[2]
- The typical mechanism of injury is a fall on an outstretched hand with the elbow in full extension.
- Patients present according to the spectrum of displacements.

Patients with minimally displaced fractures suggested only by a posterior fat pad have limitations in range of motion and tenderness.

Patients with gross displacement have bruising, skin puckering, and deformity at the elbow with possible neurovascular involvement.

- Particular attention is paid to the vascular examination.
- Supracondylar humerus fractures are classified based on Gartland's classification.[6]

Type I—undisplaced

Type II—posterior hinge

- If medial comminution is present, this suggests significant instability, and the injury should be reclassified as type III.

Type III—completely displaced (Fig. 21-7)

Type IV—displaces into extension and flexion

- Radiographic examination consists of anteroposterior and lateral views of the elbow. Additional studies are rarely needed, even in the setting of vascular injury. Several studies showed that arteriography is not helpful in vascular injury because it delays the more helpful treatment option of fracture reduction.[7] In all cases, the site of the vascular occlusion is usually at the apex of the fracture.
- Treatment is dictated by fracture type, vascular status, and any threat to the soft tissue envelope.

Patients with threatened perfusion require an emergent operative reduction with the assistance of a vascular surgeon.

Patients with a threatened soft tissue envelope require an emergent reduction.

If an open fracture is identified, open reduction and internal fixation (ORIF) is performed with appropriate débridement of bone.

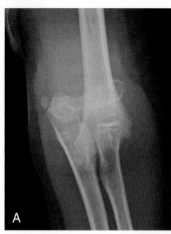
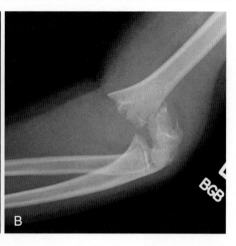

**FIGURE 21-7.** Anteroposterior **(A)** and lateral **(B)** projections of the left elbow in a 9-year-old boy who fell off playground equipment. The x-rays show a completely displaced extension-type supracondylar humerus fracture.

- Neurologic injury is relatively common in patients with displaced supracondylar humerus fractures, with most series suggesting a 10% to 20% incidence.[8,9] The AIN is the most commonly injured nerve, followed by the radial nerve and sometimes the ulnar nerve.
- Vascular injury occurs with an incidence of 10% to 20% in type III supracondylar humerus fractures.[10,11]

  A perfused hand—defined as a pink, warm hand with adequate capillary refill—in the absence of a palpable pulse requires fracture reduction, stabilization, and observation.

  A hand with poor perfusion after reduction requires operative exploration by a vascular surgeon.

- For closed fractures without neurovascular injury, the following treatment algorithm is recommended.

  Type I—cast treatment

  Type II—closed reduction and pin fixation

  - Casting may be used; however, operative treatment is preferred because there is a risk of compartment syndrome and vascular compromise when casting the elbow in hyperflexion to hold the fracture reduction.

  Type III—closed versus open reduction with pin fixation

  Type IV—closed versus open reduction with pin fixation

- Lateral Condyle Fracture
  - Lateral condyle fracture occurs through the lateral condyle and crosses the physis, ending lateral to or in the trochlea.
  - This fracture is most similar to a Salter-Harris type IV fracture of the distal humerus.
  - Injury usually results from an avulsion mechanism secondary to varus stress to the elbow with the elbow in extension. The injury may also result from a direct shear force as in a valgus injury to the elbow.

- The clinical presentation typically consists of elbow pain and loss of range of motion. In contrast to supracondylar fractures, gross deformity is notably absent, and the only irregularity may be significant lateral-sided elbow swelling.
- Radiographs of the elbow often show a small lucent line along the lateral condyle metaphysis, just proximal to the lateral condyle ossification center. An internal oblique radiograph of the elbow is invaluable for showing the true displacement of the fragment. Fractures with greater displacement are typically more obvious.
- The fracture may be classified according to Milch, who proposed a classification based on the location of the distal fracture line.

  Milch I fractures exit lateral to the trochlea, whereas Milch II fractures exit into the trochlea.

  Although the Milch classification has been found to have no direct correlation to fragment stability and does not direct operative decision making, it can indicate overall elbow stability.

  Milch II fractures compromise the ulnohumeral articulation and allow elbow dislocation or subluxation as a consequence of the fracture.

- Treatment is dictated by fracture displacement.

  Minimally displaced fractures are treated with long arm cast immobilization and close, weekly follow-up because there is a chance of displacement in these presumably stable fractures (Fig. 21-8).

  Displaced fractures, defined as a fracture gap of more than 2 mm on an internal rotation oblique view of the elbow, are treated with operative fixation, through either open or closed means (Fig. 21-9).

- A missed lateral condyle injury is common. Vigilance in early and serial follow-up of elbow injuries without a clear diagnosis is crucial to ensure that long-term function is not compromised by an unrecognized lateral condyle injury.

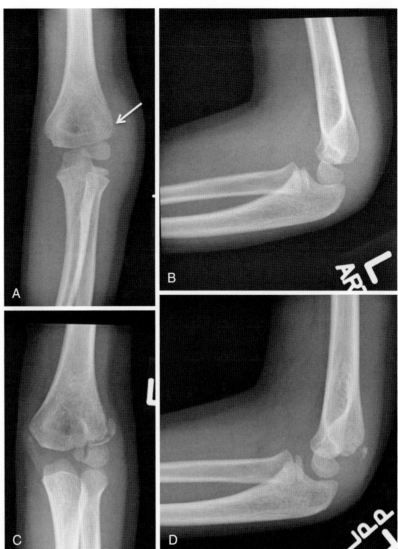

**FIGURE 21-8.** Anteroposterior **(A)** and lateral **(B)** views show a minimally displaced lateral condyle fracture *(arrow).* The patient was placed into a long arm cast. Follow-up examination 3 weeks later showed progressive displacement of the lateral condyle and early evidence of healing **(C** and **D).**

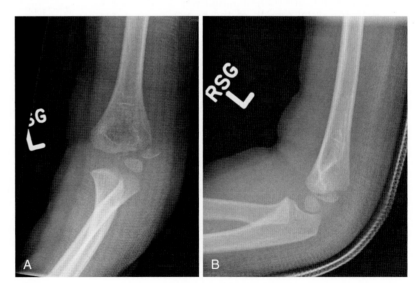

**FIGURE 21-9.** Anteroposterior with internal rotation **(A)** and lateral **(B)** views of a displaced lateral condyle fracture. The visible metaphyseal fleck is evidence of the displaced, mostly cartilaginous lateral condyle.

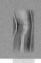

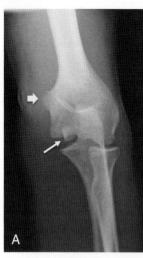

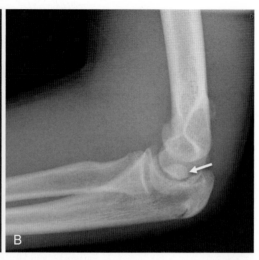

**FIGURE 21-10. A** and **B,** Incarcerated medial epicondyle fracture in a 15-year-old boy after spontaneous reduction of an elbow dislocation. The *thin white arrow* indicates the position of the medial epicondyle, and the *broad white arrow* indicates the base from which it fractured.

- Medial Epicondyle Fractures
  - Medial epicondyle fractures occur through the medial epicondylar apophysis with a peak age of 9 to 12 years.
  - Boys sustain this fracture four times more often than girls. An elbow dislocation is associated in 50% of such injuries, and in at least 15% to 18% of such injuries the fragment is incarcerated in the joint (Fig. 21-10).
  - Injury results most commonly from valgus extension stress placed on the elbow. An isolated avulsion from a forceful muscle contraction can also cause this fracture.
  - Radiographs of the elbow are adequate for diagnosis. The epicondylar fragment is usually displaced anteriorly and distally.
  - Although controversy surrounds the treatment of these injuries, most injuries may be treated closed with a simple posterior splint and initiation of range of motion at 7 to 10 days.
  - Because the epicondylar apophysis is not involved with the distal growth of the humerus, no growth consequences have been identified as a result of this injury.
  - Generally agreed on operative indications include an incarcerated medial epicondyle fragment or a displaced fracture (>5 mm) in the arm of an athlete who requires elbow stability for his or her sport.
- Olecranon Fractures
  - Isolated olecranon fractures are rare in pediatric patients. The two main fracture types are apophyseal fractures and metaphyseal fractures.
  - Apophyseal olecranon fractures are exceedingly rare and most often seen in patients with osteogenesis imperfecta.

    Clinically, patients have elbow swelling, a palpable defect, and difficulty with active extension.

    Radiographs may be subtle in the absence of the secondary ossification centers for the olecranon apophysis, which appear by 9 to 10 years of age.

    Fractures include recurrent traction injury (apophysitis), incomplete stress fracture, and complete

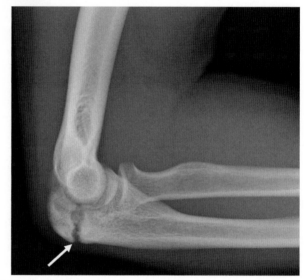

**FIGURE 21-11.** Olecranon stress fracture in a 16-year-old throwing athlete. Lateral projection shows the cortical irregularity at the site of the olecranon apophysis. The olecranon apophysis should be essentially closed at this age.

apophyseal and apophyseal-metaphyseal avulsions (Fig. 21-11).

Traction injuries or incomplete stress fractures are treated with activity modification. If healing does not progress, ORIF is performed.

Minimally displaced fractures may be treated in a long arm cast with the elbow extended.

Displaced fractures require ORIF, typically with a tension band construct.

- Metaphyseal fractures of the olecranon have an incidence of 4% to 6% in major series, with most fractures occurring in association with other forearm fractures.[12,13] The peak age for this injury is between 5 and 10 years.[14]

  Patients present with a swollen elbow, a palpable defect, or difficulty with active extension.

Radiographs usually reveal a line perpendicular to the long axis of the ulna in flexion injuries. This finding helps to distinguish the fracture from the more oblique apophyseal fracture line.

Fractures may be classified as flexion type, extension type, or shear type.

Flexion injuries are the most common type and result from a tension force along the posterior cortex of the olecranon. Minimally displaced fractures may be treated in a long arm cast, whereas displaced fractures require operative fixation.

Extension injuries result in either varus or valgus fractures of the olecranon metaphysis.

- When the child falls, the olecranon itself is locked into the olecranon fossa owing to elbow extension, and the major coronal plane bending force dictates the direction of the fracture. The fracture is often a greenstick pattern and associated with a concurrent fracture of the radial neck (valgus force) or a dislocation of the radiocapitellar joint (varus force).
- Treatment usually consists of closed reduction and cast immobilization, paying special attention to the reduction of concurrent proximal radial injury. Close serial follow-up for the first 3 weeks is necessary because progressive displacement may occur (Fig. 21-12).

- Operative fixation sometimes is needed to prevent the coronal plane deformity from recurring.

Shear injuries are the reverse of flexion injuries and occur when the anterior cortex of the olecranon fails, usually from a direct blow to the posterior olecranon. The distal fragment typically displaces anteriorly, while the radioulnar joint relationship remains as a unit.

- Treatment is typically with long arm cast immobilization in hyperflexion.
- If the fragment is unstable or the reduction cannot be maintained, operative fixation is used.

■ Radial Neck Fractures
- Radial neck fractures account for only 1% of all fractures in children.
- Fracture of the radial head is rare in a skeletally immature child. In greater than 90% of proximal radius fractures, the fracture line involves either the physis or the neck.[15]
- The median age for this injury is 9 to 10 years.[15]
- Changes in the congruency of the radioulnar articulation from disruptions in the radial neck angulation compromise the patient's supination and pronation. This result can often be seen even with minimally displaced fractures.
- Physical examination most commonly reveals tenderness over the radial head with more marked limitations in supination and pronation than with elbow

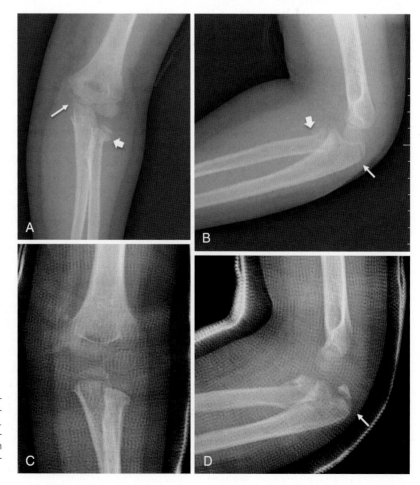

**FIGURE 21-12. A** and **B,** Minimally displaced olecranon fracture *(arrow)* in a 12-year-old boy with a concurrent radial neck fracture. The injury was treated in a cast. **C** and **D,** Progressive displacement of the olecranon fracture has occurred 3 weeks after the initial injury, with progressive subluxation of the ulnohumeral and radiocapitellar joints.

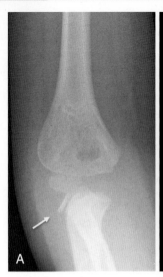
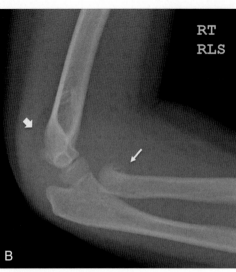

**FIGURE 21-13.** Displaced radial neck fracture. **A,** Anteroposterior projection of the elbow shows lateral tilt of the proximal radial epiphysis with incongruity of the radiocapitellar joint *(arrow).* **B,** Metaphyseal irregularity and unclear radial epiphysis morphology suggest displacement of the radial neck *(thin arrow).* There is a posterior fat pad sign *(wide arrow).*

flexion. For younger children, the primary complaint may be wrist pain because the elbow pain is sometimes referred from the wrist.

- Radiographic diagnosis may be difficult before radial head ossification. A fracture may be suggested by any radial neck metaphyseal irregularity (Fig. 21-13).
- Radial neck and head fractures may be classified into three groups according to the primary displacement and the mechanism of injury.

  Group I fractures involve a primary displacement of the radial head such that the radioulnar articulation is disrupted. These fractures may occur in association with elbow injuries or as a result of an angular force being applied to an extended elbow, as is the case during a fall.

  - This group includes the rare Salter-Harris IV injury through the radial epiphysis.
  - The most frequent fracture pattern is a Salter-Harris type I or type II injury or a metaphyseal level injury through the neck.

  Group II fractures maintain the radioulnar articulation and are usually a result of angular or torsional forces. These fractures, by definition, do not include intra-articular fracture patterns and are rare.

  Group III includes stress injuries to the radial epiphysis, most commonly from repetitive compressive loads applied during sports. Radiographically, irregular ossification of the radial epiphysis is observed along with decreased size. If the stress is chronic, angular deformity may result secondary to loads on the growth plate.

- Treatment for the rare radial head fracture (Salter-Harris type IV) involves open reduction and operative fixation.
- Treatment for radial neck fractures (metaphyseal and Salter-Harris type I or type II varieties) depends on fracture displacement and angulation.

  Fractures with less than 30 degrees of angulation and less than 3 mm of translation may be treated with a long arm cast or splint for 2 weeks.

  Fractures exceeding these criteria usually require closed versus open reduction, with or without operative fixation.

- Fractures with significant residual translation typically fare worse than fractures with moderate degrees of angulation. In addition, if an operative reduction is required, it is imperative that these fractures be approached rapidly because results worsen if the procedure is delayed more than 5 days from the time of injury. [16]
- Stress injuries of the radial head and neck usually can be treated effectively with activity restriction and a short period of immobilization.

■ "T" Condylar Distal Humerus Fractures

- The "T" or "Y" condylar distal humerus fracture involves a vertical fracture line that extends proximally from the distal humeral articular surface and separates into fracture lines that exit through the medial and lateral condyles.
- This fracture type is rare in young children, and case series are limited.
- The most common mechanisms of injury are a direct blow to the posterior elbow, usually from a fall, or a direct fall on the arm with the elbow slightly flexed.
- Classifications vary in the adult literature and are not directly applicable to pediatric patients.
- All fractures require operative reduction and stabilization. Fractures in patients older than 12 years should be managed with adult techniques, as described in Chapter 10. Fractures in younger children with widely open physes are best managed with multiple smooth Kirschner wire fixation and a 4- to 6-week period of immobilization (Fig. 21-14).

■ Elbow Dislocations

- A dislocated elbow is a pathologic spectrum that may involve dislocations of the three articulations around the elbow.

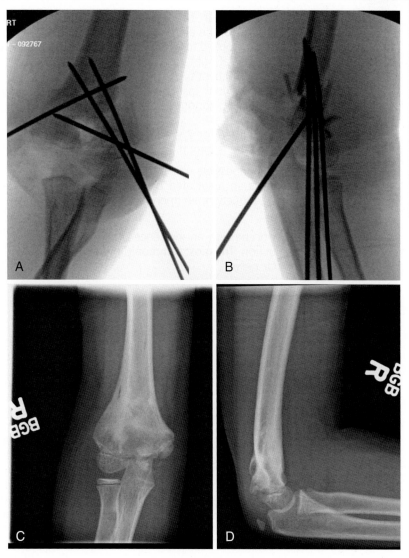

**FIGURE 21-14. A** and **B,** Open "T" condylar distal humerus fracture in a 9-year-old girl that was treated with multiple Kirschner wire fixation. Cast immobilization was used for 6 weeks with in-office removal of pins. **C** and **D,** The patient has full range of motion 1 year after injury.

Ulnohumeral joint

Radiocapitellar joint

Radioulnar joint

- Elbow dislocations in pediatric patients are rare, with a reported incidence of only 3%.[17] These injuries typically occur in the age range of 13 to 14 years, when the physes begin to close. Dislocations in younger children are often associated with a medial epicondyle fracture.
- Elbow dislocations are classified according to the position of the proximal radioulnar joint in relation to the distal humerus—posterior, anterior, medial, or lateral.
- Posterior elbow dislocation

  This injury is classified further into posteromedial or posterolateral dislocation.

  This is the most common type of dislocation.

  Posterior elbow dislocations occur with failure of the ulnar collateral ligament or medial epicondyle, the anterior joint capsule, and, laterally, the lateral collateral ligament complex.

  Symptoms can mimic a type III supracondylar humerus fracture, given the flexed position of the elbow and the swelling. However, the smooth edges of the radial head and olecranon posteriorly during palpation allow ready distinction on physical examination.

  Associated fractures can occur in 50% of posterior elbow dislocations, such as fractures of the medial epicondyle, radial head and neck, and coronoid process.[18]

  Radiographs of the elbow are distorted with considerable overlap of the distal humerus and proximal radioulnar joint. The radiographs should be scrutinized for associated osteochondral fractures because these may interfere with a concentric reduction.

  Most posterior dislocations may be reduced with a closed technique.

- With adequate sedation or intra-articular block, the forearm is supinated, the elbow is flexed, and a longitudinal force is applied to engage the radius and ulna under the distal humerus.
- After reduction, the patient's elbow should be examined for any residual instability, abnormal anatomic landmarks, or abnormal resistance to passive range of motion.
- The elbow is immobilized for 2 weeks in a splint, and progressive motion is begun.

If closed reduction is impossible, if the dislocation is open, or if there is an associated osteochondral fracture impeding reduction, an open reduction is necessary.

Nerve injuries can occur with an incidence of 10% after closed reduction. The most commonly injured nerve is the ulnar nerve.

There is no role for acute ligamentous repair in posterior elbow dislocations because most can be treated well with a closed reduction.

- Anterior elbow dislocation

These injuries are rare and account for 1% of all elbow dislocations.[17]

Anterior elbow dislocation usually results from a direct posterior blow.

The elbow is typically held in extension, and there is massive associated swelling. A careful neurovascular examination is mandatory.

Standard elbow radiographs are diagnostic.

Associated fractures of the olecranon and capitellum are common, and in children, the triceps insertion may be avulsed with a small cortical bony fragment.

Reduction is performed by applying longitudinal traction and then applying a posterior force through the elbow joint while flexing the elbow. The patient is typically splinted in partial extension for 2 weeks.

- Medial elbow dislocation

No case reports of a medial dislocation pattern for pediatric patients exist.

- Lateral elbow dislocation

This is an extremely rare injury, especially in children.

A lateral elbow dislocation may be incomplete, in which the semilunar notch articulates with the capitellum.

- In this case, despite the dislocation, the patient retains a surprising degree of elbow motion.
- Radiographs should be scrutinized. A complete lateral dislocation gives the impression of a markedly widened elbow and notably limited elbow motion.

Reduction of a lateral dislocation involves longitudinal traction with a medially directed force on the elbow. The patient should be splinted for 2 weeks in a neutral position, and motion should be subsequently begun.

- Divergent elbow dislocation

Divergent elbow dislocation is also an extremely rare injury that reflects high-energy trauma.

The diagnosis is made with a standard elbow series. Associated fractures such as radial neck, proximal ulna, and coronoid fractures are common.[19]

Closed reduction typically requires little force with articular block, conscious sedation, or, if necessary, general anesthesia as longitudinal traction is applied to the semiextended elbow and a compressive force is applied to the forearm. The elbow is splinted for 2 weeks, and elbow range of motion is begun. Patients with this injury in the absence of associated fractures are expected to regain a full range of motion.

The dislocation rarely requires open treatment. However, reports exist of interposed soft tissue blocking reduction.[20]

- ■ Nursemaid's Elbow
  - Nursemaid's elbow refers to a traction injury to the elbow where the annular ligament subluxates over the radial head, interfering with the motion of the radiocapitellar joint.
  - The typical mechanism is longitudinal traction on an extended elbow and pronated forearm; this can occur if a child is being pulled or swung by the hand. Patients with these injuries are prone to have some features of ligamentous laxity.[21]
  - The mean age of injury is 2 to 3 years, but the range may be 2 months to 7 years of age.[22] The injury is quite common, but the exact incidence is unknown because most of these injuries are treated in emergency departments or by primary care physicians.
  - Examination reveals disuse of the extremity and direct tenderness to palpation over the radial head. Motion tends to be limited at the extremes of flexion, supination, and pronation.
  - Standard elbow radiographs are necessary only if an associated injury is suspected. With a classic history, examination, and resolution of symptoms after reduction, no radiographs are needed.
  - Closed reduction is the treatment in nearly all cases.

  Direct pressure to the radial head is applied while the elbow is taken through a full range of supination and pronation and flexion.

  A palpable snap frequently occurs with reduction, and full elbow range of motion is restored.

  No immobilization is necessary after reduction if the child is comfortably using the arm. A sling may be needed if there is persistent discomfort caused by synovitis from a delayed reduction.

- If closed reduction fails, radiographs may be needed to exclude associated injury. Even if left untreated, most annular ligament subluxations reduce spontaneously.
- Parents should be informed that recurrence is quite common, and the subluxation can be reduced as described.

    The frequency of dislocations decreases when the patient reaches age 5 years secondary to spontaneous tightening of the ligaments.

    If recurrence is functionally limiting, casting for a short time may be employed.

■ Little Leaguer's Elbow
- As child participation in organized sports has increased over the past 2 decades, the incidence of injuries to the elbow has also increased. Although most reports suggest an overuse injury incidence of 30% to 50% for adolescent athletes, the incidence is likely higher because most athletes do not seek treatment. Overuse injury should be considered in a child presenting with elbow pain to the emergency department.
- Little Leaguer's elbow includes injuries such as apophysitis, osteochondral fracture, and growth abnormality of the elbow from repetitive valgus overload to the elbow.
- As repetitive valgus loads are applied to the elbow, the ulnar collateral ligament may experience microtrauma, an apophysitis may develop along the medial epicondyle, medial epicondylar growth may be slowed or accelerated, the capitellum may exhibit osteochondral injury, and the radial head and neck may experience an alteration of growth (Fig. 21-15).
- The history is usually revealing for year-long participation in sports. Symptoms may consist of dull, achy pain along the medial or lateral aspect of the elbow. The discomfort is often associated with a 10- to 15-degree elbow flexion contracture.
- Examination may reveal tenderness over the medial epicondyle, radial head, or capitellum. Limitations to extension and pronation and supination may exist. In addition, a valgus laxity may be appreciated compared with the opposite extremity.
- Standard elbow radiographs may show irregular ossification at the medial epicondyle or along the course of the ulnar collateral ligament. Osteochondral lucency at the capitellum or radial head may be present. Loose bodies may also be noted.

    Additional imaging with MRI may be necessary to define further an osteochondral defect in an older child or to evaluate further for the presence of loose bodies.

- Most treatment protocols involve a period of rest with immobilization and a subsequent therapy program. No acute surgical interventions are needed for this constellation of findings, but elective surgical interventions may be necessary to repair osteochondral lesions, to stabilize medial epicondyle fractures, or to remove symptomatic foreign bodies.

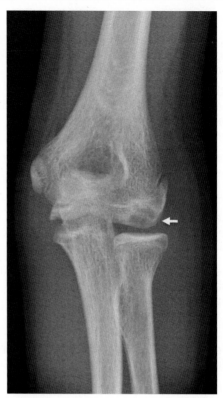

**FIGURE 21-15.** A 12-year-old boy pitcher with persistent lateral-sided elbow discomfort. Note the lateral condylar epiphyseal irregularity *(arrow)* from chronic valgus, overload stress.

## GUIDELINES FOR EMERGENCY DEPARTMENT MANAGEMENT

■ When and How Should a Specialist Be Consulted?
- All open injuries, injuries with soft tissue compromise, and injuries with associated neurovascular deficit require a bedside consultation. Consultation recommendations for isolated, closed injuries to the elbow are presented.
- Distal humeral epiphyseal separation

    A bedside consultation is required for examination and operative planning.

- Supracondylar humerus fracture

    Patients with minimally displaced fractures (type I) require only a telephone consultation.

    Patients with type II or type III supracondylar humerus fractures require a bedside consultation for closed reduction or surgical planning.

- Lateral condyle

    Patients with minimally displaced fractures require only a telephone consultation with early follow-up.

    Patients with displaced lateral condyle fractures require a bedside consultation for surgical planning.

- Medial epicondyle

  All patients with isolated medial epicondyle fractures do not require immediate consultation and may be prepared for outpatient follow-up.

  If there is an associated elbow dislocation or additional fracture, a telephone consultation is required to develop a treatment plan with the orthopedist.

  Incarcerated medial epicondyle fractures require a bedside consultation.

- Olecranon

  Patients with minimally displaced olecranon fractures require at least a telephone consultation to develop an appropriate treatment plan.

  Patients with displaced olecranon fractures require a bedside evaluation for likely closed reduction or operative planning.

- Radial neck

  Patients with minimally displaced or angulated radial neck fractures do not require formal consultation.

  A telephone consultation is required for a significantly displaced or angulated radial neck fracture or a radial head fracture to develop a treatment plan with the consultant.

- "T" condylar distal humerus fractures

  A bedside consultation is required to formalize the surgical plan.

- Elbow dislocations

  For an isolated, closed elbow dislocation with an intact neurovascular examination and no associated fracture, an experienced practitioner may perform the reduction without formal consultation.

  A bedside consultation is necessary if an associated fracture exists, if a fracture or neurologic injury develops after reduction, or if the elbow is not reducible.

- Nursemaid's elbow

  No formal consultation is required.

- Little Leaguer's elbow

  No formal consultation is required.

■ What Should Be Communicated to the Specialist?
- Presumed diagnosis or reason for consultation
- Age and gender
- Mechanism of injury
- Time of injury
- Additional injuries
- Neurovascular examination of the extremity with assessment of skin integrity (i.e., open fracture)
- Summary of radiographic findings and all studies ordered so far

■ What Analgesia or Anesthesia Should Be Used?
- Intravenous narcotic analgesia is used to maintain patient comfort. Intravenous diazepam may be used to minimize muscle spasm.
- Sedation is performed according to the standard emergency department protocol, usually with either ketamine or propofol.
- Anesthesia for operative procedures is performed in the operating room.

■ What Is Acceptable Alignment for Each Fracture?
- Distal humeral epiphyseal separation

  Extensive remodeling has been reported after these injuries, and large degrees of displacement may be acceptable. However, because most case series are limited with no long-term follow-up, anatomic reduction is recommended if diagnosed early.

- Supracondylar humerus fracture

  Anatomic reduction with varus or valgus angulation comparable to the opposite elbow and an anterior humeral line that crosses the central third of the capitellum is acceptable.

- Lateral condyle

  Anatomic reduction with less than 2 mm of displacement on an internal oblique view of the elbow is acceptable.

- Medial epicondyle

  Acceptable displacement is controversial. However, most orthopedists consider greater than 5 mm unacceptable, especially in the dominant extremity of a throwing athlete.

- Olecranon

  Anatomic alignment is desired to restore joint congruity and extensor function.

- Radial neck

  Acceptable alignment includes angulation of less than 30 degrees on any projection, less than 3 mm of displacement, and a congruent radiocapitellar articulation.

- "T" condylar distal humerus fractures

  Anatomic reduction is required for this intra-articular injury.

- Elbow dislocations

  Anatomic reduction is required.

- Little Leaguer's elbow

  For medial epicondyle stress fractures, reduction parameters for an acute medial epicondyle fracture may be used.

  For other injuries, formal reductions are not applicable.

- Nursemaid's elbow

  No radiographic criteria exist.

  Satisfactory reduction is based on the restoration of full elbow range of motion.

14. Graves SC, Canale ST: Fractures of the olecranon in children: long-term follow-up. J Pediatr Orthop 13:239–241, 1993.
15. Henrikson B: Isolated fractures of the proximal end of the radius in children epidemiology, treatment and prognosis. Acta Orthop Scand 40:246–260, 1969.
16. Blount WP, Schulz I, Cassidy RH: Fractures of the elbow in children. JAMA 146:699–704, 1951.
17. Henrikson B: Supracondylar fracture of the humerus in children: a late review of end-results with special reference to the cause of deformity, disability and complications. Acta Chir Scand Suppl 369:1–72, 1966.
18. Linscheid RL, Wheeler DK: Elbow dislocations. JAMA 194:1171–1176, 1965.
19. Carey RP: Simultaneous dislocation of the elbow and the proximal radio-ulnar joint. J Bone Joint Surg Br 66:254–256, 1984.
20. Chiboub H, Ajbar M, el Bardouni A, et al: [Divergent dislocation of the elbow in an adolescent: a case report]. Chir Main 21:51–55, 2002.
21. Amir D, Frankl U, Pogrund H: Pulled elbow and hypermobility of joints. Clin Orthop Relat Res (257):94–99, 1990.
22. Choung W, Heinrich SD: Acute annular ligament interposition into the radiocapitellar joint in children (nursemaid's elbow). J Pediatr Orthop 15:454–456, 1995.

**Chapter 22**

# Pediatric Forearm and Distal Radius and Ulna Fractures

Mark C. Lee, Silas Marshall, and John C. Brancato

INTRODUCTION
ANATOMIC CONSIDERATIONS
HISTORY
PREHOSPITAL CARE AND MANAGEMENT
PHYSICAL EXAMINATION

DIAGNOSTIC STUDIES
DIFFERENTIAL DIAGNOSIS
TREATMENT OF SPECIFIC INJURIES
GUIDELINES FOR EMERGENCY DEPARTMENT MANAGEMENT
COMMON PITFALLS

## INTRODUCTION

■ A forearm fracture includes any fracture of the radius or ulnar shaft or fracture involving both bones. Although the distal radius and ulna, including the metaphyseal flare to the level of the physis, are technically forearm fractures, they are given separate attention because surgical indications and growth impairments from this fracture pattern differ notably from forearm shaft fractures.

■ Forearm fractures can be associated with a disruption of the distal radioulnar joint (DRUJ) (Galeazzi) or a radial head dislocation (Monteggia).

■ Forearm fractures, including distal radius and ulna fractures, are considered to be the most common long bone fractures in children with an incidence of 30% to 50% of all pediatric fractures.[1-3]

■ Most forearm fractures involve the distal one third of the forearm, with an incidence rate of 70% to 80%, followed by involvement of the middle one third, with an incidence of 10% to 15%.[1-3]

■ Fractures involving the proximal one third of the forearm, including classic Monteggia fractures and variants, have less than a 5% incidence.[1-3]

## ANATOMIC CONSIDERATIONS

The forearm serves as a bridge between the humerus and the carpal bones. It is the origin for muscles that control finger movements and hand and wrist pronation and supination. A normally functioning upper extremity requires an unimpaired ulna and radial skeletal structure and uninterrupted articulations at the radioulnar joint, radiocapitellar joint, and DRUJ.

■ Bones (Fig. 22-1)
  • The radius is the main contributor to the wrist joint. Proximally, the radial head along with the radial bow allows the radius to rotate around the fixed ulna during pronation and supination. Restoration of this

anatomy is a critical component of forearm fracture care.
  • The ulna is a relatively straight bone. The proximal ulna is the main contributor to the elbow joint.
  • The radial styloid and the bicipital tuberosity maintain an essentially 180-degree relationship to each other, and this relationship is preserved through the arc of supination and pronation.

■ Physes
  • The radius has proximal and distal physes.

    Approximately 75% of longitudinal growth comes from the distal physis.[4]

    The distal radial epiphysis appears between 1 and 2 years of age, and the distal radial physis closes between 16 and 17 years of age.

  • The ulna has proximal (olecranon) and distal physes.

    Greater than 80% of longitudinal growth comes from the distal physis.[4]

    The distal ulna epiphysis begins ossification at 7 years of age, and the distal physis closes between 16 and 17 years of age.

  • The distal radial epiphysis is first to appear, followed by the proximal radius (4 to 6 years of age), the distal ulna, and finally the proximal ulna (9 years of age).

■ Joints
  • The proximal radioulnar joint allows for pronation and supination of the forearm. It is stabilized by the annular ligament, which wraps around the radial neck (Fig. 22-2).
  • The DRUJ also allows for pronation and supination of the forearm and can be disrupted in distal radius fractures or dislocated in Galeazzi injuries (radial shaft fracture with a DRUJ disruption).
  • The radiocarpal joint (wrist joint) allows for flexion and extension and radial and ulnar deviation. It is stabilized by strong palmar ligaments.

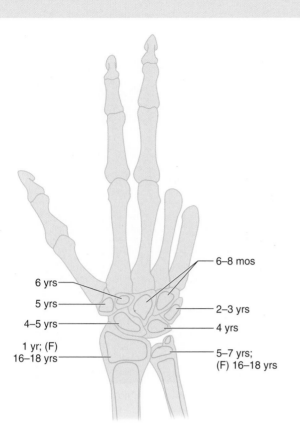

FIGURE 23-1. The order and age of appearance of the ossific nuclei in the bones of the pediatric wrist. Ossification begins at the capitate in a circular fashion, from ulnar to radial, ending at the trapezoid and then the pisiform. *(From Beaty J, Kasser J: Rockwood and Wilkins' fractures in children, ed 6, Philadelphia, 2006, Lippincott Williams & Wilkins.)*

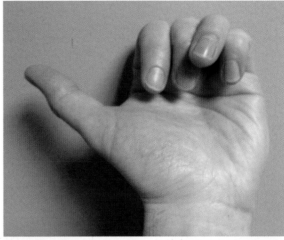

FIGURE 23-2. Rotational deformity in the ring finger of a patient with a middle phalanx malunion. Note the cascade of the unaffected fingers, which all point toward the thenar eminence in flexion.

## PREHOSPITAL CARE AND MANAGEMENT

- Initial management of a child with a hand injury includes immobilization of the hand or affected digit; this can be accomplished with a splint or splintlike material such as a tongue depressor.
- Any active bleeding including arterial bleeding should be controlled with direct pressure. Life-threatening arterial bleeding that cannot be controlled with pressure may be controlled with a temporary tourniquet.
- An amputated digit should be rinsed with clean water or sterile saline and wrapped in a moist gauze sponge or paper towel. The digit should be sealed in a plastic bag and kept on ice. Lower temperatures allow for longer viable ischemia time. Ice should not come in direct contact with the tissues.[3]

## PHYSICAL EXAMINATION

- The hand should first be examined for any signs of trauma. Erythema, edema, ecchymosis, or deformity raises suspicion for underlying injury.
- If metacarpal or phalangeal fractures are suspected, the hand should be examined for angular or rotational deformity.

- Rotational deformity is evaluated by examining the normal digital flexion cascade; all fingers in the flexed position should point to the scaphoid tubercle (Fig. 23-2).
- Although point tenderness helps to localize the injury, the close proximity of the bones in the hand makes definitive diagnosis on physical examination difficult.
- Active and passive range of motion should be checked for all digits.
  - Loss of active range of motion may indicate tendon or motor nerve injury.
  - Loss of active and passive range of motion may indicate dislocation.
- The stability of the affected IP and MCP joints should be examined. Excessive angulation with radial and ulnar deviation may indicate ligamentous or physeal injury.
- A complete neurologic examination is sometimes difficult in a pediatric patient. However, the initial examination should attempt to ascertain the strength, sensation, and vascular supply of the affected extremity.
- A thorough vascular examination to determine the perfusion to the hand and each digit is essential.

## DIAGNOSTIC STUDIES

- X-ray
  - Initial evaluation begins with a standard hand series including posteroanterior, lateral, and oblique projections. Further detail may be obtained with digit-specific images in orthogonal projections.
  - To view the scaphoid perpendicular to its long axis, a posteroanterior view of the wrist in ulnar deviation can be ordered (Fig. 23-3). An anteroposterior view with a clenched fist shows scapholunate disruption.
  - A carpal tunnel view can be ordered for suspected hook of hamate fractures (Fig. 23-4). The hand is maximally dorsiflexed, the palmar surface of wrist

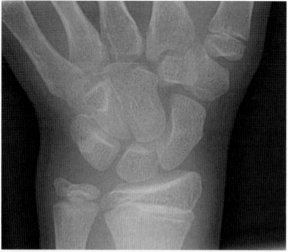

**FIGURE 23-3.** Scaphoid view x-ray. Ulnar deviation eliminates overlap of the other carpal bones and allows a view of the long axis of the scaphoid.

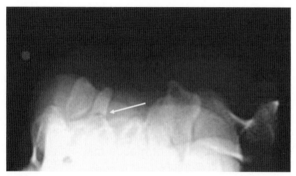

**FIGURE 23-4.** Carpal tunnel view of the wrist shows a nondisplaced fracture at the base of the hook of the hamate *(arrow)*.

rests on the cassette, and the x-ray beam is directed at the cup of the palm at an angle of 15 degrees.
- Computed Tomography (CT)
  - CT scan is infrequently part of the acute evaluation of a hand injury but may be used to delineate fractures that are difficult to visualize on plain films, such as minimally displaced hook of hamate and scaphoid fractures.
  - CT scan can be used to evaluate the extent of joint involvement in the case of intra-articular fractures.
- Magnetic Resonance Imaging (MRI)
  - MRI is infrequently used in the acute setting; however, MRI may be helpful in identifying an occult scaphoid fracture, ligamentous injury, or osteomyelitis (Fig. 23-5).
  - Whether MRI or CT is better for diagnosing suspected scaphoid fractures has been questioned.[4] MRI is preferred in pediatric patients because it avoids exposure to ionizing radiation.
- Laboratory Tests
  - In cases of suspected flexor tenosynovitis, appropriate laboratory work should be sent as outlined in Chapter 18.

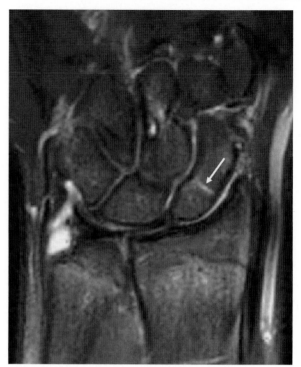

**FIGURE 23-5.** MRI shows an acute, nondisplaced scaphoid fracture.

## DIFFERENTIAL DIAGNOSIS

- The differential diagnosis for hand and finger pain and deformity is broad and depends primarily on the location of the symptoms and the mechanism of injury.
- Pain and deformity in the wrist can be caused by distal radius or ulnar fractures, fracture of the carpal bones, lunate or perilunate dislocations, ligamentous injury, and infection.
- Tenderness to palpation in the anatomic snuffbox indicates injury to the scaphoid (Fig. 23-6).
- Pain and deformity in the hand can be caused by fractures of the metacarpals, carpometacarpal (CMC) joint dislocations, MCP joint dislocations, ligamentous injury, compressive neuropathies, and infection.
- Pain and deformity in the fingers can be caused by phalangeal fractures (commonly physeal fractures), IP joint dislocations, ligamentous injuries, tendon ruptures or avulsions, compressive neuropathies, and infection.
- Loss of active and passive range of motion in any joint can be caused by dislocation and joint contracture. Joint effusion from infection or trauma can limit motion.
- Loss of active motion with maintained passive motion can be caused by tendon rupture or neuromuscular injury or can be volitional owing to pain or for some type of secondary gain.
- Loss of sensation in the hand or fingers can be caused by a compressive neuropathy or acute injury to a specific nerve. A detailed neurologic examination frequently can pinpoint the area of compression from the cervical spine roots to the hand.
- Decreased perfusion to the fingers can be caused by interruption of the blood supply, compression from swelling or a tightly applied dressing, or vasospasm.

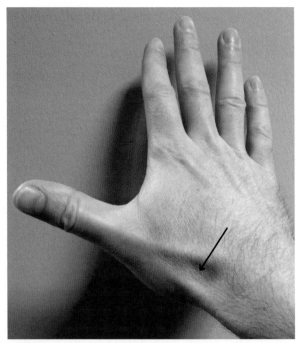

**FIGURE 23-6.** The anatomic snuffbox *(arrow)* is located between the extensor pollicis longus and extensor pollicis brevis tendons. The proximal pole of the scaphoid can be palpated in this space.

## TREATMENT OF SPECIFIC INJURIES

- Scaphoid Fractures
  - Injury to the scaphoid is the most common carpal injury seen in children.[5]
  - D'Arienzo[6] classified pediatric fractures based on the degree of ossification.

    Type I—fracture line is purely chondral and difficult to identify on x-ray; MRI is often needed to confirm the diagnosis

    Type II—fractures are osteochondral, involving part of the ossific nucleus

    Type III—fractures are primarily bony and behave similar to adult scaphoid fractures

  - The location (proximal pole, waist, and distal pole) and the displacement of the fracture are also important in determining the treatment and prognosis. Because of a distally based blood supply, distal fractures tend to heal faster and have a lower rate of nonunion than proximal fractures.[7]
  - For all scaphoid fractures, the patient should be placed in a thumb spica cast or splint. Although there is some disagreement as to whether the cast should be short arm or long arm, a short arm cast is generally used only for presumed or occult fractures and for distal nondisplaced fractures.[7]
  - Reduction of displaced scaphoid fractures should not be attempted.
  - Patients with the appropriate mechanism of injury and tenderness in the anatomic snuffbox in the setting of negative x-rays should be presumed to have an occult scaphoid fracture until proved otherwise.

Although MRI can be performed acutely to rule out a fracture, this is usually unnecessary.

The patient should be placed in a short arm thumb spica cast or splint.

At follow-up examination in 2 weeks, the cast is removed, and x-rays are obtained. If the x-rays are negative but tenderness of the anatomic snuffbox persists, a new short arm thumb spica cast is applied, and MRI is ordered.

- Nondisplaced fractures of the scaphoid usually can be treated nonoperatively in a cast.

  Patients with nondisplaced fractures of the distal pole can be placed in a short arm thumb spica cast or splint.

  Patients with a nondisplaced scaphoid waist or proximal pole fracture should be placed in a long arm thumb spica cast.

  At 3 to 4 weeks, the long arm cast is changed to a short arm thumb spica cast.

  Time to union depends on the location of the fracture. Distal pole fractures heal in 4 to 6 weeks; proximal pole fractures can take 12 weeks to heal.[7]

- Displaced scaphoid fractures require a long arm thumb spica cast regardless of the location of the fracture.

  Displaced scaphoid fractures usually require reduction and fixation in the operating room with either pins or a headless screw.

  The patient should see an orthopedic surgeon within 1 week for re-evaluation and preoperative planning.

- Hook of the Hamate Fractures
  - Fractures of the hook of the hamate are uncommon but are being seen with increasing frequency in adolescent athletes participating in sports such as baseball, golf, and hockey.[8] The fracture occurs in the hand gripping the bat, club, or stick as the wrist experiences a forceful deceleration against the object used for striking (e.g., grounding the club in golf).
  - Pain with palpation over the hook of the hamate should raise suspicion for fracture.
  - Diagnosis can be difficult because the standard hand series x-rays do not allow visualization of the hamate hook. A carpal tunnel view may be helpful, but a CT scan is most sensitive for visualizing this fracture.[8]
  - Treatment involves immobilization in a short arm cast or a volar slab splint.
  - These fractures frequently heal with a short course of immobilization; however, nonunion is common. If symptomatic, the nonunion is treated with simple excision.
  - Follow-up with a hand specialist in 3 to 4 weeks is appropriate.
- Carpal Dislocations
  - Carpal dislocations are very rare but often missed injuries in children. They are caused by high-energy

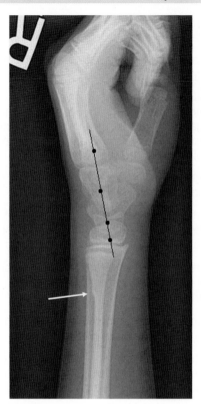

**FIGURE 23-7.** Lateral wrist x-ray after a wrist injury in a 12-year-old boy shows appropriate alignment of the distal radius, lunate, capitate, and metacarpal. Note the buckle fracture of the distal radial shaft *(arrow)*.

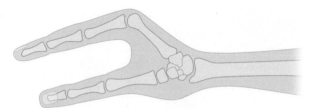

**FIGURE 23-8.** The intrinsic plus or safe position. The MCP joints are held at 70 to 80 degrees, the IP joints are in full extension, and the wrist is slightly extended.

mechanisms and can be associated with other injuries within the involved extremity, such as fractures of the distal radius, carpus, metacarpals, and phalanges.

- It is important to evaluate the lateral hand x-ray carefully to confirm that the distal radius, lunate, capitate, and middle metacarpal line up (Fig. 23-7). If there is any question of the position of the carpal bones on x-ray, a CT scan can be obtained.
- Treatment of these injuries is the same as treatment in adults and involves an urgent attempt at closed reduction under conscious sedation followed by open reduction and pinning in the operating room if closed reduction is unsuccessful.
- Intercarpal dislocations warrant a bedside consultation by the orthopedic surgeon on call.

■ Metacarpal Fractures
- The metacarpals are relatively well protected by surrounding soft tissue structures within the hand. In addition, the investing soft tissues stabilize these fractures. As a result of this stability, most metacarpal fractures can be treated nonoperatively.
- The mechanism of injury is most commonly an axial load (boxer's fractures) or a direct blow as sustained in contact sports.
- Standard hand series x-rays are usually adequate to characterize the fracture.
- Close attention should be paid to rotational deformity of the involved digit. Any amount of rotation warrants an attempt at closed reduction.

- Angulation in the coronal plane (out of the plane of motion) is rare except for the thumb and small metacarpals. Deformity out of the plane of motion is poorly tolerated and should be treated with closed reduction.
- Angulation in the plane of motion (i.e., dorsal/palmar) is better tolerated and has much better remodeling potential.
- Fractures of the distal metacarpal (e.g., metacarpal neck) have a greater acceptable range of angulation than more proximal fractures (e.g., metacarpal shaft or base).
- A hematoma block or conscious sedation should be used for closed reduction of these fractures.
- The hand should be splinted in the intrinsic plus or "safe" position with a palmar slab splint for index or middle finger metacarpals and an ulnar gutter splint for ring or small finger metacarpals (Fig. 23-8). A thumb spica splint or cast should be used for thumb metacarpal fractures.
- Metacarpal fractures are characterized in terms of their location—base, shaft, neck, intra-articular, or physeal.
- Metacarpal base fractures are usually high-energy injuries.

  Radiographs should be carefully evaluated for CMC joint dislocations or significant articular displacement.

  Thumb metacarpal base fractures warrant special mention because the thumb metacarpal has a proximal growth plate, whereas the remaining metacarpals have a distal growth plate. Closed reduction and thumb spica immobilization may be attempted for these physeal fractures. However, these injuries are frequently unstable and require operative closed reduction as opposed to open reduction and pinning.

- Metacarpal shaft fractures in isolation usually can be treated nonoperatively.

  Closed reduction should be performed to correct any amount of rotational deformity.

  Closed reduction for angulation should be attempted. However, maintenance of the reduction can be challenging owing to the pull of surrounding muscles. If acceptable alignment is not held by close reduction and splinting, operative pinning may be necessary.

- Metacarpal neck fractures are also most commonly treated nonoperatively.

  Closed reduction should be performed to correct any amount of rotational deformity.

  The most common deformity seen with metacarpal neck fractures is palmar angulation of the distal fragment.

  - Correction of this deformity can be achieved by using the Jahss maneuver.[9]
  - The MCP joint is bent to 90 degrees, and upward pressure is applied to the proximal phalanx with a downward counterforce applied dorsally to the metacarpal shaft.

  Rarely, metacarpal neck fractures are unstable and require operative pinning.

- Careful reduction of the physis is important. Significant displacement of the physis or unstable physeal fractures may require closed reduction as opposed to open reduction and pinning in the operating room.
- Follow-up with a hand specialist in 1 to 2 weeks is appropriate for stable fractures. Follow-up within 1 week is warranted for unstable fractures or fractures with unacceptable alignment.
- ■ CMC Dislocation
  - CMC joint dislocations tend to be high-energy injuries. Concomitant injuries are seen frequently.
  - It is important to evaluate the lateral hand x-ray carefully for evidence of CMC dislocation. If there is any question of the reduction of the joint on x-ray, a CT scan can be obtained.
  - Treatment of these injuries is the same as treatment in adults.

    An urgent closed reduction is performed with either a hematoma block or conscious sedation.

    Closed reduction is performed by applying gentle inline traction on the affected metacarpal, while applying a direct reduction force on the base of the metacarpal.

    The hand is splinted in the intrinsic plus position.

  - If closed reduction is unsuccessful, open reduction and pinning in the operating room should be undertaken.
  - After a closed reduction attempt, the patient should be monitored for compartment syndrome of the hand.
  - If a stable reduction is achieved, a telephone consultation with a hand surgeon to discuss further treatment and appropriate follow-up is warranted.
- ■ Phalangeal Fractures
  - Fractures of the phalanges are the most common injury in the pediatric hand with crush injuries to the distal phalanx and physeal injuries of the proximal phalanges being seen most often.[1]
  - Because of their relatively unprotected position, the index and small fingers are most prone to injury.
  - Standard hand series x-rays can be obtained to look for concomitant injury. However, an anteroposterior

and lateral view of the digit is more appropriate for isolated injuries.
- The mechanism of injury for phalangeal fractures is usually an axial load combined with an angular force.

  Crush injuries occur most often in the distal phalanx.

  Pure angular forces result in physeal injury or joint dislocation.

- Close attention should be paid to rotational deformity of the involved digit. Any amount of rotation warrants an attempt at closed reduction.
- Most phalangeal fractures can be treated nonoperatively with closed reduction and immobilization for 3 to 4 weeks.
- Unstable or irreducible phalangeal fractures require operative closed reduction as opposed to open reduction and pinning.
- Fractures of the phalanges are characterized by the specific phalanx involved (proximal, middle, or distal phalanx) and by the location of the fracture within the phalanx (physeal, shaft, neck, intra-articular, and crush).
- Physeal fractures in the phalanges are common.

  Nondisplaced or minimally displaced physeal fractures can be treated with immobilization (Aluma-Foam splint, palmar plaster splint, or buddy taping) in the safe position for 3 to 4 weeks. Care should be taken to immobilize only the affected digit or joint, allowing the unaffected digits or joints to move freely.

  Displaced physeal fractures should be treated with closed reduction using either a digital block or conscious sedation.

  - Reduction is accomplished by simply reversing the direction of the deformity.
  - For physeal fractures at the base of the proximal phalanx, a pencil or pen can be placed in the web space and used as a fulcrum to reduce the fracture (Fig. 23-9).

  Close follow-up within 1 week is appropriate for physeal fractures of the phalanges.

- Phalangeal shaft and neck fractures are treated in the same manner as fractures in adults.

  The mainstay of treatment is closed reduction and immobilization of the affected digit in the safe position.

  Phalangeal neck fractures are often unstable and may require operative closed reduction or open reduction and pinning.

  If a stable closed reduction is obtained, follow-up in 1 to 2 weeks is necessary.

- For intra-articular phalangeal fractures, near-anatomic reduction of the articular surface is mandatory.

  Nondisplaced intra-articular fractures can be treated nonoperatively. They should be immobilized in the intrinsic plus or safe position for 3 to 4 weeks.

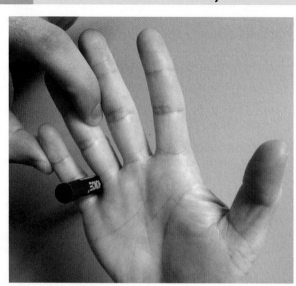

**FIGURE 23-9.** A pen or pencil can be used as a fulcrum to reduce fractures of the proximal phalanges.

Mallet finger equivalents can be both intra-articular and intraphyseal (Fig. 23-10).

- Frequently, an acceptable reduction can be obtained by extending the distal interphalangeal joint. The joint is immobilized with a mallet finger (Stax) splint (Fig. 23-11). Careful attention must be paid to the position of the joint after reduction of the fracture because subluxation is common.
- Occasionally, this fracture is open and can manifest with a nail bed injury.[1] A repair of the germinal matrix (see later) is indicated in the setting of an obvious displaced nail bed injury.
- If the fragment is irreducible by simple extension of the joint, operative reduction and pinning may be indicated.

    Displaced physeal fractures require operative closed or open reduction and pinning.

- This procedure is usually scheduled on an outpatient basis.
- In the emergency department, attempts at closed reduction are usually futile. Immobilization of the affected digit for comfort is usually all that is necessary.

    The patient should have a follow-up examination within 1 week for a displaced articular fracture in case operative planning is warranted.

- Crush injuries to the distal phalanx are one of the most common injuries in the pediatric hand.

    Crush injuries always involve some degree of soft tissue injury.

- Frequently, the distal phalanx fracture is an open fracture and should be treated as such with appropriate antibiotics and tetanus prophylaxis.
- Open wounds should be irrigated with sterile normal saline in the emergency department.

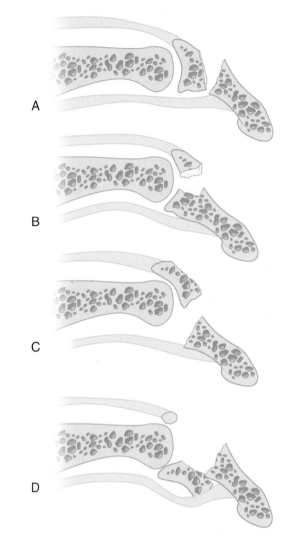

**FIGURE 23-10.** Mallet finger equivalent fractures in children involve the proximal physis of the distal phalanx. They can be intra-articular or extra-articular. *(From Beaty J, Kasser J: Rockwood and Wilkins' fractures in children, ed 6, Philadelphia, 2006, Lippincott Williams & Wilkins.)*

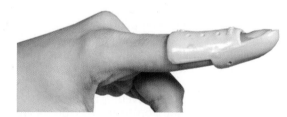

**FIGURE 23-11.** A Stax splint properly applied allows for free motion at the proximal interphalangeal joint, while keeping the distal interphalangeal joint immobilized in full extension.

- Digital block or conscious sedation allows adequate exploration of the wounds.

    Nail bed lacerations without excellent wound margin alignment should be repaired in the emergency department.

- Using a Freer elevator or small pair of dissecting scissors, the remaining nail should be removed to allow access to the germinal matrix.
- The nail bed should be irrigated with normal saline and repaired using either a 6-0 absorbable suture or surgical glue such as cyanoacrylate (Dermabond).
- After the nail bed repair, either the nail or a piece of foil from the suture pack can be cleaned with povidone-iodine (Betadine) and placed under the eponychial fold. The nail or foil can be held in place either with absorbable suture or glue.[10]

  Distal phalanx fractures should be immobilized with an Alumafoam splint that wraps around the tip. Care must be taken to avoid compressing the finger tip with this splint.

  For closed, isolated distal phalanx crush fractures, follow-up in 1 to 2 weeks is appropriate.

  For open fractures and fractures with nail bed repair, follow-up should be within 1 week.

- ◼ IP and MCP Joint Dislocations
  - The collateral ligaments and other soft tissues surrounding the IP and MCP joints in children are stronger than the physes. As a result, IP joint dislocations are much less common than phalangeal fractures through the physis.
  - IP and MCP joint dislocations are also frequently associated with concomitant physeal fractures.
  - Acute treatment of IP and MCP joint dislocations in children is similar to treatment of dislocations in adults. However, the physis must always be evaluated carefully both before and after reduction.
  - Closed reduction can be accomplished with a digital block or conscious sedation. Frequently, the joint reduces with gentle inline traction. Often, the deformity must first be exaggerated and then traction applied as the deformity is reversed.
  - MCP joint dislocations

    MCP joint dislocations are classified as simple or complex.

    Complex dislocations are irreducible by closed means because the volar plate has become interposed into the joint. These dislocations can be identified on x-ray by bayonet apposition of the proximal phalanx onto the metacarpal (Fig. 23-12). Although an attempt at closed reduction is appropriate, it is important to recognize this injury and to have a low threshold for specialist consultation.

  - IP and MCP joint dislocations that are stable after reduction require only a short period of immobilization followed by early motion.

    Immobilization can be accomplished with an Alumafoam splint or buddy taping.

    The patient should have follow-up within 1 week to remove the splint and start gentle range of motion.

  - For unstable dislocations, it is important to determine whether there is a stable range of motion.

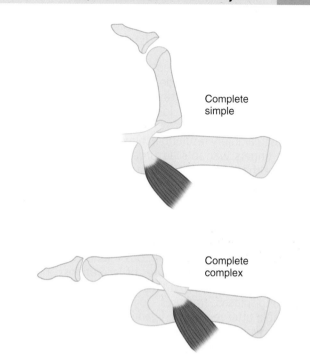

**FIGURE 23-12.** A simple MCP dislocation tends to manifest in extension. With no interposed soft tissue, this dislocation tends to be reducible. A complex MCP joint dislocation manifests with bayonet apposition. Interposed soft tissues tend to make this injury irreducible. *(From Beaty J, Kasser J: Rockwood and Wilkins' fractures in children, ed 6, Philadelphia, 2006, Lippincott Williams & Wilkins.)*

- Many dorsal dislocations that are unstable at full extension can be held reduced in flexion. In this case, a dorsal extension-block splint can be used.
- Unstable joints can be treated nonoperatively with more specialized splints.

  Operative reduction and pinning is frequently needed.

  Consultation by a hand specialist is warranted.

- ◼ Soft Tissue Injuries and Infections
  - Soft tissue injuries, including tendon lacerations or ruptures, ligament injuries, nerve lacerations, vascular injuries, and skin wounds, are treated as they are in an adult patient.
  - Infections in the pediatric hand are treated as they are in the adult hand.

## GUIDELINES FOR EMERGENCY DEPARTMENT MANAGEMENT

- ◼ When and How Should a Specialist Be Consulted?
  - Pediatric hand injuries rarely necessitate emergent intervention by a consultant. The initial care of these injuries can be delivered by the emergency staff with subsequent outpatient follow-up with a hand specialist.
  - Emergent bedside consultation by a specialist is appropriate for suspected acute carpal tunnel

syndrome, infection involving a joint, and infection within the flexor tendon sheath (flexor tenosynovitis).

- Injuries warranting bedside consultation on a less emergent basis include displaced physeal fractures, irreducible joint dislocations, tooth penetration into an IP or MCP joint ("fight bite"), and open fractures.
- Vascular injury resulting in hypoperfusion of the hand or fingers warrants an urgent bedside consultation by either a hand specialist or a vascular surgeon, depending on institutional protocol.
- Telephone consultation to discuss management and follow-up is appropriate for displaced fractures that do not involve the physis, fractures involving the articular surface, nail bed injuries, dorsal hand and finger abscesses, ligamentous injuries with resultant instability, tendon ruptures or lacerations, and nerve lacerations without vascular compromise.
- Nondisplaced fractures, joint dislocations that are stable after reduction, ligament sprains, and isolated soft tissue injuries (without associated tendon, ligament, joint, or neurovascular injury) can be treated without specialist consultation, as long as appropriate outpatient follow-up is arranged.

■ What Should Be Communicated to the Specialist?
- Presumed diagnosis or reason for consultation
- Age and gender
- Mechanism of injury
- Time of injury
- Additional injuries
- Location and degree of deformity
- Neurovascular examination of the extremity
- Summary of radiographic findings and all studies ordered so far
- Summary of interventions preformed so far (e.g., digital block, reduction attempts)

■ What Analgesia or Anesthesia Should Be Used?
- Oral non-narcotic pain medications are frequently sufficient for patients with nondisplaced fractures. These medications have the best safety profile and fewest side effects. Intravenous or oral narcotic analgesia is used to maintain patient comfort for more severe pain. Intravenous benzodiazepine may be used to minimize patient spasm for reduction.
- For most finger injuries, a digital block of the affected finger is adequate analgesia.

  This block can be performed with either 1% lidocaine or 0.5% bupivacaine (Marcaine) without epinephrine because epinephrine can theoretically lead to hypoperfusion of the digit by inducing vasospasm. Usually, 6 mL of analgesic is adequate.

  Using a 25-gauge needle, 2 mL of analgesic is infused into the web space from a dorsal approach along the radial and ulnar aspects of the digit. The needle should be directed as palmarly as possible and withdrawn dorsally during infusion. A final 1 to 2 mL of analgesic should be infused into the dorsal tissues overlying the base of the proximal phalanx.

  Before injection, aspiration of the needle should be done to ensure that the needle is not intravascular.

- A hematoma block with 2 to 3 mL of 1% lidocaine or 0.5% bupivacaine can be effective anesthesia for metacarpal fractures and many dislocations of the hand and wrist.
- For injuries proximal to the MCP joints or injuries in patients younger than 8 years, conscious sedation is often required.

■ What Is Acceptable Alignment for Metacarpal or Phalangeal Fracture or IP or MCP Joint Dislocation?
- For metacarpal and phalangeal fractures, no amount of rotation and minimal amounts of angulation in the coronal plane are acceptable for both functional and cosmetic reasons. Although children do have remodeling potential, the degree of remodeling of angulation out of the plane of motion is much less than that of dorsal or palmar angulation.
- Occasionally, acceptable alignment can be obtained but not held by closed means. These unstable fractures may require reduction and pinning in the operating room.
- A significant amount of angulation in the plane of motion can be tolerated at the metacarpal neck and shaft.

  Depending on the patient's age, varying degrees of remodeling can be expected over time.

  The more mobile rays (ring and small fingers) can tolerate greater degrees of angulation.

  Generally, the hand can tolerate 10 to 20 degrees of angulation in the index and middle fingers and 30 to 40 degrees of angulation in the ring and small fingers.[11]

- Metacarpal base fractures tend to be high-energy injuries. Rather than alignment, attention should be paid to the degree of displacement of the articular surface and the possibility of a CMC dislocation.
- Any physeal displacement warrants closed reduction.
- For phalangeal shaft fractures in children younger than 10 years, 20 to 30 degrees of angulation in the plane of motion is acceptable.
- In children older than 10 years, only 10 to 20 degrees of palmar or dorsal angulation is acceptable.[1]

■ What Initial Splinting or Immobilization Should Be Provided?
- The younger the patient, the less at risk he or she is for joint contracture after immobilization. However, every attempt should be made to immobilize only the affected bones and joints, leaving uninjured digits free to move.
- Scaphoid fractures should be immobilized in a thumb spica splint or cast. There is some controversy regarding whether a long arm or short arm cast is better. A long arm cast seems reasonable for waist, proximal, or any displaced fracture, whereas a short arm cast is adequate for nondisplaced distal fractures.

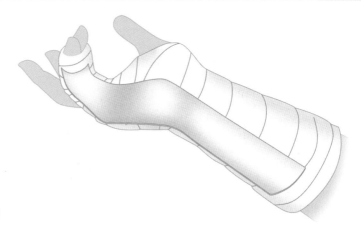

**FIGURE 23-13.** Ulnar gutter splint with the hand in the intrinsic plus or safe position.

Data suggest that there is little difference between the two casts.
- Metacarpal fractures should be immobilized with either a palmar slab or an ulnar gutter in the intrinsic plus or safe position (Fig. 23-13).
- Phalangeal fractures or IP joint dislocations can be immobilized with an Alumafoam splint, making sure to leave unaffected joints free.
- Stable phalangeal fractures and IP fractures can also be immobilized with simple buddy taping to the neighboring finger.
- Distal phalanx fractures and dislocations of the distal interphalangeal joint can be immobilized with a Stax finger splint, leaving the proximal interphalangeal joint free.

■ What Postreduction Imaging Is Necessary?
- A repeat hand series is appropriate after closed reduction of a metacarpal fracture and a carpal, CMC, or MCP joint dislocation.
- Anteroposterior and lateral views of the affected digit are appropriate after closed reduction of a phalangeal fracture or an IP joint dislocation.

■ What Is the Plan for Follow-up Care?
- The hand specialist usually requires a follow-up examination within 1 week of the injury.
- In the case of injuries requiring surgery on an outpatient basis (i.e., unstable fractures, intra-articular fractures, tendon lacerations, and nerve lacerations), the follow-up examination should be within a few days of the emergency department encounter.

■ What Are Outpatient Pain Relief Options?
- Reduction of deformity, splinting, and elevation provide excellent pain control.
- Over-the-counter ibuprofen and acetaminophen provide excellent pain relief with an excellent side-effect and safety profile.
- Oral narcotic pain medications such as hydrocodone or oxycodone are useful. A codeine/acetaminophen combination is usually adequate.

■ What Further Care Plan Should Be Discussed With the Patient?
- For infections requiring incision and drainage, it should be explained that a repeat procedure might be necessary.

- For unstable fractures, fractures with unacceptable alignment after reduction, tendon lacerations, nerve lacerations, and unstable ligamentous injuries, the possibility of operative intervention should be discussed with the hand specialist on call and communicated to the patient.
- The patient should be warned to expect stiffness in the immobilized joints.
  Stiffness usually resolves without intervention in younger patients.
  Older patients may require a course of hand therapy to regain motion.

■ Discharge or Inpatient Admission?
- Most pediatric patients with hand injuries can be discharged from the emergency department with appropriate outpatient follow-up.
- Patients who require urgent or emergent operative intervention should be admitted as inpatients. This includes patients with irreducible joint dislocations, deep infections of the palmar side of the hand (flexor tenosynovitis, web space infections, deep palmar infections), acute carpal tunnel syndrome, and fight bites.
- Patients with hand infections requiring incision and drainage in the emergency department may need to be admitted for a course of intravenous antibiotics.

■ What Is Anticipated Specialist Care Treatment or Anticipated Definitive Treatment?
- The hand specialist directs subsequent operative or nonoperative management of the patient.
- For the urgent or emergent diagnoses listed previously, operative intervention can be expected on the day of admission or the following morning.
- For injuries requiring nonurgent surgery, an outpatient procedure is planned at the initial follow-up.
- See earlier for definitive treatments of specific hand injuries.

■ Discharge Care and Instruction
- All dressings, splints, and casts should be kept clean and dry.
- The injured extremity should be elevated above the level of the heart as much as possible to reduce swelling.

- Applying an ice bag wrapped in a towel for 15-minute intervals may help with inflammation and pain control.
- Patients should have a follow-up appointment 7 to 10 days after discharge from the emergency department or the floor.
- Patients who require outpatient surgery should have the surgery scheduled within a few days after discharge from the emergency department.
- The individual surgeon determines follow-up for surgical patients. Brace or cast immobilization may or may not be a component of the postoperative protocol.
- Frequent range of motion exercises of the uninjured free joints should be emphasized.

## COMMON PITFALLS

- Occult and chondral fractures of the scaphoid are frequently missed. A short arm thumb spica cast should be placed in the emergency department if there is reason to suspect these fractures.
- Lunate or perilunate dislocations also are frequently missed. Careful evaluation of the lateral hand film is important to confirm that the distal radius, lunate, capitate, and metacarpals are colinear.
- Metacarpal base fractures tend to be high-energy injuries and are often associated with a CMC joint dislocation.
- A complex MCP joint dislocation must be recognized because closed reduction maneuvers may be futile.

- Rotational deformity should be evaluated in metacarpal and phalangeal fractures.
- Careful repair of the nail bed is essential in the case of crush injuries to the distal phalanx.
- Absorbable suture only should be used when repairing skin or nail bed injuries in the pediatric hand.

## References

1. Beaty J, Kasser J: Rockwood and Wilkins' fractures in children, ed 6, Philadelphia, 2006, Lippincott Williams & Wilkins.
2. Nafie SA: Fractures of the carpal bones in children. Injury 18:117–119, 1987.
3. Partlin MM, Chen J, Holdgate A: The preoperative preservation of amputated digits: an assessment of proposed methods. J Trauma 65:127–131, 2008.
4. Mallee W, Doornberg JN, Ring D, et al: Comparison of CT and MRI for diagnosis of suspected scaphoid fractures. J Bone Joint Surg Am 93:20–28, 2011.
5. Gholson JJ, Bae DS, Zurakowski D, et al: Scaphoid fractures in children and adolescents: contemporary injury patterns and factors influencing time to union. J Bone Joint Surg Am 93:1210–1219, 2011.
6. D'Arienzo M: Scaphoid fractures in children. J Hand Surg Br 27:424–426, 2002.
7. Anz AW, Bushnell BD, Bynum DK, et al: Pediatric scaphoid fractures. J Am Acad Orthop Surg 17:77–87, 2009.
8. Morgan WJ, Slowman LS: Acute hand and wrist injuries in athletes: evaluation and management. J Am Acad Orthop Surg 9:389–400, 2001.
9. Jahss S: Fractures of the metacarpals: a new method of reduction and immobilization. J Bone Joint Surg 20:9, 1938.
10. Strauss EJ, Weil WM, Jordan C, et al: A prospective, randomized, controlled trial of 2-octylcyanoacrylate versus suture repair for nail bed injuries. J Hand Surg Am 33:250–253, 2008.
11. Kozin SH, Thoder JJ, Lieberman G: Operative treatment of metacarpal and phalangeal shaft fractures. J Am Acad Orthop Surg 8:111–121, 2000.

**Chapter 24**

# *Pediatric Cervical Spine Fractures*

Mark C. Lee, Silas Marshall, and John C. Brancato

**INTRODUCTION**
**ANATOMIC CONSIDERATIONS**
**HISTORY**
**PREHOSPITAL CARE AND MANAGEMENT**
**PHYSICAL EXAMINATION**

**DIAGNOSTIC STUDIES**
**TREATMENT OF SPECIFIC INJURIES**
**GUIDELINES FOR EMERGENCY DEPARTMENT MANAGEMENT**
**COMMON PITFALLS**

## INTRODUCTION

Cervical spine fractures in children are rare; they account for 1% of all pediatric fractures.[1] Upper cervical spine fractures are more common in children younger than 8 years of age. As children mature, the anatomy approaches the anatomy of adults, and upper and lower cervical spine injuries become equally distributed.[2]

## ANATOMIC CONSIDERATIONS

An understanding of the normal growth and development of the pediatric spine, the ossification centers, and the closure of the typical synchondroses is important to the diagnosis and treatment of cervical spine injuries in pediatric patients.

- ■ C1 (Atlas)
  - • The atlas has three ossification centers present by 1 year of age, one for the body and one each for the neural arches (Fig. 24-1).
  - • A synchondrosis (neurocentral), essentially a bidirectional growth plate, links the vertebral body to the neural arches. The neurocentral synchondroses close by 7 years of age and may be mistaken for a fracture before closure.
  - • The anterior arch may be bifid or may develop from two centers.
  - • Posterior arches typically fuse by 3 years of age.
  - • Adult dimensions to the ring of C1 are reached by 4 years of age.
  - • Failure of C1 to segment from the skull (occipitalization of C1) can lead to narrowing of the foramen magnum and neurologic deficits and predispose to upper cervical spine instability.
- ■ C2 (Axis)
  - • The axis develops from at least four primary ossification centers, one each for the dens, the body, and the neural arches (Fig. 24-2).
  - • The neurocentral synchondroses close at 7 years of age.

- • A synchondrosis exists between the body and dens, which also closes at 7 years of age. Before closure, this synchondrosis can be mistaken for fracture. However, the location of this synchondrosis below the level of the C2 facets distinguishes this line from a fracture or an os odontoideum.
- • A separate summit ossification may exist at the tip of the dens and fuses by 12 years of age.
- • The inferior epiphyseal ring along the body may not fuse until 25 years of age.
- • Multiple congenital anomalies of the dens have been reported, with complete or partial absence of the dens leading to varying degrees of instability.[3]
- • Os odontoideum refers to a separate ossicle of the dens with no physical attachment to the C2 body, predisposing to C1-2 instability.
- ■ C3 to C7 (Lower Cervical Spine)
  - • Each of the lower cervical vertebrae form from three primary ossification centers, one each for the body and the neural arches (Fig. 24-3).
  - • The neural arches fuse by 2 to 3 years of age.
  - • The neurocentral synchondroses fuse by 3 to 6 years of age.
  - • The vertebrae are normally wedge-shaped until 8 years of age.[4]
  - • Five secondary centers of ossification can remain open until skeletal maturity, one for the spinous process, each transverse process, and each ring apophysis.
  - • The longitudinal growth of the spine occurs through the endplates, physes located between the vertebral body and the disk. The endplate is a potential area of weakness through which fractures are more likely to occur.
  - • The sagittal plane angulation of all facets in the newborn is relatively horizontal and increases in angulation with growth.

  The angle of the facet joints in the lower cervical spine for a newborn is 30 degrees.

  The angle increases to 70 degrees at maturity.

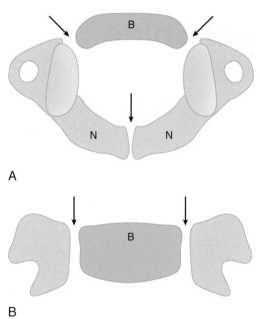

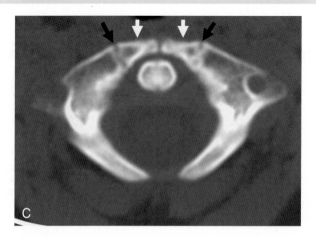

**FIGURE 24-1.** Axial **(A)** and coronal **(B)** plane diagrams of a skeletally immature C1 vertebral body. Three general ossification centers are depicted, one each for the neural arches *(N)* and one for the body *(B)*. The body often fuses from two separate ossification centers, as noted in a CT scan **(C)** in a 6-year-old boy. The *black arrows* indicate the location of the neurocentral synchondroses. The *white arrows* identify the separate ossification centers in the body forming the anterior arch.

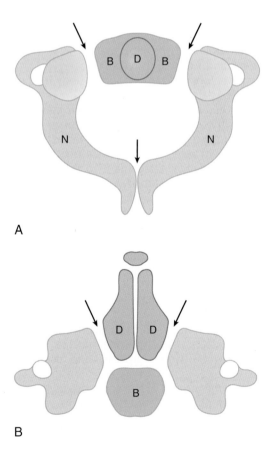

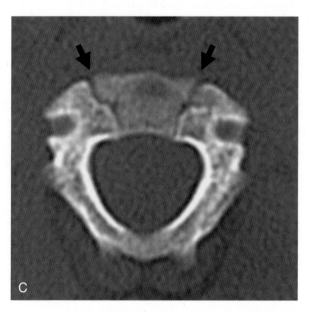

**FIGURE 24-2.** Axial **(A)** and coronal **(B)** plane diagrams of a skeletally immature C2 vertebral body with CT scan **(C)** of C2 vertebral body in a 1-year-old boy. Five ossification centers are depicted, one each for the dens *(D)*, body *(B)*, and neural arches *(N)*. The *arrows* identify the neurocentral synchondroses. Note the synchondrosis between the dens and the body, which may be confused for a fracture.

The facet orientation may make the pediatric spine more susceptible to instability with trauma.

• Generalized pediatric ligamentous laxity is also reflected in the cervical spine; flexion and extension at C2-C3 is 50% greater in children than adults.

The most mobile segment in the cervical spine proceeds distally with age: C3-C4, 3 to 8 years; C4-C5, 9 to 11 years; C5-C6, 12 to 15 years.[5]

This mobility in association with age may contribute to the greater incidence of lower cervical spine fractures with advancing age.

- Narcotic analgesics are useful.

  If a closed reduction is necessary with traction, the initial application may be in the emergency department. In these cases, an awake, alert patient is desirable, and dosing of narcotic analgesics should be monitored to allow a coherent conversation with a cooperative patient.

  For closed reduction maneuvers in young children, an operating room may be preferable because cooperation is often limited.

- What Is Acceptable Alignment?
  - Alignment after reduction is judged by the specialist.
  - The residual alignment often determines the need to proceed with operative intervention.
- What Initial Splinting or Immobilization Should Be Provided?
  - Inherently stable cervical spine injuries can be treated with a hard collar.
  - A cervical spine injury that requires closed reduction often requires halo or cast immobilization. Both are likely to be placed in the operating room for pediatric patients, although young adults tolerate a halo application in the emergency department.
  - A hard collar with appropriate head management (sandbags, contoured board to allow for relatively larger head) is minimal stabilization for a cervical spine injury and should be maintained until the protocol for spine clearance is satisfied.
- What Postreduction Imaging Is Necessary?
  - Plain radiographs and CT scan are used to assess a reduction.
- What Is the Plan for Follow-up Care?
  - Referral to an orthopedic or neurosurgical pediatric spine surgeon should occur within 7 to 10 days of injury.
- What Are Outpatient Pain Relief Options?
  - Oral narcotic pain medications such as hydrocodone or oxycodone are useful.
  - Muscle spasm is often a major symptom and may be controlled with a weight-appropriate dose of diazepam.
- What Further Care Plan Should Be Discussed With the Patient?
  - Before discharge, it must be explained to the patient that follow-up and maintenance of immobilization are important because presumably stable injuries may become unstable over time.
  - The patient is restricted from gym and sports activities until further notice. The patient may need to remain out of school until the follow-up visit.
- Discharge or Inpatient Admission?
  - The patient may be discharged from the emergency department if the patient has an inherently stable cervical spine injury by clinical and radiographic data and is alert and comfortable.
  - Patients with unstable cervical spine injuries, focal neurologic deficits, persistent neck pain despite radiographic normality, or multiple distracting injuries and an unclear examination require inpatient admission.

- What Is Anticipated Specialist Care Treatment or Anticipated Definitive Treatment?
  - If the patient is stable, simple follow-up with immobilization is needed. The injuries usually heal reliably in 3 to 6 weeks, and follow-up includes radiographs to assess stability.
  - If the patient has an unstable injury, immediate treatment may be closed reduction. For persistent instability either in the acute setting or as an outpatient, surgical stabilization may be necessary.
- Discharge Care and Instruction
  - Hard collar immobilization or halo immobilization should not be changed by the patient.
  - These patients should have a follow-up appointment 7 to 10 days after discharge from the emergency department or the hospital.
  - Patients with halos require a pin care protocol, typically a hydrogen peroxide cleansing of the pin tips daily. If the pin sites become loose or bothersome, the patient should be instructed to contact the specialist immediately.
  - The individual surgeon determines follow-up for surgical patients. Cervical immobilization may or may not be a component of the postoperative protocol.

## COMMON PITFALLS

- The radiographic variations in the pediatric cervical spine that may be confused for injury need to be recognized.
- Severe spinal cord injury can occur in pediatric patients in the absence of plain radiograph or CT scan evidence of bony or ligamentous injury.
- Child abuse must be considered in an infant or toddler with a cervical spine injury.

### References

1. Hadley MN, Zabramski JM, Browner CM, et al: Pediatric spinal trauma: review of 122 cases of spinal cord and vertebral column injuries. J Neurosurg 68:18–24, 1988.
2. Orenstein JB, Klein BL, Gotschall CS, et al: Age and outcome in pediatric cervical spine injury: 11-year experience. Pediatr Emerg Care 10:132–137, 1994.
3. Hensinger RN: Congenital anomalies of the cervical spine. Clin Orthop Relat Res 264:16–38, 1991.
4. Lawson JP, Ogden JA, Bucholz RW, et al: Physeal injuries of the cervical spine. J Pediatr Orthop 7:428–435, 1987.
5. Pennecot GF, Gouraud D, Hardy JR, et al: Roentgenographical study of the stability of the cervical spine in children. J Pediatr Orthop 4:346–352, 1984.
6. Aufdermaur M: Spinal injuries in juveniles: necropsy findings in twelve cases. J Bone Joint Surg Br 56:513–519, 1974.
7. Ghatan S, Ellenbogen RG: Pediatric spine and spinal cord injury after inflicted trauma. Neurosurg Clin N Am 13:227–233, 2002.
8. Kokoska ER, Keller MS, Rallo MC, et al: Characteristics of pediatric cervical spine injuries. J Pediatr Surg 36:100–105, 2001.
9. Zuckerbraun BS, Morrison K, Gaines B, et al: Effect of age on cervical spine injuries in children after motor vehicle collisions: effectiveness of restraint devices. J Pediatr Surg 39:483–486, 2004.
10. Evans DL, Bethem D: Cervical spine injuries in children. J Pediatr Orthop 9:563–568, 1989.
11. Nypaver M, Treloar D: Neutral cervical spine positioning in children. Ann Emerg Med 23:208–211, 1994.
12. Lally KP, Senac M, Hardin WD, Jr, et al: Utility of the cervical spine radiograph in pediatric trauma. Am J Surg 158:540–541, 1989.

13. Adelgais KM, Grossman DC, Langer SG, et al: Use of helical computed tomography for imaging the pediatric cervical spine. Acad Emerg Med 11:228–236, 2004.

14. Lerman JA, Haynes RJ: Open versus closed halo rings: comparison of fixation strengths. Spine (Phila Pa 1976) 26:2102–2104, 2001.

15. Ralston ME, Chung K, Barnes PD, et al: Role of flexion-extension radiographs in blunt pediatric cervical spine injury. Acad Emerg Med 8:237–245, 2001.

16. Cattell HS, Filtzer DL: Pseudosubluxation and other normal variations in the cervical spine in children: a study of one hundred and sixty children. J Bone Joint Surg Am 47:1295–1309, 1965.

17. Allington NJ, Zembo M, Nadell J, et al: C1-C2 posterior soft-tissue injuries with neurologic impairment in children. J Pediatr Orthop 10:596–601, 1990.

18. Flynn JM, Closkey RF, Mahboubi S, et al: Role of magnetic resonance imaging in the assessment of pediatric cervical spine injuries. J Pediatr Orthop 22:573–577, 2002.

19. Taylor AR: The mechanism of injury to the spinal cord in the neck without damage to vertebral column. J Bone Joint Surg Br 33:543–547, 1951.

20. Pang D, Pollack IF: Spinal cord injury without radiographic abnormality in children—the SCIWORA syndrome. J Trauma 29:654–664, 1989.

21. Menezes AH: Craniovertebral junction anomalies: diagnosis and management. Semin Pediatr Neurol 4:209–223, 1997.

22. Momjian S, Dehdashti AR, Kehrli P, et al: Occipital condyle fractures in children: case report and review of the literature. Pediatr Neurosurg 38:265–270, 2003.

23. Tuli S, Tator CH, Fehlings MG, et al: Occipital condyle fractures. Neurosurgery 41:368–376, 1997.

24. Papadopoulos SM, Dickman CA, Sonntag VK, et al: Traumatic atlantooccipital dislocation with survival. Neurosurgery 28:574–579, 1991.

25. Sun PP, Poffenbarger GJ, Durham S, et al: Spectrum of occipitoatlantoaxial injury in young children. J Neurosurg 93(1 Suppl):28–39, 2000.

26. Thakar C, Harish S, Saifuddin A, et al: Displaced fracture through the anterior atlantal synchondrosis. Skeletal Radiol 34:547–549, 2005.

27. Judd DB, Liem LK, Petermann G: Pediatric atlas fracture: a case of fracture through a synchondrosis and review of the literature. Neurosurgery 46:991–994, 2000.

28. Korinth MC, Kapser A, Weinzierl MR: Jefferson fracture in a child—illustrative case report. Pediatr Neurosurg 43:526–530, 2007.

29. Griffiths SC: Fracture of odontoid process in children. J Pediatr Surg 7:680–683, 1972.

30. Ries MD, Ray S: Posterior displacement of an odontoid fracture in a child. Spine (Phila Pa 1976) 11:1043–1044, 1986.

31. Odent T, Langlais J, Glorion C, et al: Fractures of the odontoid process: a report of 15 cases in children younger than 6 years. J Pediatr Orthop 19:51–54, 1999.

32. Howard AW, Letts RM: Cervical spondylolysis in children: Is it posttraumatic? J Pediatr Orthop 20:677–681, 2000.

33. van Rijn RR, Kool DR, deWitt Hamer PC, et al: An abused five-month-old girl: hangman's fracture or congenital arch defect? J Emerg Med 29:61–65, 2005.

34. Mortazavi M, Gore PA, Chang S, et al: Pediatric cervical spine injuries: a comprehensive review. Childs Nerv Syst 27:705–717, 2011.

# Chapter 25

# Pediatric Thoracolumbar Spine Fractures

## Mark C. Lee, Silas Marshall, and John C. Brancato

**INTRODUCTION**
**ANATOMIC CONSIDERATIONS**
**HISTORY**
**PREHOSPITAL CARE AND MANAGEMENT**
**PHYSICAL EXAMINATION**

**DIAGNOSTIC STUDIES**
**TREATMENT OF SPECIFIC INJURIES**
**GUIDELINES FOR EMERGENCY DEPARTMENT MANAGEMENT**
**COMMON PITFALLS**

## INTRODUCTION

■ Injuries to the thoracic and lumbar spine in pediatric patients are less frequent than injuries of the cervical spine, although they are not rare.

■ Injuries are typically described using adult classifications and may be broadly divided into four groups: compression, burst, flexion-distraction, and fracture-dislocation.

■ Treatment is dictated by the mechanism of injury, neurologic status, and associated injuries.

## ANATOMIC CONSIDERATIONS

■ Growth and ossification patterns are important for understanding potential fracture planes and for distinguishing normal anatomic variations from bony injury.

■ Development of the thoracic and lumbar vertebrae is similar to development of the lower cervical vertebrae.
  • A single primary ossification center develops during fetal life in the vertebral centrum (body) and in each neural arch (Fig. 25-1).
  • A neurocentral synchondrosis, the bidirectional physis between the primary ossification centers, closes between 3 and 6 years of age.
  • The neural arch ossification centers fuse between 2 and 4 years.
  • A vertical lucency on anteroposterior radiographs suggestive of a failure of fusion defect before age 2 years is normal.

■ Secondary ossification centers form at various times during puberty at the tips of the spinous, transverse, and mammillary processes (see Fig. 25-1).

■ The ring apophysis, the cartilaginous superior and inferior margins of the vertebral body, begins ossification during puberty as well but appears simultaneously throughout the spine (Fig. 25-2; see Fig. 25-1).

■ The vertebral body enlarges circumferentially by perichondral and periosteal apposition.
  • Vertical growth is through endochondral ossification at the vertebral endplates, which are essentially growth plates.
  • The ring apophysis, which is a cartilaginous structure contiguous with the vertebral endplate physes, does not contribute to the vertical growth of the spine.
  • The growth of the vertebral body is typically complete by the bone age of 14 years in girls and 16 years in boys, although the canal diameter is well formed by 5 years of age.

■ Ligamentous stability of the thoracic vertebrae and lumbar vertebrae is a function of longitudinal ligaments running along the anterior and posterior aspects of the vertebral bodies, the facet joint capsules, and the interspinous and supraspinous ligaments. Additional stability is conferred to the thoracic spine by the surrounding ribs.

## HISTORY

■ An adequate history may be difficult to obtain at the initial evaluation.
  • Most of the initial information may come from medical personnel at the site of the injury.
  • For all patients, it is important to gather information on the time from injury and method of immobilization because this may suggest potential medical interventions for patients with a spinal cord injury.

■ Thoracic and lumbar spine injuries in infants and young children should raise suspicions for child abuse.[1]

■ Motor vehicle accidents are the most common mechanism of thoracolumbar spine injury in all age groups.[2]
  • A lap belt without a shoulder strap or shoulder harness in a car seat predisposes to flexion-distraction–type injuries as the thoracolumbar spine flips over the restraint, causing anterior compression of abdominal contents.

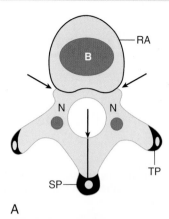

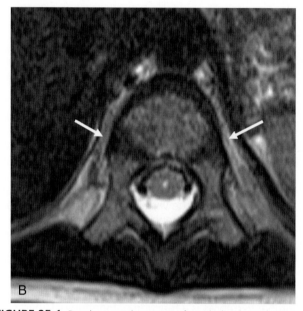

**FIGURE 25-1.** Developmental anatomy of an idealized vertebra within the thoracolumbar spine. **A,** Line diagram illustrating the vertebral body *(B)* and the neural arches *(N).* The gray centers indicate primary ossification centers. Everything colored in black indicates secondary centers of ossification, including the ring apophysis *(RA),* the transverse processes, and the spinous processes. The *arrows* indicate synchondroses. **B,** MRI of T6 vertebra in a 1-year-old girl shows the location of the neurocentral synchondroses *(arrows).*

■ Motor vehicle accidents, sports injuries, and falls from a height can produce an axial loading mechanism that results in a burst fracture or a compression fracture, depending on the degree of spine flexion at the time of impact.

■ A spine fracture in a child that results from a low-energy mechanism may suggest an insufficiency fracture of bone secondary to iatrogenic causes (steroid use), primary lesions of bone (aneurysmal bone cyst, Langerhans cell histiocytosis), or infection.

■ Communicative patients sometimes can describe neurologic deficits such as loss of sensation or motor function in the extremities. However, this history is often absent in young, uncooperative, or obtunded patients.

■ Multiple mechanistic and injury-related associations with spine fractures can help guide additional evaluations or treatments.

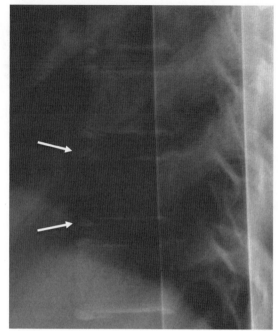

**FIGURE 25-2.** Ossification of the ring apophysis *(arrows)* in a thoracic vertebra of a 10-year-old girl.

● A spine fracture at one level is a high risk for having a spine fracture at another level.
● A lap-belt mechanism can be associated with intra-abdominal injury.
● Abdominal injuries are present in 50% of patients with Chance fractures.[3]

## PREHOSPITAL CARE AND MANAGEMENT

■ Initial management of a child with a potential spine injury is appropriate immobilization in the field. The cervical spine should be immobilized in a neutral position with access to the airways, while the remainder of the patient is placed on a rigid board.

■ The relatively larger head in a child younger than 8 years places the child's neck in relative flexion when on a typical adult rigid board.
● The head size requires that a cut-out for the head or a split-mattress technique be used to prevent excessive cervical or upper thoracic flexion.

## PHYSICAL EXAMINATION

■ After appropriate evaluation of the cardiorespiratory system using the ABCs, the spine examination is performed with appropriate spinal precautions observed.

■ Examination of the back is performed by logrolling the patient. Areas of swelling, ecchymosis, and tenderness should be identified. The overall sensitivity of the physical examination for detecting thoracolumbar spine fracture is 87%.[4]

■ A complete neurologic examination is sometimes difficult in a pediatric patient.

- The initial examination including strength, sensation, proprioception, rectal sphincter tone, bulbocavernosus reflex, and perianal sensation should be documented.
- The examination is serially repeated, and any improvement or deterioration is noted.
■ A neurologic deficit with normal computed tomography (CT) scan or plain radiographs does not exclude the possibility of a spinal cord injury with associated spinal column instability in a child.
  - Spinal cord injury without radiographic abnormality (SCIWORA) may be present in a child secondary to the relatively greater elasticity of the spinal column compared with the spinal cord.
  - Magnetic resonance imaging (MRI) is the study of choice to detect ligamentous or bony injury that is not apparent on plain radiographs or CT.

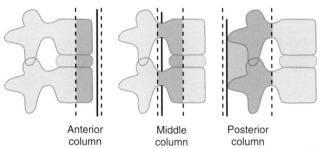

**FIGURE 25-3.** Denis classification of thoracolumbar spine injury. The spine is divided into three columns: anterior column (extending from the anterior longitudinal ligament posterior to the midportion of the vertebral body), middle column (extending from the midportion of the vertebral body to the junction of the laminopedicular junction), and posterior column (extending from the laminopedicular junction to the interspinous ligaments). Injuries with disruption of two or more columns are considered unstable. *(Adapted from Denis F: The three column spine and its significance in the classification of acute thoracolumbar spinal injuries. Spine [Phila Pa 1976] 8:817–831, 1983.)*

## DIAGNOSTIC STUDIES

■ X-ray
  - Alert, cooperative patients without a significant injury mechanism, without reported pain or tenderness, and with a normal neurologic examination do not require further imaging.
  - Plain films of the thoracolumbar spine are required in patients who are obtunded, who have spinal tenderness, or who have a distracting injury (e.g., long bone fracture, cervical spine injury, head injury) in the setting of a significant injury mechanism (e.g., motor vehicle accident, fall from >10 feet).
  - Initial radiographs should include supine anteroposterior and lateral views of the thoracolumbar spine. This film series should also be standard in any patient with a cervical spine injury. Evaluation of the films should be systematic.

    Anteroposterior radiographs—coronal plane malalignment; increase in soft tissue shadows laterally suggesting paravertebral hematoma; loss of height in the vertebral bodies suggesting compression or burst; increased interpedicular space, such as found in a fracture; increased interspinous distance from any injury causing kyphosis

    Lateral radiographs—sagittal plane malalignment, specifically any areas of focal kyphosis; anterior vertebral wedging suggesting compression; posterior element distraction or fracture

■ CT
  - CT scan has become standard in the evaluation of trauma patients and invariably provides a more detailed view of any fracture pattern.
  - CT scan is necessary only as an additional study if plain radiographs are abnormal because the CT scan information assists with decisions regarding final treatment. CT is more sensitive and more rapidly obtained than plain radiographs and helps distinguish acute from old injuries.[5]
  - The higher sensitivity of CT relates to the detection of small, stable injuries. CT scan does not identify

unstable injuries with any higher degree of accuracy than plain radiographs.
  - Axial images evaluate the integrity of the spinal canal, as in the case of a burst fracture or fracture-dislocation. The degree of spinal canal compromise is correlated with the probability of a neurologic deficit.[6]
  - Sagittal images detail vertebral body compression and posterior element distraction or fracture.
■ MRI
  - MRI evaluates all the soft tissue components of the spine and has an excellent correlation with the intraoperative findings of soft tissue disruption.[7]
  - MRI is required in a pediatric patient with a neurologic deficit. MRI allows localization of the specific cord injury level and any soft tissue or ligament injury that is not readily apparent on plain radiographs or CT scan.
  - The posterior ligamentous complex may be evaluated in burst fractures, compression fractures, and flexion-distraction injuries to understand the stability of the injury.

## TREATMENT OF SPECIFIC INJURIES

■ Denis Classification
  - The Denis classification separates the thoracolumbar spinal element into three columns—anterior column, middle column, and posterior column.[8] The classification is intended for adult spine injury but translates well for pediatric thoracolumbar trauma (Fig. 25-3).
  - The Denis classification identifies four broad categories of injury: compression fracture, burst fracture, flexion-distraction injury, and fracture-dislocation (Fig. 25-4).
  - SCIWORA and apophyseal avulsion fracture do not fit easily into the Denis classification and are discussed as separate entities.

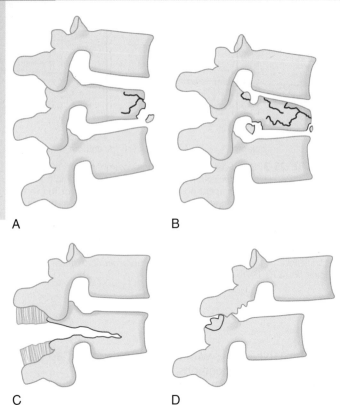

**FIGURE 25-4.** Denis classification of thoracolumbar fractures. **A,** Compression fracture. **B,** Burst fracture. **C,** Flexion-distraction injury. **D,** Fracture-dislocation.

■ General Treatment Considerations
- Treatment of spine fractures is centered on the concepts of structural stability and neurologic compromise.
- Structural stability is necessary to prevent future neurologic injury and to allow an optimal environment for the recovery of an existing neurologic deficit.
- Although the definition of structural stability continues to evolve with some injury patterns, any patient with an associated neurologic injury is likely to require surgical stabilization.

■ Compression Fracture
- This is the most common thoracolumbar spine fracture pattern.[9]
- The mechanism of injury is axial loading with flexion.
- Radiographically, the posterior wall of the vertebral body is, by definition, intact.

  CT scan may be used to rule out a burst fracture.

  MRI may be necessary if there is a suspicion of posterior ligament injury on plain radiographs.

  MRI or bone scan may distinguish a new injury from old compression fractures or vertebral wedging from developmental or metabolic conditions, such as Scheurmann kyphosis.

- Most fractures are isolated with no neurologic involvement.
- Treatment with a Jewitt brace for 4 to 6 weeks is recommended in isolated injuries without a

significant kyphotic component to provide pain relief and limit flexion across the injured segment.

  The fracture should be followed with long radiographs over the first 6 weeks to ensure no additional collapse or kyphotic degeneration.

  Activity restrictions are imposed for 12 weeks.

  Most fractures typically maintain the sagittal alignment noted at injury, and there is a modest capacity for remodeling in young children.[10]

- If the fracture is above the level of T6, a Minerva cast may be required.
- If focal kyphosis created by the single fracture or multiple compression fractures is greater than 40 degrees, surgical treatment consisting of an instrumented posterior fusion should be considered.

  Vertebral body loss of height greater than 50% is a relative indication for surgical stabilization.

  Surgical treatment is recommended in any case with an associated neurologic injury.

- Insufficiency fractures commonly manifest as multilevel compression fractures.

  Bracing is indicated.

  The root cause of the insufficiency fracture should be identified, be it metabolic or a primary bony process.

■ Burst Fracture
- Burst fracture refers to an axial compression injury that fractures the posterior wall of the vertebra.
- There is often involvement of the lamina with an increased risk of associated dural injury.[11]
- These injuries pose a higher risk of spinal cord injury.

  The risk of injury is correlated to the severity of the injury and the degree of spinal canal encroachment by retropulsed bony fragments.[11]

- The determination of stability dictates operative versus nonoperative treatments, and many classification systems have been proposed.[8,12,13]
- A useful guideline is neurologic status and posterior ligamentous integrity, as evaluated by MRI (Fig. 25-5).
- If the neurologic status is intact, and the posterior ligamentous complex is intact, thoracolumbosacral orthosis (TLSO) brace treatment is advocated.[14]

  The brace is worn for 3 months.

  Serial long film radiographs are required in the course of follow-up to ensure no subsequent instability develops.

- If the neurologic status or posterior ligamentous integrity is compromised, an instrumented fusion from an anterior or posterior approach is performed.

  The surgeon's preference dictates the use of an anterior versus a posterior approach.

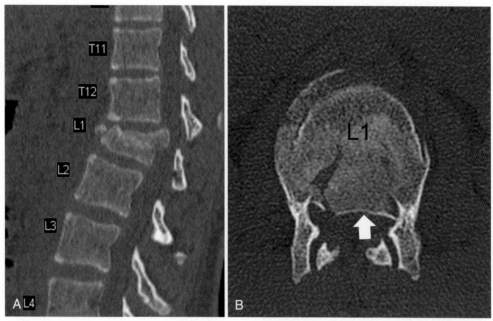

**FIGURE 25-5.** A 14-year-old boy with L1 burst fracture. **A,** Sagittal reformat CT image shows focal kyphosis at L1 with disruption of the vertebral body (anterior and middle columns). **B,** Axial CT reformat image shows a comminuted L1 body fracture with retropulsion of the central vertebral body fragment and greater than 50% intrusion into the spinal canal *(arrow)*.

Spinal cord decompression is indicated if significant (>50%) canal compromise by associated retropulsed fragments is noted.

- Flexion-Distraction Injury (Chance Fracture)
  - This is a common backseat lap belt injury in frontal crash motor vehicle accidents in which the weight of the torso is driven forward relative to a stabilized distal spine and pelvis.
  - The axis of rotation is anterior to the spinal column, causing compression of the vertebral body and distraction of the posterior elements, yielding an unstable three-column injury.
  - The posterior element disruption is either bony or ligamentous, and the path of the Chance fracture may be completely bony or completely ligamentous.

    In pediatric patients, the disk space is typically not involved in a purely ligamentous Chance fracture.

    The fracture line exits across the endplate physes either superiorly or inferiorly.[15]

  - Associated abdominal injuries and life-threatening aortic injury may exist.[16]
  - In a neurologically intact patient younger than 10 years with a bony Chance fracture and no significant associated injuries, extension casting with inclusion of a single thigh is appropriate.

    Patients older than 10 years may be managed with extension orthoses.

  - In a patient with neurologic compromise, associated abdominal injury, or inability to tolerate casting in the setting of a bony Chance fracture, instrumented

posterior fusion across the unstable level is recommended.
- For ligamentous Chance fractures, instrumented posterior fusion is necessary.

  In a young patient, postoperative immobilization may be necessary; this is at the discretion of the surgeon (Fig. 25-6).

- Fracture-Dislocation
  - Fracture-dislocation results from complex loading mechanisms in a high-energy injury. A component of shearing and rotation also exists.
  - This fracture is unstable by definition.
  - Instrumented fusion, usually through a posterior approach, with or without an associated decompression is typically required regardless of neurologic function.

    If spinal cord function is intact, instrumented fusion gives the greatest chance of neurologic recovery.

    If spinal cord function is compromised, instrumented fusion aids in the rehabilitation process by allowing early transfers and upright sitting.

  - In patients younger than 10 years with complete neurologic compromise, a long fusion should be considered because the risk of paralytic scoliosis is high.
  - After the adolescent growth spurt, the risk of progressive deformity is low.
- SCIWORA
  - SCIWORA is discussed in detail in Chapter 24.
  - MRI is necessary for evaluating the level of spinal cord injury and any associated ligamentous disruption.
  - Great care in regard to spinal instability must be taken in a patient with SCIWORA because neurologic

PART III Pediatrics

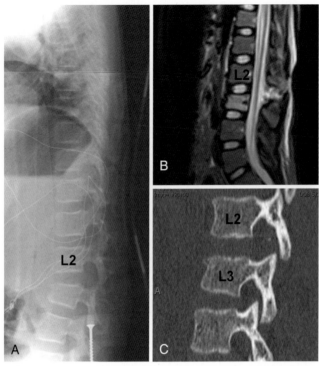

**FIGURE 25-6.** A 10-year-old girl with a ligamentous Chance fracture at L2-3. **A,** There is relative kyphosis at L1-2. **B,** CT scan shows a mild compression pattern with subluxation of the L1-2 facet joint. **C,** T2-weighted MRI shows bony edema at L2 and disruption of the posterior ligaments at L1-2, demonstrating a ligamentous Chance injury.

deficits can worsen in a delayed fashion without the appropriate initial spine precautions.[17]
- Any ligamentous instability as identified on MRI requires surgical stabilization.
■ Apophyseal Ring Avulsion
- The apophyseal ring can shear off and displace posteriorly through a flexion mechanism.
- The typical location is the lumbar spine.
- MRI is the most useful test for evaluating the injury and for planning treatment.
- The symptoms mimic symptoms of an acute disk herniation, with lower extremity radiculopathy and weakness in specific dermatomal distributions. However, the herniated material is bone and cartilage.
- Treatment is surgical excision of the disk material.

## GUIDELINES FOR EMERGENCY DEPARTMENT MANAGEMENT

■ When and How Should a Specialist Be Consulted?
- All unstable or questionably stable thoracolumbar spine injuries in pediatric patients require a bedside consultation with a spine specialist. These patients should not be discharged without a thorough examination by a specialist.
- Patients with back pain or a neurologic deficit require a bedside consultation by the spine specialist and continued evaluation as an inpatient.

- Telephone consultations with follow-up arrangements are appropriate for an isolated compression fracture with less than 50% loss of height in a coherent, cooperative patient whose pain is well controlled and without focal neurologic deficit or distracting injury.
■ What Should Be Communicated to the Specialist?
- Presumed diagnosis or reason for consultation
- Age and gender
- Mechanism of injury
- Time of injury
- Prolonged extraction or associated fatalities
- Appropriate immobilization in the field
- Distracting injuries
- Neurologic examination with reference to rectal examination or bulbocavernosus reflex
- Description of radiographic findings with reference to studies ordered so far, the level of the injury, and the degree of canal compromise or deformity
■ What Analgesia or Anesthesia Should Be Used?
- Narcotic analgesia is used to maintain patient comfort.
- Anesthesia for casting or operative reductions is performed in the operating room.
■ What Is Acceptable Alignment?
- If a reduction is necessary, operative reduction is performed, and acceptable alignment is determined by the operating surgeon.
■ What Initial Splinting or Immobilization Should Be Provided?
- Patients with isolated compression fractures without neurologic compromise may be placed in a Jewitt brace or a Minerva cast (for injury more proximal than the T6 level).
- Patients with isolated burst fractures with an intact posterior ligamentous complex and no neurologic compromise may be managed with a TLSO.
- Logroll precautions should be maintained for the remaining injury types.
■ What Postreduction Imaging Is Necessary?
- No additional imaging is required for stable compression fractures and burst fractures after application of immobilization.
■ What Is the Plan for Follow-up Care?
- Referral to an orthopedic or neurosurgical pediatric spine surgeon within 7 to 10 days of injury is required.
■ What Are Outpatient Pain Relief Options?
- Oral narcotic pain medications such as hydrocodone or oxycodone are useful.
- Muscle spasm often is a major symptom and may be controlled with a weight-appropriate dose of diazepam.
■ What Further Care Plan Should Be Discussed With the Patient?
- Before discharge, it must be explained to the patient that follow-up and maintenance of immobilization are important because presumably stable injuries may become unstable over time.
- The patient is restricted from gym and sports activities until further notice. The patient may need to remain out of school until the follow-up visit.

- Discharge or Inpatient Admission?
  - Patients may be discharged from the emergency department if they have an inherently stable thoracolumbar spine injury by clinical and radiographic data, are alert, and are comfortable.
  - Patients with unstable thoracolumbar spine injuries, focal neurologic deficits, persistent back pain despite normal radiographs, or multiple distracting injuries and an unclear examination require an inpatient admission.
- What Is Anticipated Specialist Care Treatment or Anticipated Definitive Treatment?
  - Patients with isolated compression fractures are managed with immobilization for 4 to 6 weeks and are restricted from activities for an additional 6 weeks.

    If the patient is stable, simple follow-up with immobilization is needed.

    Injuries usually heal reliably in 3 to 6 weeks; follow-up includes serial radiographs to assess stability.

  - Patients with an isolated burst fracture and no posterior ligamentous disruption by MRI are managed in a TLSO brace for 3 months.

    Serial radiographs are obtained to ensure that the injury is stable without progressive deformity.

  - If the patient has an unstable injury, treatment typically involves surgical stabilization.
- Discharge Care and Instruction
  - Brace or cast immobilization should not be removed by the patient until follow-up evaluation.
  - Patients should have a follow-up appointment within 7 to 10 days after discharge from the emergency department or the hospital.
  - Follow-up for surgical patients is determined by the individual surgeon. Brace or cast immobilization may or may not be a component of the postoperative protocol.

## COMMON PITFALLS

- Do not hesitate to obtain more advanced imaging.
- Look for additional levels of injury when a single-level spinal column injury has already been detected.
- Look for associated injuries, such as abdominal injuries in flexion-distraction patterns.
- Document the neurologic examination frequently and accurately.
- Verify all imaging findings with a detailed spine examination.
- Consider child abuse in an infant or toddler with a thoracolumbar spine injury.

## References

1. Carrion WV, Dormans JP, Drummond DS, et al: Circumferential growth plate fracture of the thoracolumbar spine from child abuse. J Pediatr Orthop 16:210–214, 1996.
2. Beaunoyer M, St-Vil D, Lallier M, et al: Abdominal injuries associated with thoraco-lumbar fractures after motor vehicle collision. J Pediatr Surg 36:760–762, 2001.
3. Mulpuri K, Reilly CW, Perdios A, et al: The spectrum of abdominal injuries associated with chance fractures in pediatric patients. Eur J Pediatr Surg 17:322–327, 2007.
4. Santiago R, Guenther E, Carroll K, et al: The clinical presentation of pediatric thoracolumbar fractures. J Trauma 60:187–192, 2006.
5. Antevil JL, Sise MJ, Sack DI, et al: Spiral computed tomography for the initial evaluation of spine trauma: a new standard of care? J Trauma 61:382–387, 2006.
6. Meves R, Avanzi O: Correlation between neurological deficit and spinal canal compromise in 198 patients with thoracolumbar and lumbar fractures. Spine (Phila Pa 1976) 30:787–791, 2005.
7. Lee HM, Kim HS, Kim DJ, et al: Reliability of magnetic resonance imaging in detecting posterior ligament complex injury in thoracolumbar spinal fractures. Spine (Phila Pa 1976) 25:2079–2084, 2000.
8. Denis F: The three column spine and its significance in the classification of acute thoracolumbar spinal injuries. Spine (Phila Pa 1976) 8:817–831, 1983.
9. Holmes JF, Miller PQ, Panacek EA, et al: Epidemiology of thoracolumbar spine injury in blunt trauma. Acad Emerg Med 8:866–872, 2001.
10. Karlsson MK, Moller A, Hasserius R, et al: A modeling capacity of vertebral fractures exists during growth: an up-to-47-year follow-up. Spine (Phila Pa 1976) 28:2087–2092, 2003.
11. Hashimoto T, Kaneda K, Abumi K: Relationship between traumatic spinal canal stenosis and neurologic deficits in thoracolumbar burst fractures. Spine (Phila Pa 1976) 13:1268–1272, 1988.
12. Gertzbein SD, Court-Brown CM: Rationale for the management of flexion-distraction injuries of the thoracolumbar spine based on a new classification. J Spinal Disord 2:176–183, 1989.
13. McCormack T, Karaikovic E, Gaines RW: The load sharing classification of spine fractures. Spine (Phila Pa 1976) 19:1741–1744, 1994.
14. Wood K, Buttermann G, Mehbod A, et al: Operative compared with nonoperative treatment of a thoracolumbar burst fracture without neurological deficit: a prospective, randomized study. J Bone Joint Surg Am 85:773–781, 2003.
15. de Gauzy JS, Jouve JL, Violas P, et al: Classification of chance fracture in children using magnetic resonance imaging. Spine (Phila Pa 1976) 32:E89–E92, 2007.
16. Swischuk LE, Jadhav SP, Chung DH: Aortic injury with Chance fracture in a child. Emerg Radiol 15:285–287, 2008.
17. Pang D, Wilberger JE, Jr: Spinal cord injury without radiographic abnormalities in children. J Neurosurg 57:114–129, 1982.

# Chapter 26   *Pediatric Fractures of the Pelvis and Acetabulum*

Mark C. Lee, Silas Marshall, and John C. Brancato

INTRODUCTION
ANATOMIC CONSIDERATIONS
HISTORY
PREHOSPITAL CARE AND MANAGEMENT
PHYSICAL EXAMINATION

DIAGNOSTIC STUDIES
DIFFERENTIAL DIAGNOSIS
TREATMENT OF SPECIFIC INJURIES
GUIDELINES FOR EMERGENCY DEPARTMENT MANAGEMENT
COMMON PITFALLS

## INTRODUCTION

- Although pelvic fractures are rare in children (<0.2%),[1,2] they are associated with injury to numerous other organ systems because they are typically the result of high-energy mechanisms.
- A pelvic fracture should be appreciated as a sign of severe whole-body injury. Patient mortality is not usually related to the pelvic fracture itself but to the associated injuries.
- Older notions of good functional outcome from non-operative treatment of pediatric pelvic fractures are not supported by more recent data,[3] and more recent emphasis is on operative treatment of unstable fractures or fractures that involve the acetabular growth plates.
- Acetabular fractures are an even rarer fracture type, constituting 6% to 17% of pediatric pelvic fractures.[1,2] The impact of such fractures on the triradiate cartilage, the growth center of the acetabulum, is the central difference between pediatric and adult acetabular injury.

## ANATOMIC CONSIDERATIONS

- Important differences exist between the pelvis of a child and an adult.
  - A child's pelvis has greater elasticity secondary to the elasticity of the joints and the bone. The child's pelvis can absorb greater energies before fracture.
  - A child's pelvis may fracture in only one location as a result of its elasticity, whereas the adult pelvic ring, because of its rigid nature, must necessarily fracture in two locations.
  - Avulsion fractures and fractures of the acetabulum through the triradiate cartilage are more frequent because the apophyseal or physeal cartilage presents a relative weak point in the pelvis.
  - Growth plate fractures can result in late deformity.
- A primary ossification center exists in each of the three bones of the pelvis: the ilium, the ischium, and the pubis. The three centers meet at the triradiate cartilage and fuse at 16 to 18 years of age (Fig. 26-1).

- The ischiopubic synchondrosis, a persistent lucent area in the bilateral inferior pubic rami, is present through late adolescence and can often be confused for a fracture.
- Secondary ossification centers are found throughout the pelvis and may be confused for fracture.
  - The iliac crest appears at 13 to 15 years and fuses at 15 to 17 years.
  - The ischial apophysis appears at 15 to 17 years and fuses by 25 years.
  - The anterior inferior iliac spine appears at 14 years and fuses at 16 years.
  - The pubic tubercle, ischial spine, and lateral wing of the sacrum all have secondary ossification centers.
- The cuplike acetabulum grows in depth through the triradiate cartilage, and its periphery enlarges through appositional growth from cartilage and periosteal new bone formation at the acetabular margin.
- At puberty, two main secondary centers of ossification appear in the cartilage surrounding the acetabulum.
  - The os acetabuli, the epiphysis of the pubis bone, appears at 8 years of age and expands to form most of the anterior acetabular wall, fusing with the pubis by 18 years.
  - The acetabular epiphysis, or the epiphysis of the ilium, follows a similar time-line for appearance and fusion and constitutes a large portion to the roof of the acetabulum.

## HISTORY

- Most pelvic fractures in children result from motor vehicle accidents, either as a pedestrian struck by a motor vehicle (60%) or as a passenger in a motor vehicle (22%).[4]
- Avulsion injuries from the pelvis are generally sports injuries.
- Isolated fractures of the pelvis in an infant or toddler may be the only indication of child abuse.[5] Pelvic radiographs are necessary for any skeletal survey.

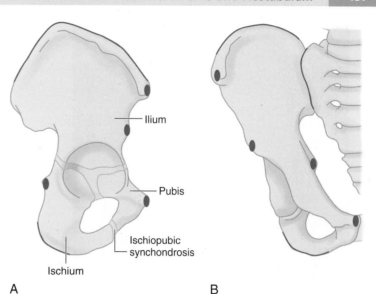

**FIGURE 26-1.** Lateral **(A)** and anteroposterior **(B)** views of the pelvis, showing the junction of the ilium, ischium, and pubis at the triradiate cartilage. The ischiopubic synchondrosis between the ischium and the pubis is apparent. The secondary ossification centers for the iliac crest, ischial apophysis, anterior inferior iliac spine, pubic tubercle, ischial spine, and lateral wing of the sacrum are illustrated. (*Adapted from Herring J: Tachdjian's pediatric orthopaedics, ed 4, Philadelphia, 2007, Saunders.*)

- Pelvic fractures in pediatric patients are associated with multiple organ system injury.
  - Associated head injury occurs in 9% to 48% of fractures[1,6] and is the leading cause of death and the major cause of long-term disability in patients with pelvic fractures.
  - Life-threatening hemorrhage from an arterial interruption is rare in pediatric patients and differs in this respect from adults[7]; bleeding is typically venous, and acute interventions to reduce pelvic volume, such as a simple pelvic wrapping, usually suffice.
  - Urogenital injury occurs in 4% to 15% of patients, although the incidence of hematuria is notably greater and can occur in 52% of patients.[8,9]
  - Vaginal and rectal lacerations may be present in 2% to 18% of patients and should be sought if a fracture has significant displacement, or perineal ecchymosis or bleeding exists.[9,10] This injury suggests an open pelvic fracture.
  - Abdominal and hollow viscera injuries range from 14% to 21%.[4,11]

    Computed tomography (CT) scan best shows injuries to the abdomen.

    Ultrasound and diagnostic peritoneal lavage may be useful adjuncts.[12]

  - Long bone fractures are present in 40% to 50% of children with pelvic fractures.[4,13]

    Long bone fractures in patients with pelvic fractures are associated with twice the frequency of death, thoracic injury, laparotomy, and nonorthopedic procedures.

    Long bone fracture is strongly associated with additional abdominal or head injury.

  - Lumbosacral plexus injury is rare and may occur in 1% to 3% of patients.[10] This injury is found in pelvic ring fractures with significant posterior displacement.
  - Acetabular fractures may result from high-energy or low-energy mechanisms.

    The fracture pattern is determined by the position of the femur at the time of impact.

    Acetabular fractures are often seen in association with pelvic fractures. Pelvic fractures, such as ramus fractures, may often propagate into the triradiate cartilage.

## PREHOSPITAL CARE AND MANAGEMENT

- Initial management of a child with a pelvic or acetabular fracture consists of board transport and immobilization of the lower extremities.
- Cervical spine stabilization should also be performed because pelvic fractures most often result from high-energy mechanisms, and additional associated injuries may be present.
- Fractures with gross bleeding should be covered with a moist saline dressing for transport. No attempts at reduction should be made before transport to the emergency department.

## PHYSICAL EXAMINATION

- Life-threatening associated injuries to the head, chest, and abdomen should be evaluated and managed before a thorough physical examination of the pelvis.
- Areas of contusion, abrasion, laceration, ecchymosis, or hematoma, especially in the perineal region (Fig. 26-2), should be inspected and documented.

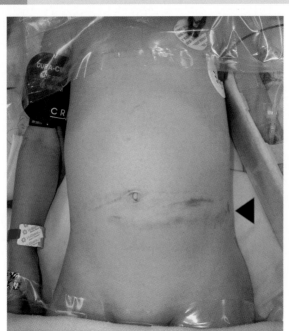

**FIGURE 26-2.** An 8-year-old boy was struck by a car. The pattern of ecchymosis *(arrowhead)* across the lower abdomen and pelvis suggests significant injury.

- Palpation should be performed only once, especially in the setting of a potentially unstable pelvic ring injury, because repeated examination can disrupt a tenuous intrinsic hemostasis process.
- Posterior pressure along the anterior superior iliac spines and medially directed compression of the iliac wings may yield crepitus, suggesting gross fracture and instability.
- Posterior pressure on the symphysis pubis may cause motion and suggest instability.
- The hip should be put through range of motion; any discomfort may suggest a proximal femur or acetabular fracture.
- A complete neurovascular examination is necessary to rule out peripheral nerve injury.
- As with any high-energy trauma, a complete spine examination is required.
- Inspection of the genitourinary system is indicated, especially if there is associated ecchymosis or hematoma along the perineum.
- Rectal examination should not be done routinely in pediatric patients but is indicated in significantly displaced fractures or with evidence of ecchymosis in the perineum to exclude a communication with the fracture site.[14]

## DIAGNOSTIC STUDIES

- X-ray
  - Evaluation and stabilization of a child with a potential pelvic ring injury precedes diagnostic studies.
  - The initial evaluation begins with a single anteroposterior projection of the pelvis.

- Any suggestion of pelvic ring instability on plain radiographs should prompt additional imaging.
- CT
  - CT scan has largely supplanted radiographs for further clarification of bony anatomy if an injury is suspected.
  - CT scan has numerous advantages over plain radiographs, including rapid acquisition, ability to reconstruct the pelvis in multiple planes, and superior sensitivity.
  - Although plain radiographs can reliably predict the need for operative intervention, the information from a CT scan can change the specific operative management.[15]
  - Most centers routinely obtain CT scan images through the abdomen in trauma patients; the addition of cuts through the pelvis may obviate screening plain radiographs.
- Magnetic Resonance Imaging (MRI)
  - In young patients, MRI examination is necessary to decipher completely any fracture lines through the triradiate cartilage or posterior wall of the acetabulum.
  - Minimally displaced fractures may be better visualized.

## DIFFERENTIAL DIAGNOSIS

- The differential diagnosis for groin or hip pain and limp in children is broad and depends on the age at presentation.
  - Infants and toddlers—differential diagnosis must include infection (septic arthritis, osteomyelitis) and transient synovitis
  - Children—differential diagnosis should include congenital coxa vara, Perthes disease or other causes of avascular necrosis, and osteochondritis dissecans lesions of the femoral head
  - Adolescents—differential diagnosis should include Perthes disease, femoral neck stress fracture, and slipped capital femoral epiphysis
- For adolescent girls, pelvic pain may be a product of ovary-related conditions (polycystic ovarian disease, ovarian torsion) or endometriosis.
- Normal growth plates or secondary ossification centers should also be considered because these are often confused for fracture (e.g., ischiopubic synchondrosis).
- Normal anatomic variants, such as apex posterior angulation of the coccyx, should not be confused for fracture.
- With an appropriate history of trauma and radiographic evidence of pelvic injury, the diagnosis is narrowed significantly.

## TREATMENT OF SPECIFIC INJURIES

- Classification Systems
  - Numerous classification systems exist for pediatric pelvic fractures. The most important information

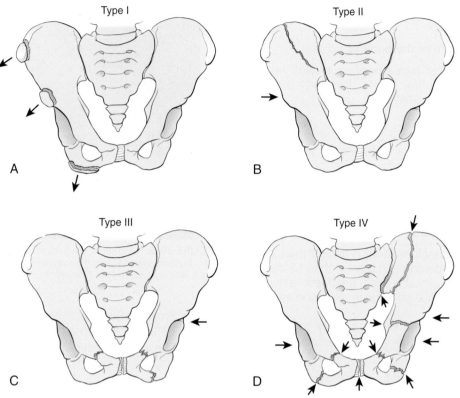

**FIGURE 26-3.** Torode and Zieg classification of pelvic ring injury. *(From Herring J: Tachdjian's pediatric orthopaedics, ed 4, Philadelphia, 2007, Saunders.)*

provided by each classification system relates to maturity and stability.

Maturity—a pelvis with an unossified triradiate cartilage (Risser O) and an open triradiate cartilage is considered immature, whereas a pelvis with a closed triradiate cartilage is considered mature; mature pelvic injuries follow adult guidelines for management

Stability—any injury with a break in the anterior and posterior pelvic ring, extreme deformity, displaced posterior ring, or displaced triradiate fracture is considered unstable and requires operative intervention

- The Torode and Zieg classification is the most commonly used for pelvic fractures in pediatric patients (Fig. 26-3).
■ Torode and Zieg Classification
  - Type I—avulsion fracture of the pelvis

    These fractures are typically associated with sports participation[16]; 50% are ischial avulsions, 23% are avulsions of the anterior superior iliac spine, and 22% are avulsions of the anterior inferior iliac spine (Fig. 26-4).

    Treatment is usually protected weight bearing with a restriction from athletics for 2 to 4 weeks.

    Rarely, significantly displaced avulsion fractures require elective surgical management.[16]

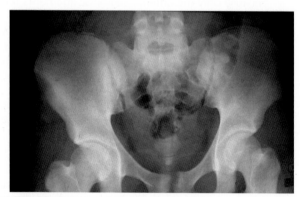

**FIGURE 26-4.** Right anterior superior iliac spine avulsion fracture in a 15-year-old boy.

- Type II—fracture of the iliac wing

    Isolated iliac wing fractures are relatively rare, constituting 5% to 12% of fractures of the pelvis, but the overall incidence is likely higher because they occur in association with other pelvic fractures.[8,17]

    Symptomatic treatment for closed iliac wing fractures is usually all that is required because these fractures heal regardless of displacement. Protected weight bearing is instituted, and the expectation is healing within 4 to 6 weeks.

Open fractures may require operative débridement and stabilization.

- Type III—fracture of the pubis or ischium

  Usually a result of high-energy injury with frequent associated injuries, these fractures constitute approximately 50% of pelvic injuries in children.[4,8]

  Stable injuries consist of fractures of the ipsilateral superior and inferior pubic ramus and fractures of the body of the ischium near the acetabulum. Both are managed symptomatically with protected weight bearing.

  Fractures near the symphysis pubis or a dislocation of the symphysis pubis may be unstable.

  - If the radiographic diastasis is greater than 2.5 cm or rotational deformity is greater than 15 degrees, the injury is unstable, and treatment is typically with external fixation or open reduction and internal fixation.[18]
  - CT scan is required before surgery to exclude a concurrent sacroiliac or triradiate cartilage fracture.

  Stable injuries are treated symptomatically with progressive weight bearing.

  Fractures near the sacroiliac joint or dislocations of the sacroiliac joint are rare in children.

  - These injuries are unusually stable in children because only the anterior sacroiliac ligaments tend to tear incompletely.
  - The rarity of such an isolated injury allows no formal examination of treatment options. The largest series in the literature suggested an operative approach for patients with gross instability and associated neurologic injury.[19]
  - Some patients with gross instability in the absence of other symptoms may be treated with protected weight bearing.

- Type IV—unstable fracture pattern consisting of a ring disruption

  Bilateral superior and inferior pubic ramus fractures or a fracture of the pubis and a symphysis disruption are inherently unstable.

  - If displacement is not great or the pubic symphysis diastasis is limited and no posterior injuries exist, these fractures may be treated symptomatically, and excellent remodeling should occur in a pediatric patient.
  - If there is significant displacement or posterior injuries, surgical stabilization is required.

  Dual breaks in the pelvic ring, anterior and posterior to the acetabulum, are inherently unstable and more often associated with abdominal injury and bleeding than other pelvic fracture types (Fig. 26-5).

  The first step in treatment is to achieve hemodynamic stability of the patient through a multispecialty approach.

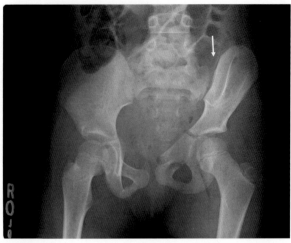

**FIGURE 26-5.** Pelvic fracture in a 9-year-old girl. Note the left sacroiliac joint disruption *(arrow)* and the superior pubic ramus fracture, suggesting a Torode and Zieg type IV injury.

- Provisional stabilization of an unstable injury may be achieved with a pelvic binder.
- The pelvic binder should be quickly replaced by traction or external fixation.

  Definitive treatment of type IV injuries is dictated by the age of the patient, fracture displacement or stability, and associated injuries.

  - Younger patients (<5 years old) with minimally displaced fractures may be treated with spica casting.
  - Patients with severe fracture instability, associated visceral or soft tissue injuries, or significant displacement (>1 cm) should undergo operative stabilization.

- Open Pelvic Fractures
  - Open pelvic fractures are relatively uncommon constituting approximately 13% of all pediatric pelvic fractures.[20]
  - Suspicion of an open injury should be maintained in fractures with significant comminution or in a fracture with associated vaginal or rectal bleeding.
  - Open pelvic fractures require débridement and operative stabilization.[20]
- Fractures of the Sacrum
  - Fractures of the sacrum are rare and are found in 5.4% of pediatric patients with pelvic fractures.[4]
  - Most sacral fractures are minimally displaced and treated symptomatically.
  - Sacral fractures extending vertically through the ala or foramina may represent the posterior disruption of a type IV pelvic injury and require operative stabilization.
  - Sacral fractures with significant displacement may disrupt the sacral level nerve roots and result in bowel and bladder dysfunction. These fractures require decompression and operative stabilization.
- Fractures of the Coccyx
  - Fractures of the coccyx are treated symptomatically.
  - Pain typically improves over 4 to 6 weeks, but discomfort may last 1 year.

- Fractures of the Acetabulum
  - The goal of treatment of fractures of the acetabulum is to restore the normal acetabular architecture and prevent growth abnormalities in the triradiate cartilage.
  - Although no extensive series exists, outcomes in both regards are thought to be optimized if surgical fixation is used in displaced acetabular fractures.[18]
  - Minimally displaced fractures may be treated nonoperatively with a 6- to 8-week period of protected weight bearing.
  - Premature closure of the triradiate cartilage may result in acetabular dysplasia and hip subluxation. This possibility must be included in any discussion with caretakers regarding a possible treatment plan.

## GUIDELINES FOR EMERGENCY DEPARTMENT MANAGEMENT

- When and How Should a Specialist Be Consulted?
  - Pelvic fractures in a child with an associated high-energy mechanism of injury or other associated injury should involve a bedside consultation with a pediatric orthopedic surgeon.
  - Acetabular fractures should involve a bedside consultation with a pediatric orthopedic surgeon.
  - Stable pelvic fractures with low-energy mechanisms of injury and without associated organ system injury (e.g., avulsion fracture) require a telephone consultation with a pediatric orthopedic surgeon.
- What Should Be Communicated to the Specialist?
  - Presumed diagnosis or reason for consultation
  - Age and gender
  - Mechanism of injury
  - Time of injury
  - Open or closed fracture
  - Additional injuries
  - Neurovascular examination of the extremity or both extremities in the case of a pelvic fracture
  - Summary of radiographic findings and all studies ordered so far
- What Analgesia or Anesthesia Should Be Used?
  - Intravenous narcotic analgesia is used to maintain patient comfort.
  - Intravenous diazepam may be used to minimize patient spasm.
  - Anesthesia for operative procedures is performed in the operating room.
- What Is Acceptable Alignment?
  - Acceptable alignment for a pelvic fracture is determined both by fracture displacement and the stability of the fracture pattern.

    Wide displacements may be acceptable in a stable pelvic injury.

    In an unstable pelvic injury, even minor displacements may be unacceptable.

  - Acetabulum fracture alignment is acceptable only if the displacement is minimal and the joint surface appears to be congruous.

Any significant displacement is likely to require operative stabilization.

- What Initial Splinting or Immobilization Should Be Provided?
  - An unstable pelvic fracture should be placed into a pelvic binder as initial management to tamponade potential sites of venous bleeding.
  - No splinting is necessary for stable pelvic fractures or avulsion fractures from the pelvis.

    Restricted weight bearing on the side of the injury may be necessary.

  - No splinting is necessary for fractures of the acetabulum.

    Restricted weight bearing is imposed on the side of the injury.

- What Postreduction Imaging Is Necessary?
  - Plain radiographs and CT scan may be used to evaluate a pelvic or acetabular fracture after operative reduction.
  - MRI may be necessary to define the reduction of acetabular fractures in pediatric patients or pelvic fractures that extend into the acetabulum because the posterior wall of the acetabulum may not yet be ossified or triradiate cartilage injury exists.
- What Is the Plan for Follow-up Care?
  - The pediatric orthopedic surgeon usually requires a follow-up appointment within 7 to 10 days of injury.
- What Are Outpatient Pain Relief Options?
  - Oral narcotic pain medications such as hydrocodone or oxycodone are useful.
  - Muscle spasm is often a main symptom and may be controlled with a weight-appropriate dose of diazepam.
- What Further Care Plan Should Be Discussed With the Patient?
  - For unstable pelvic fractures, the operative treatment plan is discussed with the patient's caretakers by the pediatric orthopedic surgeon.
  - For stable pelvic fractures and pelvic avulsion fractures, the patient may require weight-bearing restrictions on one or both legs for comfort.
  - The patient is restricted from gym and sports activities until further notice. The patient may need to remain out of school until the follow-up visit.
- Discharge or Inpatient Admission?
  - Patients with pelvic ring fractures with a high-energy mechanism of injury or associated injury require an inpatient admission.
  - Patients with pelvic ring fractures with a low-energy mechanism of injury, a stable pattern, and no associated injury may be discharged to home.
  - Patients with pelvic avulsion fractures may be discharged to home.
  - Patients with acetabulum fractures require an inpatient admission.
- What Is Anticipated Specialist Care Treatment or Anticipated Definitive Treatment?
  - The pediatric orthopedic surgeon directs the subsequent surgical management of a patient with

an acetabulum fracture or an unstable pelvic ring injury.

- Patients with stable pelvic ring injuries or pelvic avulsion fractures typically are managed with restricted weight bearing for comfort and early follow-up with an orthopedic surgeon.
- Discharge Care and Instruction
  - Patients younger than 5 years are placed into a spica cast for treatment of the pelvic ring injury. Patients are instructed on care of the spica cast by the floor nurses and by the surgeon's office.
  - Patients should have a follow-up appointment within 7 to 10 days after discharge from the emergency department or the hospital.
  - Follow-up for surgical patients is dictated by the individual surgeon. Brace or cast immobilization may or may not be a component of the postoperative protocol.
  - Stable pelvic fractures and avulsion injuries to the pelvis require crutches or a wheelchair to restrict weight bearing for comfort.

## COMMON PITFALLS

- The secondary ossification centers of the pelvis must be recognized and not confused for fracture.
- Patients with a pelvic fracture should be examined for other fracture or other organ system injury.
- A pelvic binder is necessary in unstable pelvic ring injuries to decrease the pelvic volume and assist in decreasing blood loss.
- MRI may be necessary to define the full extent of a pediatric acetabular fracture.

## References

1. Grisoni N, Connor S, Marsh E, et al: Pelvic fractures in a pediatric level I trauma center. J Orthop Trauma 16:458–463, 2002.
2. Silber JS, Flynn JM: Changing patterns of pediatric pelvic fractures with skeletal maturation: implications for classification and management. J Pediatr Orthop 22:22–26, 2002.
3. Upperman JS, Gardner M, Gaines B, et al: Early functional outcome in children with pelvic fractures. J Pediatr Surg 35:1002–1005, 2000.
4. Silber JS, Flynn JM, Koffler KM, et al: Analysis of the cause, classification, and associated injuries of 166 consecutive pediatric pelvic fractures. J Pediatr Orthop 21:446–450, 2001.
5. Prendergast NC, deRoux SJ, Adsay NV: Non-accidental pediatric pelvic fracture: a case report. Pediatr Radiol 28:344–346, 1998.
6. Tile M: Pelvic ring fractures: should they be fixed? J Bone Joint Surg Br 70:1–12, 1988.
7. Hauschild O, Strohm PC, Culemann U, et al: Mortality in patients with pelvic fractures: results from the German pelvic injury register. J Trauma 64:449–455, 2008.
8. Reed MH: Pelvic fractures in children. J Can Assoc Radiol 27:255–261, 1976.
9. Tarman GJ, Kaplan GW, Lerman SL, et al: Lower genitourinary injury and pelvic fractures in pediatric patients. Urology 59:123–126, 2002.
10. Reichard SA, Helikson MA, Shorter N, et al: Pelvic fractures in children—review of 120 patients with a new look at general management. J Pediatr Surg 15:727–734, 1980.
11. Musemeche CA, Fischer RP, Cotler HB, et al: Selective management of pediatric pelvic fractures: a conservative approach. J Pediatr Surg 22:538–540, 1987.
12. Chia JP, Holland AJ, Little D, et al: Pelvic fractures and associated injuries in children. J Trauma 56:83–88, 2004.
13. Rieger H, Brug E: Fractures of the pelvis in children. Clin Orthop Relat Res 336:226–239, 1997.
14. Shlamovitz GZ, Mower WR, Bergman J, et al: Poor test characteristics for the digital rectal examination in trauma patients. Ann Emerg Med 50:25–33, 2007.
15. Burgess AR, Eastridge BJ, Young JW, et al: Pelvic ring disruptions: effective classification system and treatment protocols. J Trauma 30:848–856, 1990.
16. Rossi F, Dragoni S: Acute avulsion fractures of the pelvis in adolescent competitive athletes: prevalence, location and sports distribution of 203 cases collected. Skeletal Radiol 30:127–131, 2001.
17. McIntyre RC, Jr, Bensard DD, Moore EE, et al: Pelvic fracture geometry predicts risk of life-threatening hemorrhage in children. J Trauma 35:423–429, 1993.
18. Karunakar MA, Goulet JA, Mueller KL, et al: Operative treatment of unstable pediatric pelvis and acetabular fractures. J Pediatr Orthop 25:34–38, 2005.
19. Heeg M, Klasen HJ: Long-term outcome of sacroiliac disruptions in children. J Pediatr Orthop 17:337–341, 1997.
20. Mosheiff R, Suchar A, Porat S, et al: The "crushed open pelvis" in children. Injury 30(Suppl 2):B14–B18, 1999.

# Chapter 27    *Pediatric Fractures and Dislocations of the Hip*

Mark C. Lee, Silas Marshall, and John C. Brancato

## INTRODUCTION

- Hip fractures and dislocations are relatively rare in children accounting for less than 1% of all fractures and less than 5% of all dislocations.[1,2]
- Hip fractures and dislocations are usually the result of high-energy mechanisms, and 30% of patients have associated injuries to other organ systems.
- The pediatric hip is unique in the interplay of its various growth plates and its susceptibility to potential avascular necrosis. The impact of both injury and treatment on the future growth of the hip must be carefully considered.

## ANATOMIC CONSIDERATIONS

- Bones
  - Ossification

    Ossification of the femoral shaft occurs in at 7 weeks of age.

    The femoral head begins ossification between 3 and 6 months of age.

    The greater trochanter begins ossification at 4 years of age.

  - Growth of the proximal femur occurs at three growth plates: the proximal femoral physis, the trochanteric physis, and a physis along the lateral femoral neck (Fig. 27-1).

    The proximal femoral physis contributes to femoral neck length.

    The trochanteric physis contributes to greater trochanteric height.

    The lateral femoral neck physis contributes to femoral neck width and length.

  The greater trochanter and the femoral head grow by appositional growth.

  - Fusion of the proximal femoral and trochanteric physes occurs at 14 years of age in girls and 16 years in boys.
  - The cuplike acetabulum grows through the triradiate cartilage. Growth of the acetabulum is thought to be complete near the onset of puberty, at which point the triradiate cartilage closes.
  - The continued interaction of the femoral head and the acetabulum is crucial for the normal development of both anatomic structures.

  Deformity of the femoral head and acetabulum results from a developmentally dislocated hip.

  Traumatic dislocations and traumatic deformity in early childhood have profound effects on this femoral head–acetabulum couple.

- Vascular Supply
  - The vascular supply to the femoral head in a growing child is unique.
  - The metaphyseal blood supply present at birth essentially stops by age 4, when the proximal femoral physis becomes fully developed.
  - The intracapsular lateral epiphyseal vessels, originating from the medial circumflex artery and branching from the medial circumflex at the level of the trochanteric notch, run along the femoral neck and are the dominant blood supply to the femoral head until physeal closure (Fig. 27-2).
  - The ligamentum teres contributes no clinically significant blood supply to the femoral head throughout extrauterine life.
- Hip Capsule
  - The hip capsule is thick and fibrous in a child and unlikely to be disrupted by trauma.
  - The hip capsule can contain a traumatic hematoma and create significant intra-articular pressures,

potentially compromising the lateral epiphyseal blood supply.

## HISTORY

■ Almost all hip fractures in children are caused by high-energy trauma.[3]

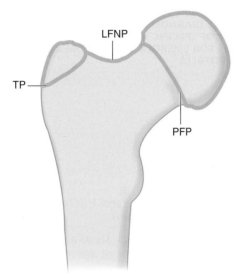

**FIGURE 27-1.** The blue coloring identifies the various growth plates at the level of the proximal femur. Only three growth plates contribute to longitudinal growth: the proximal femoral physis *(PFP)*, trochanteric physis *(TP)*, and lateral femoral neck physis *(LFNP)*. The remaining growth plates contribute to appositional enlargement of the femoral head and the greater trochanter.

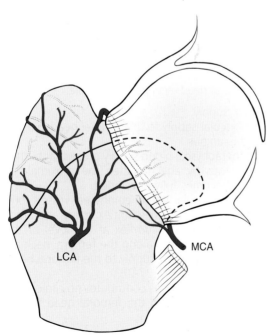

**FIGURE 27-2.** Blood supply to the femoral head. The major blood supply derives from the medial circumflex vessels and enters the intracapsular space as the lateral retinacular sheath along the superolateral aspect of the femoral neck. *(From Herring J: Tachdjian's pediatric orthopaedics, ed 4, Philadelphia, 2007, Saunders.)*

■ If a low-energy mechanism is offered, one should suspect a pathologic process, insufficiency fracture from metabolic disease, sickle cell disease, or a developmental condition such as slipped capital femoral epiphysis (SCFE).

■ Cooperative patients typically report difficulty or an inability to ambulate with severe groin or knee pain.

■ Hip dislocations usually involve low-energy mechanisms in patients younger than 6 years. The typical mechanism is a simple fall while at play.[4]

■ Hip dislocations in older patients usually involve high-energy mechanisms, such as football and motor vehicle accidents.[4]

■ Posterior dislocations occur most commonly (90%) and occur when a force is applied axially to the leg when the hip is flexed and adducted.[4]

■ Rarer directions of dislocation include anterior and inferior directions.

## PREHOSPITAL CARE AND MANAGEMENT

■ Initial management of a child with a hip fracture or dislocation consists of board transport and immobilization of the lower extremities.

■ Cervical spine stabilization should also be performed because hip fractures or dislocations most often result from high-energy mechanisms and can have additional associated injuries.

## PHYSICAL EXAMINATION

■ An infant with a hip fracture holds the extremity flexed, abducted, and externally rotated. Pseudoparalysis of the extremity is noted.

■ The affected leg in an older child with a hip fracture is usually held in a shortened, externally rotated position.

■ Patients with acute, displaced fractures exhibit a significantly limited range of motion on examination.

■ Patients with subtle stress fractures around the femoral neck present with a slight limp with discomfort only at the extremes of rotation.

■ Patients with a dislocated hip most commonly present with the hip held adducted, flexed, and internally rotated.

■ In dislocations, associated injuries are frequently identified including fractures of the acetabulum or other long bone, sciatic nerve injury, femoral nerve or vessel injury, and concomitant knee pain secondary to bony bruising or internal derangement.[5]

■ A complete neurologic examination is sometimes difficult in a pediatric patient. However, the initial examination should attempt to ascertain best the strength, sensation, and vascular supply of the affected extremity.

■ Examination of the spine and distal lower extremity should be routine in uncooperative or noncommunicative children because a pathologic process in the axial skeleton or in the lower extremity distal to the hip joint can also lead to pseudoparalysis.

# DIAGNOSTIC STUDIES

■ Initial evaluation begins with an anteroposterior projection of the pelvis and a cross-table view of the affected hip to minimize unnecessary motion.

■ The hip evaluation in an infant is best done with ultrasound. Ultrasound allows visualization of the scantily ossified femoral epiphysis, the proximal femoral physis, and any associated effusions in the hip joint.

■ If a joint effusion is present, further diagnostic testing includes hip aspiration in the operating room with an associated arthrogram.
   • If the hip aspiration is bloody, a traumatic etiology is likely.
   • A serous aspirate makes toxic synovitis more likely.
   • A purulent aspirate confirms septic arthritis.

■ Subtle insufficiency or stress fractures may be delineated on computed tomography (CT) scan or bone scan.

■ The most sensitive additional imaging study for detecting subtle fracture is magnetic resonance imaging (MRI).
   • The fracture line appears as a black line with surrounding bony edema on T2-weighted films (Fig. 27-3B).
   • MRI can detect an occult hip fracture in the first 24 hours after injury.[6]
   • Pathologic fractures should be additionally evaluated with MRI to assess bony involvement if plain radiographs are unclear and to assess any associated soft tissue component to the lesion that may prove to be high yield on biopsy and clarify the differential diagnosis.
   • MRI can help to exclude osteomyelitis as a cause of hip pain and early avascular necrosis of various etiologies.

■ In patients with hip pain and without clear evidence of fracture, a complete blood count and C-reactive protein should be done to evaluate for the possibility of infection.

■ Hip dislocations are typically evaluated with plain radiography. Occasionally, hip dislocations in children can spontaneously reduce, and only a subtle difference in joint congruency remains (Fig. 27-4A).[7]

■ Further evaluation of subtle fracture or interposed osteocartilaginous or soft tissue is best performed with MRI (Fig. 27-4B).

# DIFFERENTIAL DIAGNOSIS

■ The differential diagnosis for hip pain and limp in children is broad and depends on the age at presentation.
   • Infants and toddlers—differential diagnosis must include infection (septic arthritis, osteomyelitis), transient synovitis, and developmental dislocation of the hip
   • Children—differential diagnosis should include congenital coxa vara, Perthes disease or other causes of avascular necrosis, and osteochondritis dissecans lesions of the femoral head
   • Adolescents—differential diagnosis should include Perthes disease, stress fracture, and SCFE.

■ Dislocation of the hip may occur voluntarily, in the setting of generalized ligamentous laxity or hyperlaxity, excessive anteversion of the femur and acetabulum, and coxa valga.[8]

■ Snapping iliotibial band syndrome—a dramatic rub of the iliotibial band against the greater trochanter with certain motions of the leg—is often confused for a dislocating hip.
   • The distinction from a true hip dislocation may be made by radiographs because the hip joint remains congruent before and after the snap.

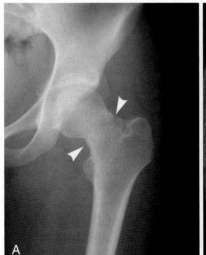
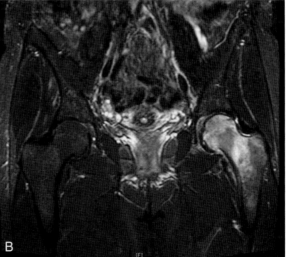

**FIGURE 27-3. A,** Anteroposterior projection of the left hip in a 14-year-old female track athlete. The lucency across the femoral neck *(arrows)* identifies a femoral neck stress fracture. **B,** Corresponding coronal plane pelvic T2-weighted MRI shows significant surrounding bony edema with a signal void at the level of the fracture.

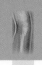
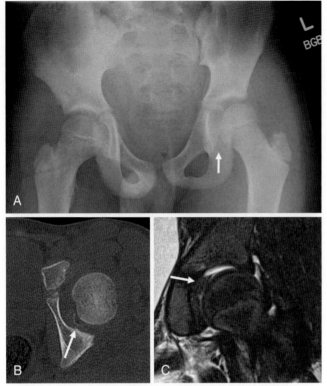

**FIGURE 27-4. A,** Anteroposterior projection of the pelvis after a traumatic hip dislocation with spontaneous reduction in a 9-year-old boy. Note the increased joint space in the left hip compared with the right hip *(arrow)*. **B,** Axial CT scan shows a small osteochondral fragment *(arrow)*. **C,** T2-weighted MRI shows interposed soft tissue *(arrow)*. During surgery, the patient was found to have a ligamentum teres avulsion with a small head fragment connected to the ligamentum.

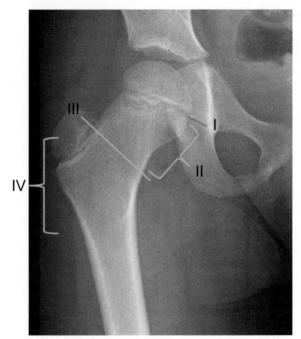

**FIGURE 27-5.** Delbet classification of proximal femur fractures in children.

## TREATMENT OF SPECIFIC INJURIES

- Traumatic Proximal Femoral Fractures
  - Traumatic proximal femoral fractures are classified according to Delbet and are divided into four general types (Fig. 27-5).[9]
  - More significant rates of avascular necrosis and growth arrest are noted in type I and type II injuries, and greater rates of varus malunion are noted in type III and type IV injuries.
  - Type I

    Type I is a transphyseal fracture of the proximal femur.

    - Approximately 50% of these fractures are type IA, where the femoral epiphysis remains located.
    - The other 50% are type IB, where the femoral head is dislocated.

    This injury can be distinguished from an unstable SCFE in that acute transphyseal fractures occur in young children after high-energy trauma, whereas most SCFEs occur after minor trauma in obese adolescents with prodromal hip or knee pain.

    - Transphyseal fractures lack the mild to severe femoral neck deformity on plain radiographs often identified in patients with SCFE.

Iatrogenic type I fractures may result from attempted reduction of a hip dislocation.[10,11]

Type IA fractures have a dismal prognosis, with invariable osteonecrosis and growth arrest.[9]

Treatment is typically in the operating room.

For patients younger than 2 years with minimal displacement, a spica cast is applied with early follow-up examination to ensure no subsequent displacement of the fracture occurs.

- If the fracture is displaced, gentle manual reduction may be performed with or without smooth wire fixation and casting. Close follow-up is mandatory.

For older patients, operative stabilization with reduction is usually necessary.

Fixation necessarily crosses the proximal femoral physis. After the age of 10, threaded fixation is preferred because the residual growth would have little impact on leg length differences.

- Type II

  Type II is an intracapsular femoral neck fracture that occurs between the physis and the intertrochanteric line. This is the most common proximal femoral fracture type (50%).[12]

  The rate of associated avascular necrosis is approximately 28%; patients with displaced fractures and children older than 10 years have higher rates than young children and patients with minimal displacement.[13]

A presumed contributor to avascular necrosis in minimally displaced fractures is the potential compromise in lateral epiphyseal vessel circulation by the increased intracapsular pressure that develops from a fracture hematoma in the child's thick hip capsule.

Treatment is operative anatomic reduction with stable fixation.

- Spica casting may be used in the rare patients with minimally displaced and demonstrably stable fractures.
- Fixation typically crosses the physis because this placement significantly decreases the risk of nonunion and coxa vara.[14]
- Despite the risk of early physeal closure and greater trochanteric overgrowth with this placement, avoiding the complications of avascular necrosis and nonunion is primary.

Routine release of the hematoma from the hip capsule is recommended.

Most patients younger than 8 years may require supplemental spica casting after fixation.

- Type III

Type III is an extracapsular femoral neck fracture that is located proximal to the anterior intertrochanteric line. This is the second most common type of hip fracture in children (34%).[12]

Treatment is similar to type II fractures.

- Fixation for the fracture can often stop before crossing of the proximal femoral physis.
- Type IV (Fig. 27-6)

Type IV is an intertrochanteric fracture that has the lowest rate of avascular necrosis, approximately 5%.[13] However, coxa vara and premature physeal closure have been reported.[15]

Children younger than 4 years are treated in a spica cast with frequent repeat evaluation to ensure no settling of the fracture into varus.

- The cast is maintained for 8 to 12 weeks, as determined by evidence of radiographic healing.

Children older than 3 years should be treated with internal fixation after anatomic closed reduction.

- A pediatric proximal femur locking plate and sliding screw with side plate are effective approaches.

■ Stress Fracture of the Femoral Neck
- Stress fracture of the femoral neck is an extremely rare diagnosis in children.[16]
- Fracture is usually a product of cyclic loading of the hip, often associated with intensifying running sports. It can also be a product of an underlying metabolic disorder.
- The female athletic triad (amenorrhea, anorexia, and osteoporosis) is associated with the development of stress fractures of the femoral neck.[17]
- Ambulatory patients present with a mild limp and relatively unrestricted range of motion. MRI is valuable for early detection (see Fig. 27-3B).
- Fracture is classified as compression type and tension type (Fig. 27-7).

Compression type—along the inferior femoral neck

- This type may be managed with 6 weeks of non–weight bearing.
- Surgical fixation is recommended if pain does not resolve or varus deformity or displacement occurs.

Tension type—along the superolateral neck of the femur

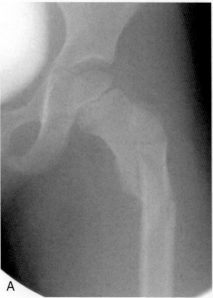
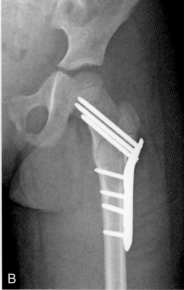

**FIGURE 27-6. A,** Anteroposterior image of the left hip in a 6-year-old girl shows a Delbet type IV proximal femur fracture. **B,** Anteroposterior image of the same hip 1 week after open reduction and internal fixation.

- This type requires operative fixation because it is inherently unstable.
- ▪ Hip Dislocation
  - Hip dislocation is classified in children with open growth plates according to the associated fractures.
  - The Stewart-Milford classification identifies four grades.

    Grade I—dislocation without fracture or a small associated posterior acetabular rim fracture

    Grade II—dislocation with a posterior rim fracture and stable hip after reduction

    Grade III—posterior rim fracture with an unstable hip after reduction

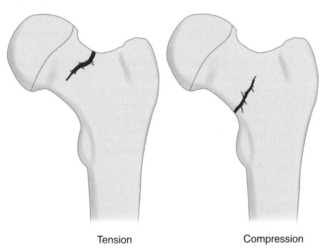

Tension                    Compression

**FIGURE 27-7.** Simple classification of femoral neck stress fractures.

Grade IV—dislocation with an associated femoral head or neck fracture (Fig. 27-8)

- Treatment for hip dislocations generally involves emergent reduction.

  Reduction within 6 hours of the dislocation minimizes the risk of osteonecrosis.

  Reductions must be performed in a controlled fashion in the emergency department with adequate analgesia and an expeditious radiographic evaluation after reduction to exclude the possibility of iatrogenic femoral neck fracture through the physis or residual joint incongruity.

- Hip dislocations with associated femoral head fractures are a relative contraindication to reduction in the emergency department, although this dislocation should be managed as an emergent surgical case.

  An open approach to reduction and fixation of this fracture type is preferred.

  Closed reduction invariably leads to joint incongruity with interposed fragments.

- Surgical approaches to a dislocated hip that fails closed reduction or has significant residual incongruity are classically dictated by the direction of dislocation—a posterior approach for posterior dislocations and an anterior approach for anterior dislocations.
- A surgical hip dislocation approach can afford wide access to the femoral head and acetabulum in the setting of a hip dislocation with an associated femoral head fracture.[18]

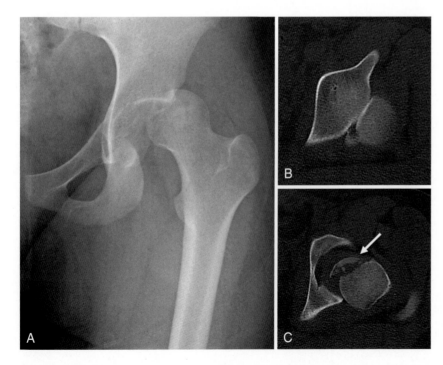

**FIGURE 27-8.** Stewart-Milford grade IV hip dislocation. **A,** Anteroposterior projection of the left hip in a 14-year-old girl involved in a motor vehicle accident. The overlap of the femoral head along the superior edge of the acetabulum suggests a dislocation. **B** and **C,** CT scan axial images at the sourcil level **(B)** and acetabulum level **(C)** show a superoposterior dislocation with a large associated femoral head fracture *(arrow)*.

# GUIDELINES FOR EMERGENCY DEPARTMENT MANAGEMENT

■ When and How Should a Specialist Be Consulted?
  • A bedside consultation with a pediatric orthopedist is indicated for any hip fracture or hip dislocation in a child with or without an associated fracture.
  • Simple telephone consultations or follow-up arrangements are inadequate.
■ What Should Be Communicated to the Specialist?
  • Presumed diagnosis or reason for consultation
  • Age and gender
  • Mechanism of injury
  • Time of injury
  • Prolonged extraction or associated fatalities
  • Additional injuries
  • Neurovascular examination of the extremity
  • Summary of radiographic findings and all studies ordered so far
■ What Analgesia or Anesthesia Should Be Used?
  • Intravenous narcotic analgesia is used to maintain patient comfort.
  • Intravenous diazepam may be used to minimize patient spasm.
  • A standard conscious sedation protocol can be used to effect a closed reduction of a hip dislocation in the emergency department.
  • Anesthesia for operative procedures is performed in the operating room.
■ What Is Acceptable Alignment for a Hip Fracture or Hip Dislocation?
  • For hip fractures, fracture alignment and acceptability of a possible reduction are determined in the operating room by the surgeon.
  • For hip dislocations, the reduction is acceptable if the hip appears congruent on plain radiographs, and more advanced imaging such as CT or MRI reveals no bony or soft tissue components interposed in the joint space.
■ What Initial Splinting or Immobilization Should Be Provided?
  • No specific initial splinting regimen is indicated for hip fractures or dislocations.
  • For intracapsular hip fractures or fracture-dislocations, patient comfort and expeditious management in the operating room are priority.
■ What Postreduction Imaging Is Necessary?
  • Plain radiographs, CT, or MRI may be used to evaluate a hip dislocation after reduction.
  • For all reductions performed in the operating room, postreduction imaging is performed intraoperatively, postoperatively, or in subsequent follow-up.
■ What Is the Plan for Follow-up Care?
  • The orthopedic pediatric surgeon usually requires a follow-up appointment within 7 to 10 days of injury.
■ What Are Outpatient Pain Relief Options?
  • Oral narcotic pain medications such as hydrocodone or oxycodone are useful.
  • Muscle spasm often is a main symptom and may be controlled with a weight-appropriate dose of diazepam.
■ What Further Care Plan Should Be Discussed With the Patient?
  • For operative hip fractures, the risk of avascular necrosis and the possibility of additional surgeries or treatments if such a complication occurs should be explained to the patient.
  • The patient is restricted from gym and sports activities until further notice. The patient may need to remain out of school until the follow-up visit.
■ Discharge or Inpatient Admission?
  • Most hip fractures should be managed on an inpatient basis because of the need to execute the appropriate diagnostic examinations.
■ What Is Anticipated Specialist Care Treatment or Anticipated Definitive Treatment?
  • The pediatric orthopedic surgeon directs the subsequent surgical management of the patient.
■ Discharge Care and Instruction
  • Patients younger than 10 years old are likely to have additional spica cast immobilization after treatment of the hip fracture.
  • Patients are instructed on care of the spica cast by the floor nurses and by the surgeon's office.
  • Patients should follow-up in 7 to 10 days after discharge from the emergency department or the hospital.
  • The individual surgeon determines follow-up for surgical patients. Brace or cast immobilization may or may not be a component of the postoperative protocol.
  • After successful closed reduction of a hip in the emergency department, an older patient may be immobilized in a hip abduction orthosis with total hip precautions for 4 to 6 weeks.
  • For younger patients, a spica cast may be applied for 4 to 6 weeks.

## COMMON PITFALLS

■ Spica cast immobilization is usually required for patients younger than 10 years treated for hip fractures because fixation is typically in weaker bone and patient cooperation with postoperative protocols sometimes can be suboptimal.
■ Stable fixation across the physis should not be sacrificed for preservation of proximal physeal growth because stability is more important than residual growth at the proximal femur in any pediatric hip fracture at any age.
■ A dislocated hip requires urgent reduction. An expeditious reduction within 6 hours of injury is critical to minimizing the risk of avascular necrosis.
■ Hip dislocations may spontaneously reduce and have apparently normal radiographs. The original injury must be correctly identified, and any residual joint incongruity should be assessed with MRI or CT.

## References

1. Beaty JH: Fractures of the hip in children. Orthop Clin North Am 37:223–232, 2006.
2. Macfarlane I, King D: Traumatic dislocation of the hip joint in children. Aust N Z J Surg 46:227–231, 1976.

3. Shrader MW, Jacofsky DJ, Stans AA, et al: Femoral neck fractures in pediatric patients: 30 years experience at a level 1 trauma center. Clin Orthop Relat Res 454:169–173, 2007.

4. Herrera-Soto JA, Price CT: Traumatic hip dislocations in children and adolescents: pitfalls and complications. J Am Acad Orthop Surg 17:15–21, 2009.

5. Schmidt GL, Sciulli R, Altman GT: Knee injury in patients experiencing a high-energy traumatic ipsilateral hip dislocation. J Bone Joint Surg Am 87:1200–1204, 2005.

6. Ingari JV, Smith DK, Aufdemorte TB, et al: Anatomic significance of magnetic resonance imaging findings in hip fracture. Clin Orthop Relat Res 332:209–214, 1996.

7. Price CT, Pyevich MT, Knapp DR, et al: Traumatic hip dislocation with spontaneous incomplete reduction: a diagnostic trap. J Orthop Trauma 16:730–735, 2002.

8. Song KS, Choi IH, Sohn YJ, et al: Habitual dislocation of the hip in children: report of eight additional cases and literature review. J Pediatr Orthop 23:178–183, 2003.

9. Canale ST, Bourland WL: Fracture of the neck and intertrochanteric region of the femur in children. J Bone Joint Surg Am 59:431–443, 1977.

10. Boardman MJ, Herman MJ, Buck B, et al: Hip fractures in children. J Am Acad Orthop Surg 17:162–173, 2009.

11. Herrera-Soto JA, Price CT, Reuss BL, et al: Proximal femoral epiphysiolysis during reduction of hip dislocation in adolescents. J Pediatr Orthop 26:371–374, 2006.

12. Hughes LO, Beaty JH: Fractures of the head and neck of the femur in children. J Bone Joint Surg Am 76:283–292, 1994.

13. Moon ES, Mehlman CT: Risk factors for avascular necrosis after femoral neck fractures in children: 25 Cincinnati cases and meta-analysis of 360 cases. J Orthop Trauma 20:323–329, 2006.

14. Morsy HA: Complications of fracture of the neck of the femur in children: a long-term follow-up study. Injury 32:45–51, 2001.

15. Ratliff AH: Fractures of the neck of the femur in children. Orthop Clin North Am 5:903–924, 1974.

16. Devas MB: Stress fractures in children. J Bone Joint Surg Br 45:528–541, 1963.

17. Haddad FS, Bann S, Hill RA, et al: Displaced stress fracture of the femoral neck in an active amenorrhoeic adolescent. Br J Sports Med 31:70–72, 1997.

18. Ganz R, Gill TJ, Gautier E, et al: Surgical dislocation of the adult hip a technique with full access to the femoral head and acetabulum without the risk of avascular necrosis. J Bone Joint Surg Br 83:1119–1124, 2001.

**TABLE 28-1** Accepted Parameters for Closed Reduction

| Age | Varus/Valgus Angulation (degrees) | Anterior/Posterior Angulation (degrees) | Shortening (cm) | Rotation* (degrees) |
|---|---|---|---|---|
| Infants | 30 | 40 | 3 | 20 |
| 1-5 yr | 20 | 30 | 2 | 10 |
| 6-10 yr | 10 | 15 | 2 | 10 |
| 11 to maturity | 5 | 10 | 1 | 10 |

*External rotation is better tolerated than internal rotation.

Although recommendations vary, generally accepted parameters for closed reduction are listed in Table 28-1.

- Traction before application of a spica cast may be necessary in a child with excessive shortening.

  In young children, shortening of 2 to 3 cm is acceptable.

- In larger children at the upper end of this age limit, flexible intramedullary rods may be considered.

■ Age 4 to 11 Years
  - As children get older, successful closed treatment becomes less reliable; although a spica cast may be appropriate in smaller children with minimally displaced fractures, this age group usually requires operative fixation.
  - External fixation may be chosen for patients with fractures with significant soft tissue injury or patients who are too unstable to tolerate longer operative procedures.
  - Intramedullary nailing with crossed, flexible, titanium rods is the most common mode of fixation for this age group (Fig. 28-8). These nails are placed in a retrograde fashion.

    Patients with transverse fracture patterns can bear weight immediately.

    Patients with more oblique fractures should remain non–weight bearing or touchdown weight bearing while the fracture heals.

    For unstable fracture patterns, a spica cast may be necessary for the first 4 weeks to avoid shortening or malalignment.

  - Open reduction and internal fixation with a plate and screw construct can also be considered in this age group (Fig. 28-9).

    This treatment offers the benefit of anatomic reduction without need for a spica cast in patients with unstable patterns.

    This method of fixation has the potential of stress fracture through the screw holes after plate removal.

■ Age 11 Years to Skeletal Maturity
  - As children approach skeletal maturity, and the anatomy allows, rigid intramedullary rod fixation becomes more common (Fig. 28-10).

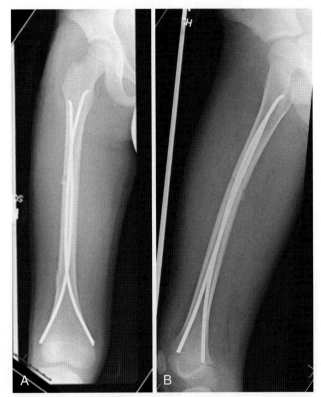

**FIGURE 28-8.** Example of intramedullary stabilization of a midshaft femur fracture in an 8-year-old boy.

- Intramedullary rods are typically placed through the greater trochanter to avoid possible vascular compromise from a piriformis fossa entry.
- This method of fixation offers the benefit of improved angular and rotational alignment and avoids the potential of fracture shortening.
- Weight bearing may be begun sooner than with the flexible rods.

## GUIDELINES FOR EMERGENCY DEPARTMENT MANAGEMENT

■ When and How Should a Specialist Be Consulted?
  - Most patients with femoral shaft fractures require bedside consultation by the orthopedist on call.
  - For infants younger than 6 months with nondisplaced femoral fractures, application of a long leg

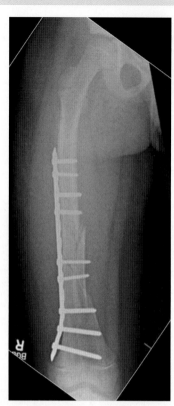

**FIGURE 28-9.** Comminuted femoral shaft fracture in a 9-year-old boy fixed with a plate and screw construct.

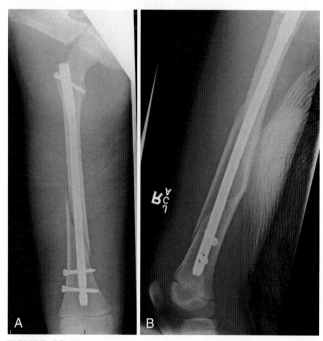

**FIGURE 28-10.** Anteroposterior **(A)** and lateral **(B)** x-rays of rigid intramedullary fixation of the fracture seen in Figure 28-2.

spica splint or a Pavlik harness with an Ace wrap around the thigh and subsequent orthopedic follow-up within 1 week may be acceptable.

■ What Should Be Communicated to the Specialist?
- Presumed diagnosis or reason for consultation
- Age and gender
- Mechanism of injury
- Time of injury
- Additional injuries
- Neurovascular examination of the extremity with assessment of skin integrity (i.e., open fracture)
- Summary of radiographic findings and all studies ordered so far

■ What Analgesia or Anesthesia Should Be Used?
- Intravenous narcotic analgesia is used to maintain patient comfort.
- Intravenous diazepam may be used to minimize muscle spasm.
- Anesthesia for operative procedures is performed in the operating room.

■ What Is Acceptable Alignment for a Femoral Shaft Fracture?
- Acceptable alignment for a femoral shaft fracture is detailed in Table 28-1.
- Generally, more sagittal plane deformity is tolerated than coronal plane deformity.
- Shortening at the fracture site of 2 cm is well tolerated.
- Parameters for distal deformity are stricter than parameters for proximal deformity.

■ What Initial Splinting or Immobilization Should Be Provided?
- A long posterior splint extending to the buttock and including the leg may be applied on the field.
- For younger children, wrapping the affected extremity to the opposite extremity loosely with bandage material is adequate.
- Splints that do not include the pelvis are useless and do not provide adequate immobilization of a femoral shaft fracture. No significant attempts should be made in the emergency department to reapply such a splint because little benefit is afforded, and discomfort is greatly increased.
- Skeletal traction may be applied if definitive stabilization is delayed as a result of distracting injury.

■ What Postreduction Imaging Is Necessary?
- Anteroposterior and lateral plain radiographs of the femur are adequate to evaluate the femur after reduction or definitive stabilization.
- In patients with spica casts, a lateral radiograph is best to evaluate fracture shortening.

■ What Is the Plan for Follow-up Care?
- Patients with femoral shaft fractures treated in a spica cast need follow-up within 7 to 10 days for clinical and radiographic evaluation.
- Patients with operative fixation for a femoral shaft fracture need follow-up within 7 to 10 days for clinical and radiographic evaluation.

■ What Are Outpatient Pain Relief Options?
- Oral narcotic pain medications such as hydrocodone or oxycodone are useful.
- Muscle spasm is often a main symptom and may be controlled with a weight-appropriate dose of diazepam.

■ What Further Care Plan Should Be Discussed With the Patient?
- Patients treated with closed reduction and a spica cast should be warned that repeat manipulation of

the fracture may be needed if the fracture alignment is unsatisfactory at follow-up examination.

- Patients treated with intramedullary implants are likely to require removal of the hardware at a later date.

■ Discharge or Inpatient Admission?
- Patients who receive a spica cast in the emergency department for treatment of a femoral shaft fracture may be discharged on the same day.
- Patients requiring operative stabilization need inpatient admission.

■ What Is Anticipated Specialist Care Treatment or Anticipated Definitive Treatment?
- Femoral shaft fractures in children younger than 5 years can typically be managed through closed means.

  Patients should have frequent follow-up for repeat radiographs to ensure maintenance of fracture alignment.

  Immobilization may be discontinued in 4 to 6 weeks or when there is evidence of circumferential callus.

  A limp is anticipated for 3 to 6 months after the fracture in toddlers.

- Femoral shaft fractures in older children are typically managed with operative stabilization.

  Weight bearing and additional immobilization are dictated by the method of fixation, the fracture pattern, and the age of the patient.

  Healing typically occurs over 4 to 6 weeks.

  Hardware removal is usually required because the implants migrate along the femoral shaft over time and create potential weak areas along the bone.

■ Discharge Care and Instruction
- A patient treated with a spica cast can be discharged from the emergency department as long as adequate

teaching for spica cast care is provided and the parents are instructed to observe for perfusion in the affected extremity and signs of potential compartment syndrome.

  For child safety, arrangements should be made for a car seat that accommodates the spica cast.

- Postoperative patients with increasing pain, fevers, or drainage from the operative site should contact the operating surgeon or return to the emergency department.

## COMMON PITFALLS

■ Particular attention should be paid to associated fractures around the knee or the hip, particularly the femoral neck.
■ Radiographs should be scrutinized for evidence of a pathologic fracture.
■ Children younger than 3 years with a femoral shaft fracture require an evaluation by Child Protective Services.

### References

1. Beaty J, Kasser J: Rockwood and Wilkins' fractures in children, Philadelphia, 2006, Lippincott Williams & Wilkins.
2. Lovell W, Winter R, Morrissy R, et al: Lovell and Winter's pediatric orthopaedics, Philadelphia, 2006, Lippincott Williams & Wilkins.
3. Rihn JA, Groff YJ, Harner CD, et al: The acutely dislocated knee: evaluation and management. J Am Acad Orthop Surg 12:334–346, 2004.
4. Tornetta P 3rd, Kain MS, Creevy WR: Diagnosis of femoral neck fractures in patients with a femoral shaft fracture: improvement with a standard protocol. J Bone Joint Surg Am 89:39–43, 2007.

# Chapter 29 — *Fractures of the Pediatric Knee*

Mark C. Lee, Silas Marshall, and John C. Brancato

## INTRODUCTION

- Most lower extremity growth occurs around the knee.
- Children who sustain injuries to the growth plates of the distal femur and proximal tibia may experience significant limb deformity with growth.
- Accurate, timely treatment and meticulous follow-up of these injuries are crucial to optimize the growth function of the lower extremity and to prevent later disability.
- Intra-articular injuries of the knee that do not involve direct physeal trauma include tibial spine fractures, osteochondral fractures, and various ligament and meniscal disruptions; although previously thought to be rare, these injuries are being seen with increased frequency likely as a result of increased participation of children in sports.

## ANATOMIC CONSIDERATIONS

- Bones (Fig. 29-1)
  - The bones of the knee include the distal femur, patella, proximal tibia, and proximal fibula.
  - The distal femur consists of the medial and lateral epicondyles (insertion sites for the medial collateral ligament [MCL] and lateral collateral ligament [LCL]), the medial and lateral condyles (articular portions of the distal femur), and the trochlear groove (located between the condyles and makes up the femoral side of the patellofemoral joint).
  - The patella forms in the quadriceps tendon and is the largest sesamoid bone in the body. It functions to increase the lever arm of the extensor mechanism at the knee.
  - The proximal tibia consists of the medial and lateral plateaus, the medial and lateral tibial spines, and the tibial tubercle (insertion point for the patellar tendon).

- Physes and Secondary Centers of Ossification
  - The distal femoral physis accounts for approximately 70% of longitudinal growth of the femur.

    The distal femoral physis is weaker than the ligaments of the knee.

    Varus or valgus stress at the knee is more likely to produce a physeal fracture than a collateral ligament injury.

  - The proximal tibial and fibular physes account for approximately 60% of longitudinal growth of the tibia.[1]

    The proximal tibial growth plate contributes approximately 55% of the length of the tibia; it averages approximately 6 mm of growth per year.[2]

    The growth plate closes between 13 and 15 years of age in girls and between 15 and 18 years of age in boys.

    The popliteal artery is particularly susceptible to injury or compression with displaced fractures of the proximal tibial physis (Fig. 29-2).

  - The tibial tubercle apophysis closes between 13 and 15 years in girls and between 15 and 19 years in boys.[3]

    The proximal tibial physis is continuous with the tibial tubercle apophysis, contributing to longitudinal growth of the bone and the development of the tubercle.

    The tubercle apophyseal ossification center appears between 7 and 9 years of age.

    The proximal tibial epiphysis and the ossification center of the tibial tubercle eventually fuse at 13 to 15 years in girls and 15 to 19 years in boys.[2]

- Osteochondritis dissecans
- Dislocations of the knee

  The rare knee or tibiofemoral dislocation should be distinguished from the more common patellar dislocation.

  Knee dislocations are high-energy injuries, are commonly posterior, and manifest with the knee in a fixed extended position with some potential associated neurologic compromise.

  Patellar dislocations occur commonly in adolescent girls, who present with the knee in a fixed flexed or semiflexed position. There is often a history of prior dislocations.
- Discoid meniscus
- Juvenile rheumatoid arthritis
- Benign or malignant bone lesion
- Vascular malformation
- Osteomyelitis
- Septic arthritis
- Prepatellar bursitis

  In prepatellar bursitis, the bursa anterior to the patella is infected or inflamed.

  In contrast to septic arthritis, erythema and edema exist anterior to the patella, and knee effusion is typically absent.

  Patients are usually able to bear weight in extension; they have minimal pain in the middle ranges of motion but severe pain with deeper flexion.

  Patients may or may not present with fevers or elevated inflammatory markers.
- Lyme arthritis

  In endemic regions, *Borrelia burgdorferi* infection causing Lyme arthritis needs to be distinguished from septic arthritis because it is not a surgical emergency.

  The effusion from knee involvement is believed to have no significant long-term effects on the articular cartilage of the knee.

  Antibiotics are the primary treatment for this condition.

## TREATMENT OF SPECIFIC INJURIES

- Distal Femur Fracture
  - Fractures of the distal femur in children usually involve the distal femoral physis.
  - Salter-Harris type III and type IV fractures of the distal femur warrant special consideration. In contrast to Salter-Harris type I and type II fractures, these fractures involve the articular surface, and anatomic reduction is imperative.
  - Salter-Harris injuries of the distal femur are typically sustained in high-energy injuries such as a motor

vehicle collision, pedestrian struck by a car, or sports injuries.
- Hyperextension force at the knee in a child more often leads to anterior distal femoral epiphyseal displacement than to a knee dislocation (Fig. 29-7).
- All Salter-Harris injuries around the distal femur have a potential for growth arrest; 40% to 50% of patients with such injuries experience a growth disturbance, often manifested as progressive angular deformity.[5]
- Initial immobilization of the fracture may be provided by a knee immobilizer or long leg splint.
- Nondisplaced Salter-Harris type I and type II distal femur fractures in a patient younger than 4 years may be treated with closed reduction and application of a spica cast.

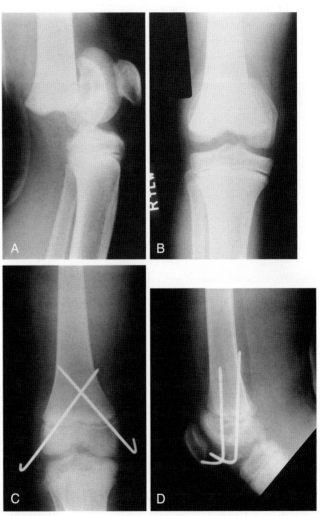

**FIGURE 29-7.** Salter-Harris type I fracture of the distal femoral physis of a 13-year-old boy. The patient sustained a hyperextension injury of the knee without any neurovascular injury. **A,** Lateral radiograph of the knee shows a completely displaced type I physeal injury of the distal end of the femur with anterior displacement of the femoral condyles. **B,** Anteroposterior radiograph of the same knee shows displacement of the condyles. **C,** Anteroposterior radiograph after closed reduction and percutaneous pinning shows anatomic restoration of the fracture. The pins are smooth and have crossed the physis. **D,** Lateral radiograph of the knee shows anatomic reduction of the fracture. *(From Green N, Swiontkowski M: Skeletal trauma in children, ed 4, Philadelphia, 2008, Saunders.)*

PART III Pediatrics

- Fixation is generally indicated in all age groups to minimize the possibility of subsequent displacement.
- Operative reduction and fixation is generally recommended for all patients with displaced Salter-Harris fractures of the distal femur (Fig. 29-8).
■ Knee Dislocation
- Dislocations of the knee joint are very rare in patients with open growth plates.[3] More frequently, pediatric patients sustain a fracture through the distal femoral or proximal tibial physis.
- Knee dislocations in children are treated similarly to dislocations in adults (see Chapter 14).
- Because of the high incidence of vascular injury with this injury, a careful vascular examination and close monitoring over the first 24 to 48 hours are warranted.
■ Tibial Spine Fracture
- In children, tensile forces in the ACL tend to displace the weak cartilage-bone interface of the anterior tibial spine rather than tear the ligament itself.

- These injuries tend to be seen in children 8 to 14 years old.
- The mechanism of injury is the same as an ACL injury in an adult.

    Hyperextension and external rotation or valgus load and external rotation cause increased tension on the ACL.

    The classic injury is a fall from a bicycle.[2]

- Fractures of the tibial spine are classified according to the degree of displacement and the continuity of the posterior bony margin (Fig. 29-9).
- Anteroposterior and lateral radiographs of the knee are the primary means of diagnosing this injury (Fig. 29-10).
- Careful attention should be paid to the degree of displacement and the integrity of the posterior portion of the fragment.
- MRI can be used to identify the extent of the injury better (Fig. 29-11).

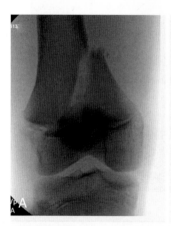
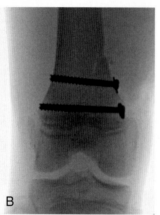

**FIGURE 29-8. A,** Anteroposterior fluoroscopic view of a Salter-Harris type II distal femur fracture in a 14-year-old boy. **B,** Fixation of the fracture using two cannulated screws.

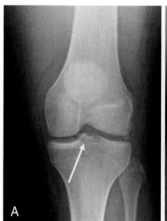
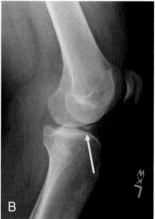

**FIGURE 29-10.** Anteroposterior **(A)** and lateral **(B)** radiographs of a type II tibial spine avulsion in a 15-year-old boy *(arrow).*

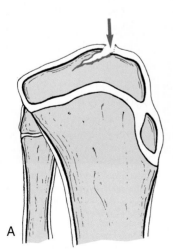
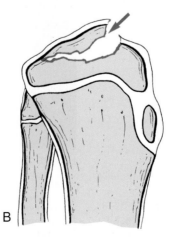
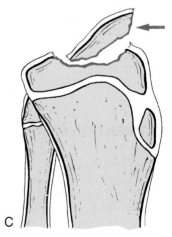

**FIGURE 29-9.** Meyers and McKeever classification of fractures of the anterior tibial spine. **A,** Type I fracture with no displacement of the fracture. **B,** Type II fracture with elevation of the anterior portion of the anterior tibial spine, but with the fracture posteriorly reduced. **C,** Type III fracture, which is totally displaced. *(From Green N, Swiontkowski M: Skeletal trauma in children, ed 4, Philadelphia, 2008, Saunders.)*

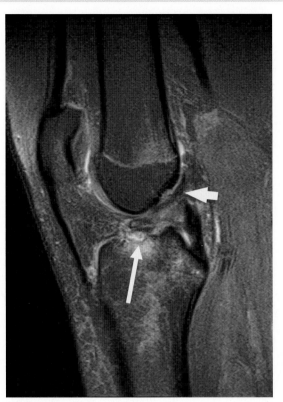

**FIGURE 29-11.** Sagittal MRI of the fracture shown in Figure 29-10. The intact ACL *(broad arrow)* is still attached to the avulsed fragment *(thin arrow)*.

- Minimally displaced fractures in the setting of a stable knee examination may be definitively treated in a long leg cast with the knee in 20 degrees of flexion.
- Displaced fractures with an unstable knee examination require operative reduction and stabilization, usually through an arthroscopic approach.
- Intra-articular Extraphyseal Knee Injury
  - Other than tibial spine fractures, most osteochondral, ligamentous, or meniscal injuries may be managed initially with a knee immobilizer.
  - In the setting of a normal neurovascular examination, no urgent surgical intervention is required.
  - The various injuries, their classification, and their surgical management are beyond the scope of this text.
- Tibial Tubercle Fractures
  - The same mechanisms that lead to quadriceps and patellar tendon avulsions in adults lead to avulsion fractures of the much weaker tibial tubercle apophysis in children.
  - Flexion of the knee occurs against a contracted quadriceps, or a violent contracture of the quadriceps occurs against a fixed tibia.
  - These injuries most commonly occur in boys between 12 and 17 years of age engaged in sports.
  - Symptoms include pain over the tibial tubercle, a large knee effusion, and inability to extend the knee actively in displaced fractures.
  - Rarely, patients with tibial tubercle avulsions may present with symptoms of compartment syndrome

secondary to tearing of the anterior tibial recurrent artery.
- Fractures of the tibial tubercle are classified according to which portion of the proximal tibial physis is affected and the degree to which it is displaced (Fig. 29-12).
- The lateral radiograph of the knee is the primary means of diagnosing this injury.

  Careful attention should be paid to the degree of displacement and any articular involvement.

  Oblique x-rays of the knee can help to define better any intra-articular involvement.

  CT scan and MRI are not very useful in diagnosing this injury.

- Most displaced fractures of the tibial tubercle require operative treatment; nondisplaced fractures may be treated in a long leg cast (Fig. 29-13).

  Operative treatment is typically nonemergent as long as no neurovascular deficit exists or a break in skin integrity is identified.

  Patients may be provisionally managed with a knee immobilizer.

- Patella Fracture
  - Fractures of the patellar body with adult fracture patterns (e.g., transverse) are managed similarly to their adult counterparts.
- Patellar Sleeve Fracture
  - The patellar sleeve fracture is an avulsion of the distal pole of the patella with a large sleeve of the distal articular surface (Fig. 29-14).
  - Results from the mostly cartilaginous nature of the skeletally immature patella, which predisposes to failure at the bone-apophyseal cartilage interface and not at the level of the patellar ligament.
  - The mechanism of injury is the same as a tibial tubercle fracture.

    Either hyperflexion of the knee or rapid contraction of the quadriceps against a bending knee causes avulsion of the patellar sleeve.

  - Symptoms include anterior knee pain, a large knee effusion, inability to bear weight, and loss of active extension of the knee.
  - On examination, the patella may be palpable in a more superior location than the contralateral side. A palpable defect is frequently felt just distal to the patella.
  - Anteroposterior and lateral radiographs of the knee are the primary means of diagnosing this injury.

    Careful attention should be paid to the degree of displacement.

    The patella is usually noted to be high riding (patella alta) relative to the uninjured side.

  - MRI can be used to identify the extent of the articular injury better but is usually unnecessary.
  - Minimally displaced fractures are treated with a knee immobilizer with the knee in full extension.

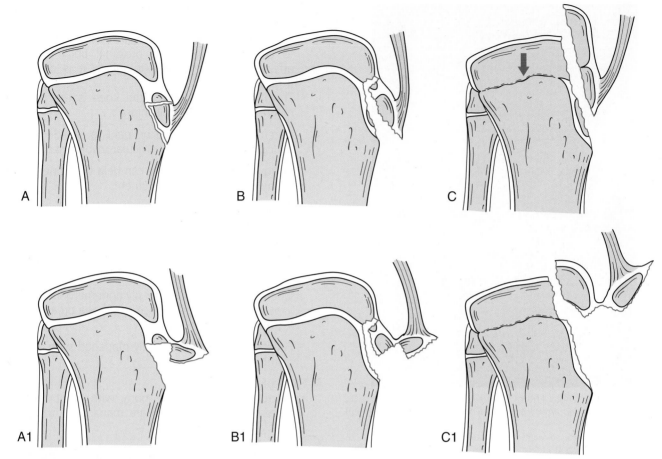

**FIGURE 29-12.** Avulsion fractures of the tibial tubercle. **A,** Type I fracture. The fracture line is through the secondary ossification center. In subtype A, the displacement is minimal. In subtype B, the fragment is hinged anteriorly and proximally. **B,** Type II fracture. The fracture occurs through the junction of the ossification centers of the proximal end of the tibia and the tuberosity. In subtype A, the fragment is not comminuted. In subtype B, the fragment is comminuted and may be more proximally displaced. **C,** A type III fracture is a true Salter-Harris type III injury that is intra-articular. In subtype A, the tubercle and anterior part of the proximal tibial epiphysis form a single unit. In subtype B, the fragment is comminuted, with the site of fragmentation at the junction of the ossification centers of the proximal end of the tibia and the tuberosity. *(From Green N, Swiontkowski M: Skeletal trauma in children, ed 4, Philadelphia, 2008, Saunders.)*

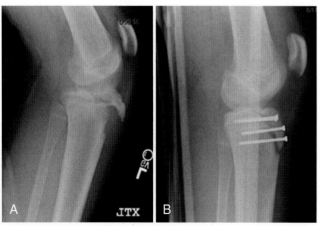

**FIGURE 29-13. A,** Lateral radiograph of a type III tibial tubercle fracture in a 16-year-old boy. **B,** The fracture was reduced and fixed with cannulated screws.

- Displaced or open fractures require operative fixation to restore the extensor mechanism.
- Fracture patterns similar to adults, such as a transverse patellar fracture, are treated with similar operative methods.

■ Proximal Tibia Fractures

- Fractures of the proximal tibia include intra-articular fractures, proximal tibial physeal fractures, and proximal tibial metaphysis greenstick fractures.
- Most proximal tibial physis fractures occur with a hyperextension force.

  These fractures should be distinguished from a displaced tibial tubercle avulsion fracture that extends through the proximal tibial physis.

- Intra-articular tibial plateau fractures result from high-energy axial loading of the knee, as occurs in motor vehicle crashes or falls from a height.
- Valgus greenstick fracture of the proximal tibial metaphysis (also known as Cozen fracture) usually occurs with low-energy injuries such as falls from playground equipment or from a bicycle.[6]

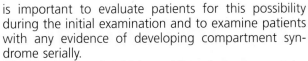

is important to evaluate patients for this possibility during the initial examination and to examine patients with any evidence of developing compartment syndrome serially.

■ Close attention should be paid to the neurovascular examination in patients with displaced distal femoral fractures.

■ Skin tenting by bone fragments, as in tibial tubercle fractures, may lead to blanching and subsequent necrosis. Failure to assess the soft tissue envelope adequately or reduce emergently a deformity that compromises the soft tissue envelope significantly complicates the treatment of the injury.

■ A concurrent patellar tendon rupture or quadriceps rupture may exist with a tibial tubercle fracture; this must be noted during the examination, as palpable defects in the soft tissue integrity of these structures, or intraoperatively, if the patellar relationship with the remainder of the knee fails to be restored after realignment of the tibial tubercle fracture.

■ Tibial spine fractures can be subtle on radiographic examination and can result in chronic knee instability.

■ Associated patellar tendon or quadriceps ruptures may exist with a patella fracture. It is important to examine the soft tissue integrity surrounding the patella after patella fracture repair.

■ Bipartite patella, an anatomic variant, may be incorrectly diagnosed as a fracture.

■ Incompletely fused ossification centers should be distinguished from true fractures in the proximal tibia.

■ Proximal tibia fractures through the metaphysis in a growing child may result in progressive valgus angulation. Parents should be warned that the progressive valgus malalignment is likely to worsen over 1 to 2 years, but that most cases spontaneously correct.

## References

1. Lovell W, Winter R, Morrissy R, et al: Lovell and Winter's pediatric orthopaedics, Philadelphia, 2006, Lippincott Williams & Wilkins.
2. Green N, Swiontkowski M: Skeletal trauma in children, Philadelphia, 2008, Saunders.
3. Beaty J, Kasser J: Rockwood and Wilkins' fractures in children, Philadelphia, 2006, Lippincott Williams & Wilkins.
4. Jackson DW, Evans NA, Thomas BM: Accuracy of needle placement into the intra-articular space of the knee. J Bone Joint Surg Am 84:1522–1527, 2002.
5. Riseborough EJ, Barrett IR, Shapiro F: Growth disturbances following distal femoral physeal fracture-separations. J Bone Joint Surg Am 65:885–893, 1983.
6. Cozen L: Fracture of the proximal portion of the tibia in children followed by valgus deformity. Surg Gynecol Obstet 97:183–188, 1953.

**Chapter 30**

# Pediatric Tibia and Fibular Shaft and Ankle Fractures

Mark C. Lee, Silas Marshall, and John C. Brancato

**INTRODUCTION**
**ANATOMIC CONSIDERATIONS**
**HISTORY**
**PHYSICAL EXAMINATION**
**DIAGNOSTIC STUDIES**

**DIFFERENTIAL DIAGNOSIS**
**TREATMENT OF SPECIFIC INJURIES**
**GUIDELINES FOR EMERGENCY DEPARTMENT MANAGEMENT**
**COMMON PITFALLS**

## INTRODUCTION

- Tibia and fibula shaft fractures are the third most common long bone injury.
- The prevalence of these injuries has been increasing since 1950, but the frequency of occurrence does not change significantly with age.
- Rotational mechanisms account for most tibia fractures yielding spiral or short oblique fractures.
  - Patients younger than 4 years old typically sustain isolated spiral or short oblique fractures, with bicycle spoke injuries peculiar to this age group.
  - Older adolescents sustain fractures most commonly along the distal third of the tibia and most often during sporting events.
- Distal tibia and fibula fractures (ankle fractures) most commonly result from sports or recreational activities.
- Although only 4% of all pediatric ankle fractures involve a physis, these injuries constitute one third of all growth plate–level injuries in pediatric patients.

## ANATOMIC CONSIDERATIONS

- Bones (Fig. 30-1)
  - The tibia is divided into the proximal tibia, the tibial shaft, and the distal tibia.

    The proximal tibia (discussed in Chapter 29) consists of the tibial plateaus, tibial spines, and tibial tubercle.

    The tibial shaft is divided into the proximal, middle, and distal third.

  - The tibial diaphysis in children has a thick periosteal layer that lends stability and healing potential to fractures of this bone.
  - In younger children 9 months to 6 years old, the tibia is susceptible to failure in torsion.
    - Torsional injuries such as tripping while running or twisting the ankle as a result of stepping on a toy may lead to a so-called *toddler's fracture*.

  - A toddler's fracture is a spiral fracture of the distal tibial shaft and is nondisplaced and frequently not visible on plain radiographs.
  - As children grow, the strength of the cortical bone in the tibial diaphysis increases, and consequently higher energy is necessary to fracture the bone, resulting in fractures of both the tibia and the fibula.

  The distal tibia consists of the medial malleolus, the posterior malleolus, and the tibial plafond.

  - The fibula consists of the head and neck, the shaft, and the lateral malleolus. The fibula bears only 6% to 17% of body weight.[1]
  - The dome of the talus forms the distal articular surface of the ankle joint.
- Physes
  - The distal tibial and fibular physes account for approximately 40% of longitudinal growth of the bones.
  - Injury to the fibular physis is far more common than lateral ankle sprain because of a relative weakness of the growth plate compared with the ligaments.
  - The distal tibial physis closes at around 12 to 13 years of age in girls and 13 to 14 years in boys.
- Growth Plate
  - The growth plate closes asymmetrically, starting centrally, progressing medially, and then fusing laterally (Fig. 30-2).
  - This sequence plays a role in two of the transitional fractures of the distal tibia (fractures that occur during the transition between open and closed growth plates).
- Joints
  - The ankle joint (mortise) allows for dorsiflexion and plantar flexion at the ankle.

    The ankle joint is created by articulations between the tibia and talus and between the fibula and the talus.

    Stability is provided by multiple structures, including the deltoid ligament medially, the lateral ligamentous complex (anterior talofibular ligament,

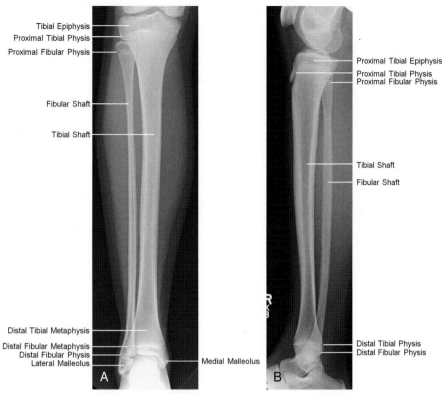

Tibial Epiphysis
Proximal Tibial Physis
Proximal Fibular Physis

Fibular Shaft

Tibial Shaft

Distal Tibial Metaphysis

Distal Fibular Metaphysis
Distal Fibular Physis
Lateral Malleolus

Medial Malleolus

A

Proximal Tibial Epiphysis
Proximal Tibial Physis
Proximal Fibular Physis

Tibial Shaft
Fibular Shaft

Distal Tibial Physis
Distal Fibular Physis

B

**FIGURE 30-1.** Anteroposterior **(A)** and lateral **(B)** views of the tibia and fibula illustrating the bony anatomy in a child.

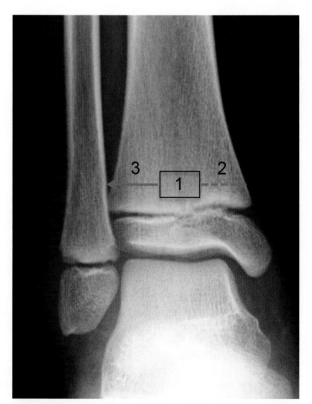

**FIGURE 30-2.** Anteroposterior radiograph of a child's ankle illustrating the direction of closure of the distal tibial physis. The physis closes centrally first *(1)*, then proceeds medially *(2)*, and later advances laterally. The closure pattern gives rise to some of the specific injury patterns for pediatric ankle fractures.

posterior talofibular ligament, and calcaneofibular ligament), and dynamic stabilization from muscles crossing the ankle (see later).

- The distal tibiofibular joint is formed by the articulation of the fibula sitting in a groove on the distal lateral tibia known as the incisura fibularis.

  Stability of this joint is provided by the syndesmotic ligaments.

- Multiple ligaments at the ankle contribute to stability of the joint (Fig. 30-3).

  Skeletally immature patients rarely sustain ankle sprains (injury to the ligaments); rather, they sustain avulsion-type fractures through the growth plate (see later).

- Muscles of the Leg
  - The muscles of the leg are contained in four myofascial compartments (see Fig. 20-4).
  - The anterior compartment contains the tibialis anterior (dorsiflexes and everts the foot), extensor hallucis longus (extends the great toe), extensor digitorum longus (extends the lesser toes), and peroneus tertius (a weak dosiflexor and evertor of the foot).
  - The lateral compartment contains the peroneus longus and the peroneus brevis, which are both evertors of the foot.
  - The superficial posterior compartment contains the gastrocnemius, soleus, and plantaris, all of which are plantar flexors of the foot. The tendons of the soleus

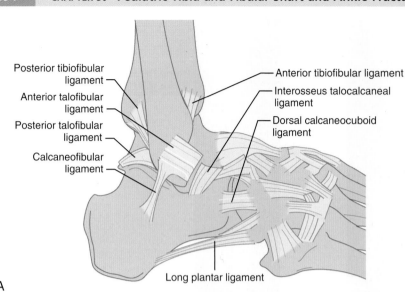

A

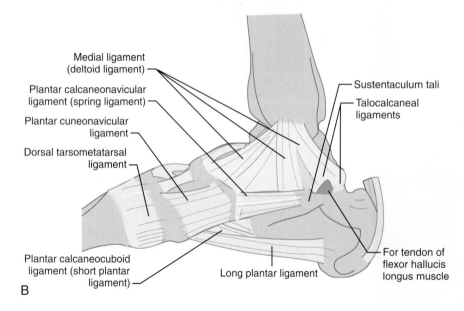

B

**FIGURE 30-3.** Illustration of the stabilizing ligaments of the ankle. *(From Bogart BI, Ort VH: Elsevier's integrated anatomy and embryology, St Louis, 2007, Mosby.)*

and the gastrocnemius combine to form the Achilles tendon.

- The deep posterior compartment contains the tibialis posterior (inverts and plantar flexes the foot), flexor hallucis longus (flexes the great toe), and flexor digitorum longus (flexes the lesser toes).
- The confined space within each compartment contributes to the relatively high rate of compartment syndrome associated with tibial shaft fractures.

The symptoms of compartment syndrome are related to compression of neurovascular structures running through each compartment.

■ Vascular Structures
- The anterior tibial artery and vein are branches of the popliteal artery and vein and run in the anterior compartment. The artery terminates as the dorsalis pedis in the foot and is palpable just lateral to the extensor hallucis longus.

- The posterior tibial artery and vein are also branches of the popliteal artery and vein and run in the deep posterior compartment. The artery is palpable at the ankle just posterior to the medial malleolus.
- The peroneal artery and vein are branches of the posterior tibial artery and vein and run in the deep posterior compartment.
- The great saphenous vein is a secondary vascular outflow from the leg. It runs with the saphenous nerve directly across the medial malleolus at the ankle.

■ Neurologic Structures
- The deep peroneal nerve is a branch of the common peroneal nerve. It runs in the anterior compartment and innervates the muscles of that compartment.
- The superficial peroneal nerve is a branch of the common peroneal nerve. It runs in the lateral compartment and innervates the muscles of that compartment.

- Displacements greater than 2 mm require operative reduction and fixation.[2]
- A CT scan should be obtained in the emergency department to confirm intra-articular displacement after cast immobilization of intra-articular fractures (i.e., Tillaux fracture, triplane fracture).

Open fractures or fractures with neurovascular compromise require operative fixation and may be managed with splinting after gentle reduction of any gross deformity.

Closed fractures with significant displacement such that the bony fragments threaten the skin integrity require an emergent closed reduction with provisional splinting.

## GUIDELINES FOR EMERGENCY DEPARTMENT MANAGEMENT

- ■ When and How Should a Specialist Be Consulted?
  - Minimally displaced, closed, extra-articular fractures of the tibial shaft or ankle in the presence of a normal neurologic examination may be splinted and scheduled for appropriate outpatient follow-up without an orthopedic consultation. This includes the subtype of toddler's fractures.
  - Any displaced or intra-articular fracture of the tibial shaft or distal tibia requires at minimum a telephone consultation so that the orthopedist may review the films and determine the need for a subsequent bedside consultation and a reduction.
  - Any fracture of the tibial shaft or ankle that is open, involves neurovascular compromise, or potentially threatens the skin requires a bedside consultation by the pediatric orthopedist.
- ■ What Should Be Communicated to the Specialist?
  - Presumed diagnosis or reason for consultation
  - Age and gender
  - Mechanism of injury
  - Time of injury
  - Additional injuries

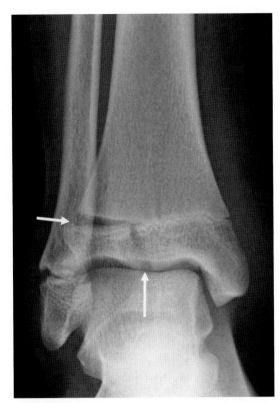

**FIGURE 30-9.** Tillaux fracture in a 12-year-old boy with characteristic distal, lateral tibial epiphyseal fragment.

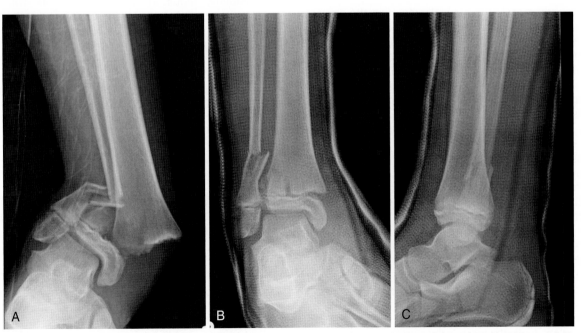

**FIGURE 30-10.** Anteroposterior **(A)** radiograph of a significantly displaced Salter-Harris type II fracture of the right ankle with an associated fibula fracture. Mortise **(B)** and lateral **(C)** radiographs of the ankle after closed reduction and bivalved cast application.

- Neurovascular examination of the extremity with assessment of skin integrity (i.e., open fracture)
- Summary of radiographic findings and all studies ordered so far

■ What Analgesia or Anesthesia Should Be Used?
- Intravenous narcotic analgesia is used to maintain patient comfort. Intravenous diazepam may be used to minimize muscle spasm.
- Provisional splinting of the leg is possible with intravenous narcotic analgesics and muscle relaxation.
- Closed reduction may be attempted with a hematoma block of 10 mL of 0.5% bupivacaine into the ankle joint.
- Conscious sedation is often necessary in a pediatric patient both for patient comfort and to effect an adequate reduction.
- Anesthesia for operative procedures is performed in the operating room.

■ What Is Acceptable Alignment for a Tibia Shaft Fracture or Distal Tibia Fracture?
- Acceptable alignment for tibia fractures is detailed in Table 30-1.
- Near-anatomic alignment is required for distal tibia fractures because remodeling potential is limited in this region.
- Intra-articular fractures of the distal tibia are acceptable if the articular gap is less than 2 mm.

■ What Initial Splinting or Immobilization Should Be Provided?
- Fractures of the tibial shaft should be immobilized by either a long leg splint or a cast.

  The splint should consist of a posterior slab extending from the toes to the proximal thigh.

  The knee should be flexed 20 to 30 degrees and the foot slightly plantar flexed to avoid displacement of the fracture by the gastrocnemius.

- Although a cast should ideally maintain the ankle at neutral dorsiflexion to prevent Achilles tendon contracture, preoccupation with foot position can sometimes cause recurvatum at the fracture site. Focus should first be on anatomic reduction of the fracture and then on the foot position because pediatric patients tolerate a poor foot position well.
- Distal tibia fractures can be provisionally immobilized in a short leg splint.
- Fractures may be definitively treated in a short leg cast.

■ What Postreduction Imaging Is Necessary?
- Anteroposterior and lateral plain radiographs of the tibia are adequate to evaluate a tibial shaft fracture after reduction.
- Anteroposterior, lateral, and mortise views of the ankle are adequate to evaluate extra-articular fractures of the distal tibia.
- CT scan is necessary to evaluate the residual articular displacement after reduction of an intra-articular distal tibia fracture.
- For all reductions performed in the operating room, imaging is performed intraoperatively, postoperatively, and in subsequent follow-up.

■ What Is the Plan for Follow-up Care?
- Patients with tibia fractures treated with a splint or cast, with or without a reduction, are toe-touch weight bearing on that extremity with crutches.

  Follow-up with an orthopedic specialist should occur within 7 to 10 days.

- Patients with distal tibia fractures treated with a splint or cast, with or without reduction, are non–weight bearing on that extremity with crutches.

  Follow-up with an orthopedic specialist should occur within 7 to 10 days.

- Patients with operative injuries maintain precautions as outlined by the operating surgeon.

  The orthopedic pediatric surgeon usually requires follow-up within 7 to 10 days of the injury.

■ What Are Outpatient Pain Relief Options?
- Oral narcotic pain medications such as hydrocodone or oxycodone are useful.
- Muscle spasm is often a major symptom and may be controlled with a weight-appropriate dose of diazepam.

■ What Further Care Plan Should Be Discussed With the Patient?
- Physeal injuries may result in partial or complete growth arrest. This possibility should be discussed with the patient and caretakers before the initiation of any treatment.
- Patients treated with closed reduction and casting should be warned that repeat manipulation of the fracture or surgical treatment of the fracture may be needed if the fracture alignment is unsatisfactory in follow-up.

■ Discharge or Inpatient Admission?
- Patients requiring nonoperative care for fracture management and whose discomfort can be adequately controlled with oral pain medication may be discharged.
- Patients requiring operative fracture care or in whom there is significant concern for a developing compartment syndrome require an inpatient admission.

■ What Is Anticipated Specialist Care Treatment or Anticipated Definitive Treatment?
- Tibial shaft fractures treated with casting typically require 5 to 6 weeks to heal in adolescent patients and less time in younger patients.

  Partial weight bearing in a long leg cast usually can be allowed at 3 to 4 weeks in most tibia fractures.

  Activity restrictions are required for 3 months.

- Toddler's fractures heal quickly, usually after a 3-week period of immobilization. Patients may be allowed to resume activities after immobilization.
- Distal tibia fractures treated in a cast require 5 to 6 weeks to heal in adolescent patients and less time in younger patients.

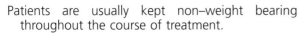

Patients are usually kept non–weight bearing throughout the course of treatment.

Activity restrictions are imposed for 3 months.

- Postoperative management is directed by the operating surgeon.

Most adolescents with tibia fractures stabilized with rigid intramedullary nails may be mobilized quickly.

Intra-articular fractures treated operatively require an extended period of non–weight bearing.

- Discharge Care and Instruction
  - Splints and casts should be maintained clean, dry, and intact.
  - The leg should be elevated above the level of the heart for the first 7 days after injury.
  - Ice can be applied to the splint or cast over the fracture site for 20-minute intervals three times daily for the first 7 days after injury.
  - If the patient has increasing pain in the lower extremity after closed treatment that is unrelieved by oral narcotics or accompanied by paresthesias, the patient should return to the emergency department.
  - Postoperative patients with increasing pain, fevers, or drainage from the operative site should contact the operating surgeon or return to the emergency department.

## COMMON PITFALLS

- Compartment syndrome can develop in patients with open or closed tibia fractures.
  - It is important to evaluate patients for the possibility of developing compartment syndrome during the initial examination and to perform serial examinations in patients admitted to the hospital with any evidence of developing compartment syndrome.
- Skin tenting by the bone fragments may lead to blanching and subsequent necrosis. Failure to assess the soft tissue envelope adequately or reduce emergently a deformity that compromises the soft tissue envelope significantly complicates the treatment of the injury.
- Articular injury cannot be adequately evaluated on radiographs.
- CT scan distinguishes operative from nonoperative injures better and evaluates the quality of a reduction.

## References

1. Browner BD, Jupiter JB, Levine AM, et al, editors: Skeletal trauma: basic science, management, and reconstruction, ed 4, Philadelphia, 2008, Saunders.
2. Karrholm J: The triplane fracture: four years of follow-up of 21 cases and review of the literature. J Pediatr Orthop B 6:91–102, 1997.

Chapter 31  ## *Pediatric Foot*

Mark C. Lee, Silas Marshall, and John C. Brancato

INTRODUCTION
ANATOMIC CONSIDERATIONS
HISTORY
PREHOSPITAL CARE AND MANAGEMENT
PHYSICAL EXAMINATION

DIAGNOSTIC STUDIES
DIFFERENTIAL DIAGNOSIS
TREATMENT OF SPECIFIC INJURIES
GUIDELINES FOR EMERGENCY DEPARTMENT MANAGEMENT
COMMON PITFALLS

## INTRODUCTION

- Foot fractures account for less than 10% of all pediatric fractures. Of these, 61% involve the metatarsals.[1]
- Most pediatric foot fractures are isolated injuries, but one series found that 21 of 125 (17%) patients with foot and ankle injuries from high-energy trauma also had injury to the axial or appendicular skeleton.
- More recent reports suggest an increase in the incidence of foot injuries, including fractures, in children wearing rubber clogs on escalators.[2]

## ANATOMIC CONSIDERATIONS

- The foot is generally divided into the forefoot, midfoot, and hindfoot.
  - The forefoot consists of the metatarsals and phalanges.
  - The forefoot is divided from the midfoot by the Lisfranc (tarsometatarsal [TMT]) joint.
  - The midfoot comprises the cuboid, navicular, and cuneiform bones.
  - The midfoot is separated from the hindfoot by the Chopart (transverse tarsal) joint.
  - The hindfoot comprises the talus and calcaneus (Fig. 31-1).
- Large portions of the foot remain cartilaginous in early childhood.
  - At birth, only the talus, calcaneus, cuboid, and phalanges have ossified.
  - Secondary ossification centers progress through childhood with the last one, the calcaneus, appearing at around 10 years of age.
- Accessory ossification centers may be confused for fractures on plain radiographs.
  - Os trigonum—present in 13% of the population and often mistaken for an avulsion fracture of the talus
  - Os vesalianum—present in 0.1% to 1% and adjacent to the base of the fifth metatarsal

- Os tibiale externum—present in 10% and medial to the navicular (Fig. 31-2)

## HISTORY

- The typical mechanism is a fall from a height or a crush injury from falling objects or motor vehicle accidents.
- Injuries in adolescents result from higher energy mechanisms than injuries in younger children.
- Patients typically present with pain and inability to bear weight.
- Patients injured by falls from a significant height or in motor vehicle accidents may have associated complaints of back pain, pelvic pain, or lower extremity pain and should be evaluated further.

## PREHOSPITAL CARE AND MANAGEMENT

- After appropriate prehospital stabilization, all foot injuries can be provisionally stabilized in a posteriorly applied short leg splint with appropriate gauze dressing applied to open wounds.
- Gross deformity should be reduced at the scene, if possible.
- Gross wound contamination can be removed at the scene, but efforts should be made to avoid detailed débridement in the field.
- The color and vascularity of the foot should be recorded before and after the application of the splint.

## PHYSICAL EXAMINATION

- The foot often is swollen around the dorsum or the ankle, depending on the location of the injury.
- Ecchymosis should be noted because plantar ecchymosis sometimes suggests a ligamentous injury.

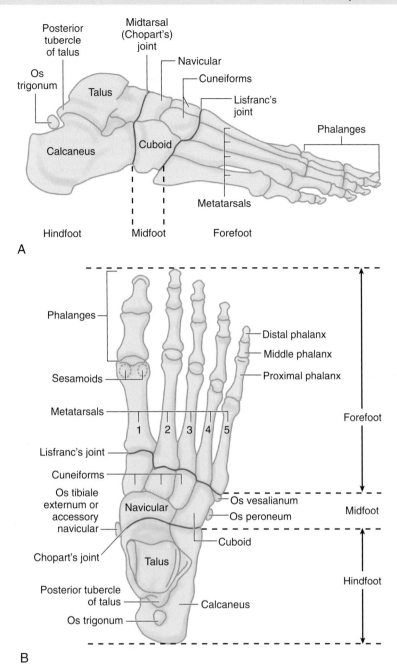

**FIGURE 31-1.** Bony anatomy of the foot.

- Lacerations or loss of soft tissue coverage should be identified.
- Palpation should be performed with reference to the bony anatomic landmarks.
  - The tuber calcanei, malleoli, talonavicular joint, calcaneocuboid joint, metatarsals, and phalanges should be systematically inspected.
- A standard neurovascular examination of the foot is performed.
  - Paresthesias distal to the zone of injury may reflect a circumferential crush injury or a progressive compartment syndrome.

## DIAGNOSTIC STUDIES

- X-ray
  - X-ray is the primary imaging modality for identifying foot injuries.
  - A standard series comprising anteroposterior, lateral, and oblique views is adequate for most foot injuries.
  - Talar fractures may be best visualized with anteroposterior, lateral, and mortise views of the ankle and a Canale view of the talus (for the Canale view, the foot is placed into equinus and pronated

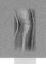

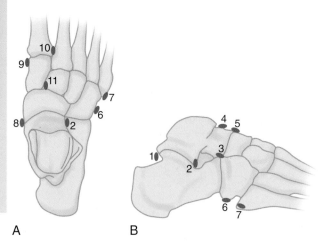

**FIGURE 31-2.** Diagram of accessory ossification centers of the foot in anteroposterior **(A)** and lateral **(B)** projections. *1*, Os trigonum; *2*, os sustentaculi; *3*, os calcaneus secondarius; *4*, secondary astralgus; *5*, supranavicular; *6*, os peroneum; *7*, os vesalianum; *8*, os tibiale externum; *9*, sesamoid tibiale anterius; *10*, os intermetatarsum; *11*, os intercuneiforme. *(From Jay RM: Pediatric foot and ankle surgery, Philadelphia, 1995, Saunders, p 11.)*

approximately 15 degrees with the beam of the x-ray angled 45 degrees horizontally).

- Calcaneal fractures may additionally require an axial view.
- Computed Tomography (CT)
  - CT scan of the foot is critical for further clarifying complex intra-articular injuries, such as a comminuted calcaneal fracture, to facilitate definitive care.
  - CT is useful for assisting with subtle diagnoses such as a Lisfranc injury or other midfoot injury when plain radiographs are inconclusive in a pediatric patient.
- Magnetic Resonance Imaging (MRI)
  - MRI is used for further classifying osteochondritis dissecans lesions along the talus.
  - MRI is useful for identifying ligamentous disruptions as in the case of a Lisfranc injury.
- Ultrasound
  - Ultrasound is rarely used for the diagnosis of bone trauma to the pediatric foot.

## DIFFERENTIAL DIAGNOSIS

- Apophysitis (calcaneal)
- Achilles tendinitis
- Juvenile rheumatoid arthritis
- Infection
  - Osteomyelitis
  - Septic arthritis
  - Cellulitis
  - Digital pulp infection
  - Plantar warts
- Tumor
- Ankle sprain
- Stress fracture
- Symptomatic flatfoot
- Plantar fasciitis
- Symptomatic toe deformity (e.g., hammer toe)

**TABLE 31-1** Modified Hawkins Classification of Talar Neck Fractures

| Type | Description | AVN Risk |
|---|---|---|
| I | Nondisplaced neck fracture (<2 mm) | Rare |
| II | Mildly displaced neck fracture with subluxation of subtalar joint | 15% |
| III | Moderately displaced neck fracture with subluxation of subtalar and tibiotalar joints | 33% |
| IV | Significantly displaced talar neck fracture with subluxation of the subtalar, ankle, and talonavicular joints | 80%-90% |

*AVN,* Avascular necrosis.
From Metzger MJ, Levin JS, Clancy JT: Talar neck fractures and rates of avascular necrosis. J Foot Ankle Surg 38:154–162, 1999.

**TABLE 31-2** DeLee Classification of Talar Body Fractures

| Type | Description |
|---|---|
| I | Transchondral dome fracture |
| II | Sagittal, horizontal, or coronal plane shear fractures with simple fracture line |
| III | Posterior tubercle fracture |
| IV | Lateral process fractures |
| V | Crushed, comminuted fracture |

From Early JS: Management of fractures of the talus: body and head regions. Foot Ankle Clin 9:709–722, 2004.

## TREATMENT OF SPECIFIC INJURIES

- Talar Fractures
  - The talus has an unusually large articulating surface area and is supplied principally by retrograde arterial flow. The limited blood supply tends to prolong fracture healing and results in a tendency for osteonecrosis in cases of talar neck and body fractures.
  - Axial loading (as in falls from a height) with forced dorsiflexion is the common mechanism of injury for talar fractures. In a series of pediatric patients, 60% of injuries resulted from motor vehicle accidents, and approximately 33% resulted from falls from a height.[3]
  - The patient typically presents with massive ankle and foot swelling with difficulty bearing weight. Dorsiflexion causes significant discomfort.
  - Radiographs consist of anteroposterior, lateral, and oblique views of the ankle and a Canale view of the talus.
  - CT scan may be necessary to define the fracture pattern further.
  - Talar fractures are broadly divided into neck or body fractures.

    Neck fractures can be classified using a modified Hawkins classification system (Table 31-1).[4]

    Body fractures can be classified using the DeLee classification system (Table 31-2).[5]

- Talar fractures in children may be classified best according to age.

  Fractures in children younger than 6 years have a generally good prognosis and are typically treated nonoperatively.

  Fractures in patients older than 6 years have a poorer prognosis and are frequently treated operatively.

- Talar neck fracture treatment

  Nondisplaced fractures (<2 mm of displacement) in a child of any age may be placed in a non–weight bearing cast for 2 months.

  Displaced talar neck fractures in young children without subluxation of the tibiotalar or subtalar joints may benefit from closed reduction and casting.

  Adolescents with displaced talar neck fractures should undergo operative reduction and fixation.

  Close monitoring for evidence of osteonecrosis is important. A positive Hawkins sign (subchondral lucency in the talar dome, usually apparent by 8 weeks after injury) is suggestive of adequate blood flow and no osteonecrosis.

- Talar body fracture treatment

  Talar body fractures are much less common than talar neck fractures in adults and children.

  Most fractures are nondisplaced and can be treated with 6 to 8 weeks of cast immobilization.

  Displaced talar body fractures (type II) require operative fixation because there is a high risk of post-traumatic degeneration in displaced fractures treated nonoperatively.

  Lateral process fractures of the talus (type IV) result from a dorsiflexion and inversion moment and have become increasingly recognized secondary to a snowboarding injury.

  Minimally displaced fractures may be treated in a short leg cast; displaced fractures require operative reduction.

- ■ Osteochondritis Dissecans (Osteochondral Fracture) of the Talus
  - Osteochondritis dissecans, or an osteochondral fracture of the talus, is an important but relatively rare cause of joint pain in active adolescents.
  - The etiology is thought to be either an interruption of the blood supply to a segment of subchondral bone, as in other types of avascular necrosis, or direct trauma.
  - The most common sites are the posteromedial or anterolateral aspects of the talar dome.
  - Pain, swelling, and decreased range of motion may be present. The patient may present after an acute traumatic event or with a history of chronic, nonspecific ankle pain.
  - Careful evaluation of plain x-rays is essential.

    A subtle lucency under the articular surface may be present, and a joint effusion may be seen.

    Later findings may include more obvious changes in density (lucency and sclerosis), an irregular cortical surface, or a frank bony fragment.

  - Plain radiographs and MRI are used to characterize the lesion fully with reference to the modified Berndt and Hardy classification (Fig. 31-3; Table 31-3).[6]
  - Treatment is dictated by the stage of the lesion (see Table 31-3).

**TABLE 31-3** Modified Bernt and Hardy Classification of Osteochondral Fractures of the Talus

| Type | Description |
| --- | --- |
| I | Subchondral trabecular compression fracture, absent on plain radiographs but identified on MRI |
| II | Incomplete avulsion or separation of a fragment |
| IIa | Same as II, with MRI finding of subchondral cyst |
| III | Complete avulsion without displacement |
| IV | Detached and rotated fragment |

From Anderson IF, Crichton KJ, Grattan-Smith T, et al: Osteochondral fractures of the dome of the talus. J Bone Joint Surg Am 71:1143–1152, 1989.

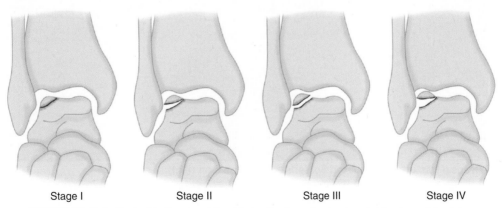

| Stage I | Stage II | Stage III | Stage IV |

**FIGURE 31-3.** Radiographic (Bernt and Hardy) classification of osteochondral fracture of the talus.

For all type I to III lesions in children, nonoperative management is recommended initially with 6 weeks of non–weight bearing in a short leg cast.

When nonoperative treatment fails and for type IV lesions, surgical drilling or drilling and repair of the lesion may be required.

- Osteochondral fractures in children and adolescents generally have a better prognosis than these injuries in adults. Bauer et al.[7] reported on long-term follow-up of patients with talar osteochondritis dissecans. Although only five patients were children, their average age was 10 years at diagnosis and almost 33 at the time of final follow-up. Four of the five pediatric patients had regression or healing of the lesions; the fifth patient did not progress. None of the five patients had osteoarthritis at follow-up.

■ Calcaneal Fractures

- Calcaneal fractures account for a small percentage (approximately 2%) of all pediatric foot fractures.
- The injury is most commonly due to axial loading, as in a fall from a height.

    Children younger than 10 years typically sustain the fracture from falls of less than 4 feet.

Children older than 10 years experience high-energy injuries with falls greater than 14 feet.[8]

A high-energy mechanism of injury frequently leads to other associated injuries, such as vertebral fractures or pelvic fractures.

- A history of a fall with pain, swelling, and localized tenderness over the heel is the common presentation.
- A standard series to evaluate the calcaneus includes lateral, axial, anteroposterior, and oblique views.
- Lateral radiographs allow measurement of Bohler angle (normal 25 to 40 degrees) (Fig. 31-4). An angle less than 20 degrees suggests a calcaneal fracture with depression of the posterior facet.
- Conservative management with casting and non–weight bearing is indicated in most pediatric calcaneal fractures.
- Operative intervention is required in the case of a displaced intra-articular fracture in an adolescent or young adult.
- The diagnosis in younger patients is often missed because radiographs may not show the injury. Although a bone scan may be used to identify the

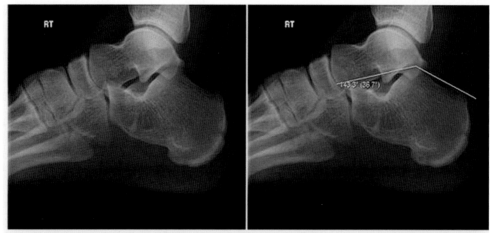

Normal calcaneus with normal Bohler's angle (shown on right)

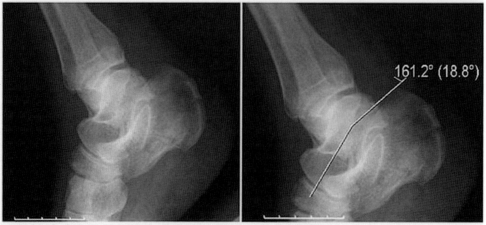

Calcaneal fracture with reduced Bohler's angle (shown on right)

**FIGURE 31-4.** Lateral radiographs of the foot illustrating Bohler angle, the angle subtended by a line from the superior point on the posterior calcaneal facet to the superior point of the calcaneal tuberosity and a line drawn from the anterior process to the highest aspect of the posterior articular surface.

fracture further, a short period of immobilization with repeat radiographs in the absence of more advanced imaging is acceptable definitive treatment for subtle injury.

■ Metatarsal Fractures
• This is the most common fracture of the foot in children, accounting for 15% of all foot injuries.[9]
• Mechanisms of injury include axial loading, inversion, and direct trauma, such as a crush injury from a falling object or a motor vehicle.
• When multiple fractures are present or there is extensive soft tissue swelling, compartment syndrome is a significant concern; this is heralded by pain out of proportion to the injury and physical examination findings such as pain with passive manipulation of the toes.
• The specific metatarsal bones involved in fractures vary by age. Two series of pediatric patients with metatarsal fractures showed a predominance of fractures of the fifth metatarsal (45% and 40%), similar to the adult population. However, fractures of the first metatarsal in these two studies (22% and 38%) were much more common than in adults.[10,11]
• In children, involvement of the first metatarsal is most frequently seen in younger children less than 5 years old. The fracture is typically a fracture of the base of the first metatarsal.
• Metatarsal stress fractures are second in frequency only to fractures of the tibia. Most (80% to 90%) involve the second and third metatarsal bones.
• Anteroposterior, lateral, and oblique radiographs of the foot are needed to assess alignment of the fracture.
• Proximal injuries should be evaluated carefully for involvement of the Lisfranc joint.
• Treatment is generally conservative.

A short period of casting with weight bearing as tolerated is appropriate for fractures with less than 20 degrees of angulation and variable quantities of medial or lateral displacement, as long as the fracture is extra-articular.

A short leg splint is preferred when significant soft tissue swelling is noted.

• Closed reduction is recommended for fractures with significant apex dorsal angulation (>20 degrees).
• Operative reduction and fixation is typically reserved for fractures in which reduction cannot be maintained, for open fractures, or for fractures with intra-articular involvement.

■ Fifth Metatarsal Fractures
• Fracture of the fifth metatarsal is often caused by repetitive stress, inversion, or direct injury.
• The prognosis varies with the exact location.
• The base of the fifth metatarsal may be divided into three zones (I, II, and III) based on its vascular anatomy (Fig. 31-5).
• Most (approximately 70%) are proximal fractures (zone I), either avulsion fractures at the apophysis or fractures with intra-articular extension. Apophyseal fractures generally respond to conservative

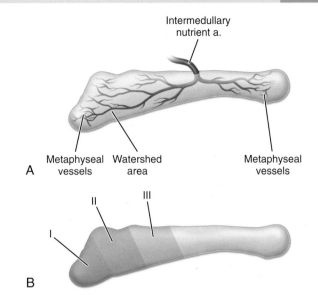

**FIGURE 31-5. A,** Vascular supply of the fifth metatarsal. The nutrient artery and metaphyseal vessels are positioned such that a watershed area exists between the two circulations. Fractures in this watershed region, at the metaphyseal-diaphyseal junction, are more prone to slow healing or nonunion. **B,** Zone II defines the previously noted watershed region and exists anatomically at the articulation between the fourth and fifth metatarsals. (*From Herring J: Tachdjian's pediatric orthopaedics, ed 4, Philadelphia, 2007, Saunders.*)

management with a weight-bearing cast for 4 to 6 weeks. One study reported a significantly longer healing time for fractures displaced more than 2 mm (average 58 days versus 37 days).[11]
• Zone II fractures are true Jones fractures—transverse fractures at the metaphyseal/diaphyseal junction first described by Sir Robert Jones in 1902.

These fractures account for approximately 15% of fifth metatarsal fractures.

The location of fracture at a poorly vascularized area increases the recovery time and the risk of incomplete healing (see Fig. 31-5).

• Zone III fractures are typically stress fractures with no anticipated delays in healing after conservative treatment.
• A well-padded short leg splint or cast for 4 to 6 weeks is used to treat most fifth metatarsal fractures.

Zone I fractures may be treated with weight bearing.

Zone II and zone III injuries are treated with non–weight bearing.

• Operative intervention for a fifth metatarsal fracture is indicated in cases of delayed union, nonunion, or refracture. A Jones fracture in an athlete is a relative indication for operative fixation.

■ Lisfranc Injuries
• Although the exact incidence is unknown, Lisfranc injuries are uncommon in children.

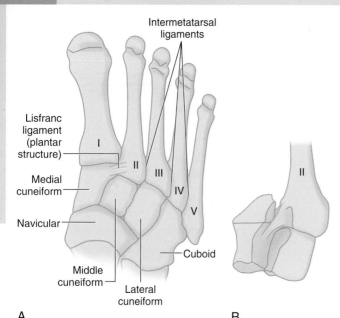

**FIGURE 31-6. A,** The Lisfranc joint complex is composed of the articulations of the medial, intermediate, and lateral cuneiforms with the cuboid and the corresponding metatarsal bases. The Lisfranc ligament is a plantar ligament between the base of the second metatarsal and the medial cuneiform (yellow band). **B,** Dorsal exposure of the Lisfranc ligament between the base of the second metatarsal and the medial cuneiform after removal of sections of the bases of the first and second metatarsals and the medial and intermediate cuneiforms.

- The Lisfranc or TMT joint comprises the articulations of the medial, middle, and lateral cuneiform bones and the cuboid with the metatarsals (Fig. 31-6).
- Dorsal, plantar, and intermetatarsal ligaments provide stability.

  The recessed position of the base of the second metatarsal in the cuneiform arch and the strong supporting plantar ligaments, including the Lisfranc ligament, make the second metatarsal–middle cuneiform articulation the most stable (see Fig. 31-6). Because of this, a fracture of the base of the second metatarsal should raise suspicion for an adjacent injury at the TMT joint.

  Because the first metatarsal–cuneiform joint is not as stable, it is more prone to injury.

- Common mechanisms of injury include forced plantar flexion (as in tripping), falls from a height (e.g., falls from bunk beds), and trauma from objects falling directly onto the foot.
- High-energy mechanisms have a high associated incidence of compartment syndrome.
- Diagnosis is notoriously difficult, especially in children.

  Patients present with dorsal foot swelling and inability to bear weight despite normal radiographs.

  Plantar ecchymosis along the midfoot in the absence of radiographic abnormality is suggestive of occult injury to the Lisfranc ligament.

- Anteroposterior, lateral, and oblique views of the foot should be obtained.

  Radiographically, separation of the bases of the first and second metatarsals by more than 2 mm should raise the possibility of TMT injury.

  The medial base of the second metatarsal should be in alignment with the medial border of the middle cuneiform on the anteroposterior radiograph, and the medial base of the fourth metatarsal should align with the medial border of the cuboid on oblique radiographs.

- A CT scan or MRI may be helpful to define more subtle injury further.
- Patients with minimally displaced Lisfranc fractures (<2 mm) or injuries that reduce anatomically can be treated nonoperatively.

  The foot is initially splinted in a bulky dressing and later converted to a non–weight bearing short leg cast 1 week later.

  The total period of immobilization is 6 weeks.

- Outcomes are generally good in pediatric patients with nonoperative treatment for minimally displaced fractures (<2 mm). In a case series of eight pediatric patients treated with short leg immobilization and followed for 32 months after injury, seven of eight patients had no limitations.[12] One patient (age 10) had midfoot pain with extended running and radiographic evidence of degenerative changes across the TMT joint.
- Fractures with greater than 2 mm displacement generally require open reduction and internal fixation.

■ Phalangeal Fractures

- Phalangeal fractures are common in children. In one series, they accounted for 18% of foot fractures (64% proximal, 29% distal, 7% middle phalanx). Incidence is likely higher because of the number of injuries for which medical attention is not sought.
- Physeal fractures most frequently are Salter-Harris type I or type II.
- The nail bed dermis is connected to the periosteum of the distal phalanx at the nail root in proximity to the physis. Fractures through the physis are likely to be open even in the absence of an overt laceration (Fig. 31-7).
- One retrospective series of five patients with "stubbed" great toes showed that all five (boys 9 to 11 years old) recalled blood around the base of the nail.[13] Three patients presented with osteomyelitis 5 to 14 days after the injury. The other two patients presented at the time of injury and were treated with oral antibiotics. Four of the five had later evidence of partial or full growth arrest but without gross deformity 10 months later.

  A plain radiograph should be obtained in patients with "stubbed" toes with bleeding. If a fracture is identified, the fracture is considered open.